PROGRESS IN BASIC AND CLINICAL IMMUNOLOGY

ADVANCES IN EXPERIMENTAL MEDICINE AND BIOLOGY

Recent Volumes in this Series

Volume 486
PURINE AND PYRIMIDINE METABOLISM IN MAN X
Edited by Esther Zoref-Shani and Oded Sperling

Volume 487
NEUROPATHOLOGY AND GENETICS OF DEMENTIA
Edited by Markus Tolnay and Alphonse Probst

Volume 488
HEADSPACE ANALYSIS OF FOODS AND FLAVORS: Theory and Practice
Edited by Russell L. Rouseff and Keith R. Cadwallader

Volume 489
HEMOPHILIA CARE IN THE NEW MILLENNIUM
Edited by Dougald M. Monroe, Ulla Hedner, Maureane R. Hoffman, Claude Negrier, Geoffrey F. Savidge, and Gilbert C. White II

Volume 490
MECHANISMS OF LYMPHOCYTE ACTIVATION AND IMMUNE REGULATION VIII
Edited by Sudhir Gupta

Volume 491
THE MOLECULAR IMMUNOLOGY OF COMPLEX CARBOHYDRATES—2
Edited by Albert M. Wu

Volume 492
NUTRITION AND CANCER PREVENTION: New Insights into the Role of Phytochemicals
Edited under the auspices of the American Institute for Cancer Research

Volume 493
NEUROIMMUNE CIRCUITS, DRUGS OF ABUSE, AND INFECTIOUS DISEASES
Edited by Herman Friedman, Thomas W. Klein, and John J. Madden

Volume 494
THE NIDOVIRUSES (CORONAVIRUSES AND ARTERIVIRUSES)
Edited by Ehud Lavi, Susan R. Weiss, and Susan T. Hingley

Volume 495
PROGRESS IN BASIC AND CLINICAL IMMUNOLOGY
Edited by Andrzej Mackiewicz, Maciej Kurpisz, and Jan Żeromski

---

PROGRESS IN BASIC AND CLINICAL IMMUNOLOGY

Edited by

Andrzej Mackiewicz
University School of Medical Sciences
GreatPoland Cancer Center
Poznan, Poland

Maciej Kurpisz
Institute of Human Genetics
Polish Academy of Sciences
Poznan, Poland

and

Jan Żeromski
University School of Medical Sciences
Department of Immunology
Poznan, Poland

Kluwer Academic / Plenum Publishers
New York, Boston, Dordrecht, London, Moscow

Library of Congress Cataloging-in-Publication Data

Progress in basic and clinical immunology/edited by Andrzej Mackiewicz, Maciej Kurpisz, and Jan Zeromski.
p. ; cm. — (Advances in experimental medicine and biology, ISSN 0065-2598; v. 495)
"Proceedings of the 14th European Immunology Meeting (EFIS 2000) held September 23–27, 2000, in Poznan, Poland"—T.p. verso.
Includes bibliographical references and index.
ISBN 0-306-46656-2
1. Immunology—Congresses. 2. Clinical immunology—Congresses. I. Mackiewicz, Andrzej. II. Kurpisz, Maciej. III. Zeromski, Jan, 1938- IV. European Immunology Meeting (14th: 2000: Poznan, Poland) V. Series.
[DNLM: I. Immunity, Cellular—Congresses. 2. Autoimmunity—Congresses. 3. Dendritic Cells—physiology—Congresses. 4. Receptors, Immunologic—Congresses. 5. T-Lymphocytes—physiology—Congresses. QW 568 P964 2001]
QR180.3 .P76 2001
616.07′9—dc21

2001038777

Proceedings of the 14th European Immunology Meeting (EFIS 2000), held September 23–27, 2000, in Poznan, Poland

ISSN: 0065 2598

ISBN 0-306-46656-2

233 Spring Street, New York, New York 10013

http://www.wkap.nl

10 9 8 7 6 5 4 3 2 1

A C.I.P. record for this book is available from the Library of Congress

Printed in the United States of America

Contributors

Supporters

- The State Committee for Scientific Research
- Olympus Optical Polska Sp. z o.o.

Contributors

- Association for Fight Against Cancer "Genes For Life"
- Becton Dickinson
- CARL ZEISS Sp. z o.o.
- GlaxoWellcome
- GreatPoland Cancer Center
- LOT - Polish Airlines
- PPS Airpol Sp. z o.o.
- Talex SA
- The Leopold Kronenberg Foundation
- University School of Medical Sciences – Poznań
- Wielkopolski Bank Kredytowy – WBK S.A.

Participants

- Alexis Corporation
- Nature Publishing Group
- Preussen Electra Polska
- SARSTEDT Sp. z o.o.
- Sigma Aldrich Sp. z o.o.

List of Exhibitors

- Abott Laboratories Poland
- ADIS International Ltd.
- Becton Dickinson
- Bellco Biomedica Polska Sp. z o.o.
- Biker PTiO
- Biocom Systems s.c.
- Biomibo
- Bio-RAD Laboratories GmbH, Prospecta Sp. z o.o.
- Birkhauser Publishers
- Caltag Laboratories Inc.
- CARL ZEISS Sp. z o.o.
- DAKO Polska Sp. z o.o.
- Elsevier
- EFIS 2003
- ICN Biomedicals, Inc.
- Inter Medic Sp. z. o.o
- KARGER AG
- Kendro Sp. z.o.o.
- Miltenyi Biotec GnbH.
- MPW Med-instruments Sp. Pracy
- Nature Publishing Group
- Olympus Optical Polska Sp. z.o.o.
- Oxford University Press
- Polaton OBRI
- R + D Systems Europe Ltd.
- SARSTEDT Sp. z o.o.
- Science International
- Schering-Plough Central Europe AG
- Stem Cell Technologies
- Wiley-Vch Verlags GmbH
- Wisepress Ltd.

Preface

Progress in Basic and Clinical Immunology is a result of the 14th European Immunology Meeting - EFIS 2000 held in Poznań, Poland on 23-27 September 2000. EFIS 2000 gathered over 1400 immunologists from all over the world. It was an exceptionally memorable meeting for a number of reasons: 1) it was held in the last year of the century and the millennium, thus provoking conclusions of past achievements of immunology and projections for the future; 2) it was held in Poland, a country that is a symbol of struggle for freedom for a large number of scientists originating from the "Eastern Bloc" countries and 3) EFIS celebrated its 25th anniversary at this occasion.

The scientific program included: Key Note Lecture by Peter Krammer (Germany), 9 State-of-Art Lectures including Rolf M. Zinkernagel (Switzerland) - Nobel Prize Laureate - lecture entitled "Immunity 2000", 14 Meet an Expert Sessions, 80 Plenary Lectures and 47 Workshops. Altogether 875 communications were presented. The philosophy of the scientific program did not follow the usual routine of immunology meetings. Topics of the plenary sessions were selected on the basis of recent developments rather than historical background. On the other hand Workshops were designed on the basis of abstracts submitted. We invited 117 authors to submit their presentations for publication in *Progress in Basic and Clinical Immunology* - 62 were received and are included in this book. Most of the papers are related to the tumour immunology and immunotherapy that reflects a major focus of submitted abstracts for EFIS 2000. Of course, not all the very valuable communications could be included in the volume. However, we trust that the selection that we have offered will be at least in part representative of the meeting and will pave the way for further developments.

Andrzej Mackiewicz
Maciej Kurpisz
Jan Żeromski

Contents

T-CELLS

IMMUNE RECEPTORS

ANTIGEN PRESENTATION / DENDRITIC CELLS

CYTOKINES

IMMUNODEFICIENCES

AUTOIMMUNITY

ALLERGY / INFLAMMATION

IMMUNOTHERAPY

VACCINES

TUMOR IMMUNOLOGY

CANCER IMMUNOTHERAPY

Introduction

ANDRZEJ MACKIEWICZ, JAN ZEROMSKI, and MACIEJ KURPISZ

Progress in Basic and Clinical Immunology contains 62 chapters grouped into 11 sections: T-cells, Immune receptors, Antigen presentation/Dendritic cells, Cytokines, Immunodeficiences, Autoimmunity, Allergy/Inflammation, Immunotherapy, Vaccines, Tumor immunology and Cancer immunotherapy. The best represented is Cancer immunotherapy section which contains 16 chapters. About one half of all chapters were prepared by invited speakers, and the second half by authors of workshop presentations. The selection of workshop communications was done on the basis of workshop chairmen recommendations and in a small part on geographical localization. Each section contains both types of papers, those prepared by invited speakers and those submitted by workshop contributors. Some chapters, especially those prepared by invited speakers are of the state-of-art type reviews, while other present original experimental data. We were unfortunately unable to include all communications from EFIS 2000 in this volume. However, abstracts of all the works are published in a Special issue of *Immunology Letters* 73:75-302, 2000 the official journal of the European Federation of Immunological Societies.

We would like to acknowledge the help of Dr Piotr Wysocki in the preparation of this volume.

T-CELLS

CD3-dependent regulation of early TCRβ gene expression in mainstream αβ and NKαβ T cell development

NICOLE BAUR and KLAUS EICHMANN
Max-Planck-Institut für Immunbiologie, Stübeweg 51, D-79108 Freiburg, Germany

1. INTRODUCTION

During development in the thymus, mainstream αβ lineage thymocytes repeatedly pass through checkpoints at which they are selected for molecular properties that make them useful for further maturation. Selection of a useful repertoire of specific αβ T cell receptors (TCR) takes place at the $CD4^{+}8^{+}$ double positive (DP) stage, i.e. relatively late in thymic development (reviewed in [1,2]). Earlier checkpoints which select cells for generic functions occur in the $CD4^{-}8^{-}$ double negative (DN) stage of thymocyte maturation (reviewed in [3,4]). This stage is divided sequentially into the subsets DN1 ($CD44^{+}25^{-}$), DN2 ($CD44^{+}25^{+}$), DN3 ($CD44^{-}25^{+}$), and DN4 ($CD44^{-}25^{-}$) [5]. Most of TCRβ locus VDJ rearrangement takes place in DN3 [6]. TCRβ polypeptide chains are then synthesized and assemble with pre-Tα 7,8 and the clonotype independent CD3 complexes (CIC) 9 to form the pre-TCR which signals $TCR\beta^{+}$ cells to continue maturation to the DP stage, a process referred to as "β-selection" (reviewed in [4,10-12]). A number of mouse strains genetically manipulated to have severe defects in the molecular composition or signaling function of the pre-TCR/CD3 complex have drastically reduced numbers of cells in DN4, suggesting a block at the DN3 stage. Moreover, we have previously shown that expression of TCRβ polypeptide chains is impaired in DN3 cells of mice deficient in CD3 and/or $p56^{lck}$ (Lck) [13,14]. While TCRβ locus rearrangement appeared to proceed independently of

CD3 signaling, TCRβ mRNA and protein levels were 5-10 fold reduced in DN cells of CD3 signaling-deficient mice [13-15]. These observations suggested that early TCRβ gene expression requires upregulation by CD3-associated signals. Subsequently, a discussion arose whether TCRβ expression is upregulated by the pre-TCR or by CD3 signaling prior to expression of TCRβ proteins, i.e. by CIC [13,16]. Because the entry of DN3 cells into the cell cycle is so far the earliest evidence of pre-TCR activity [17,18]., we investigated in this report CD3 dependent TCRβ gene upregulation in relation to cell cycle status of DN3 cells.

We also investigated TCRβ expression in NK1.1$^+$αβT cell development. NK1.1$^+$ αβT (NKT) cells represent a minor subset of lymphoid cells expressing αβTCR as well as markers of the natural killer (NK) cell lineage (reviewed in [19, 20]). The repertoire of αβTCR of these NKT cells is dominated by a single TCRα chain (Vα14-Jβ281) and a limited choice of TCRβ chain families (Vβ8 family, mostly Vβ8.2, and Vβ7, Vβ2). NKT cell development is impaired in mice bearing a variety of genetic defects, including the CD3 associated signaling molecules CD3ζ 21, p56lck (Lck), and p59fyn 22, 23. The dependence on molecules associated with CD3 complex signaling is consistent either with a requirement of positive repertoire selection in NKT cell development, or with a pre-TCR-dependent checkpoint equivalent to β-selection of mainstream αβT cells. The latter possibility is supported by the absolute requirement of pre-Tα for NKT development [24]. However, the developmental stage at which NKT cell development is arrested in pre-Tα deficient mice has not been chraracterized. Here we show that NKT cell development in CD3ζ/Lck double-deficient mice is completely arrested at a pre-NKT cell-like stage. Moreover, the results suggest an absolute dependence of initial TCRβ gene expression on CD3 signaling in pre-NKT cells, in contrast to mainstream pre-αβT cells that exhibit a low CD3 independent level of TCRβ gene expression.

2. RESULTS

2.1 Regulation of TCRβ expression in DN3 cells prior to cell cycle entry

To define the developmental timing of TCRβ upregulation, we studied intracellular (IC) TCRβ protein levels in DN thymocytes in relation to cell cycle, using four color FCM. The population comprising both DN3 and DN4 cells was first gated as $CD4^-CD8^-CD44^-CD3\varepsilon^-NK1.1^-$. The $CD25^+$ population (DN3) was then analysed for intracellular (IC) TCRβ and for DNA content by staining with 7AAD. As shown in Fig.1, mice double deficient for CD3ζ and Lck (ζ/Lck-dd mice) and mice double deficient for CD3ε and CD3ζ (ζ/ε-dd mice) generate reduced numbers of DN4 cells compared to B6 wildtype (wt) mice. Neither of the two ko strains generates any DP thymocytes (data not shown). About 75% of DN3 cells of wt mice are in G0/G1 and contain about 18% of $TCR\beta IC^+$ cells. About 25% of wt DN3 cells are in the S/G2/M phases in which the proportion of $TCR\beta IC^+$ cells is increased to about 60%. In contrast, only about 10% DN3 cells of ζ/Lck-dd mice or of ζ/ε-dd mice are in S/G2/M phases of the cell cycle and are depleted rather than enriched for $TCR\beta IC^+$ cells. As previously shown, DN3 cells of ζ/Lck-dd mice [13] and CD3ε deficient mice [15] exhibit about 5-10 fold lower levels of intracellular TCRβ mRNA and protein than wt DN3 cells. The results in Fig. 1 demonstrate that this is also the case for DN3 cells of ζ/ε-dd mice, suggesting that inefficient TCRβ gene expression is general for DN3 cells of mice with compromized CD3 complex signaling. Most importantly, DN3 cells of wt mice in G0/G1 show 5-10fold higher levels of TCRβIC staining compared to DN3 cells of ζ/Lck-dd mice or of ζ/ε-dd mice. As most of wt DN3 cells with diploid DNA content are likely to be still in G0 (see discussion), these results suggest that CD3 signals upregulate TCRβ gene expression in wt DN3 cells prior to their entry into the cell cycle.

2.2 CD3-dependent regulation of TCRβ gene expression in NKT cells

Total numbers of $CD44^+NK1.1^+$ cells per thymus in ζ/Lck-dd mice and TCRα deficient mice are about 10fold lower than in wt mice (B6, 3.0-6.3 x 10^5; TCRα ko, 0.2-0.7 x 10^5, ζ/Lck-dd, 0.4-1.0 x 10^5). In agreement with previous reports [21-25], these results confirm that the development of NKT cells in the thymus is dependent on TCRα genes and on CD3 complex signaling. To assess a putative CD3 dependence of TCRβ gene expression in NKT cells, we analyzed intracellular and cell surface TCRβ protein levels and TCRβ rearrangements in NKT cells of wt, ζ/Lck-dd mice, and TCRα deficient mice. As shown in Fig. 2, the vast majority of NKT cells of wt mice express TCRβ both intracellularly (ic) and at the cell surface (sf). TCRα-deficient mice generate $CD44^+NK1.1^+$ thymocytes with TCRβ VDJ rearrangements but without surface αβTCR expression, similar to ζ/Lck-dd mice. $CD44^+NK1.1^+$ cells of ζ/Lck-dd mice are almost entirely devoid of intracellular TCRβ protein. In contrast, intracellular TCRβ protein is seen at high levels in about one-fourth of the $CD44^{+}NK1.1^{+}$ thymocytes of TCRα-deficient mice. TCR Vβ8 and Vβ5 family members have rearranged in the $CD44^{-}NK1.1^{+}$ populations of wt mice, TCRα deficient mice, and ζ/Lck-dd mice. However, while $CD44^{+}NK1.1^{+}$ cells of wt mice and TCRα deficient mice contain mRNA for TCRVβ8 or TCRVβ5, that of ζ/Lck-dd mice are devoid of either mRNAs (data not shown). The presence of TCRβ rearrangements suggest that the $TCR\beta IC^{-}CD44^{+}NK1.1^{+}$ population in ζ/Lck-dd contains precursors of NKT cells. The generation of $TCR\beta IC^{+}$ immature NKT cells appears to be dependent on the functional CD3 complex that is present in TCRα deficient mice but not in ζ/Lck-dd mice.

While TCRβ VDJ rearrangements take place in pre-NKT cells of ζ/Lck-dd mice. the rearranged TCRβ genes are not expressed. To determine whether the $TCR\beta IC^{-}$ pre-NKT cells of ζ/Lck-dd mice contain productive TCRβ VDJ rearrangements, Vβ8DJ and Vβ5DJ junctions in sorted $CD44^{+}NK1.1^{+}$ populations were amplified by PCR, randomly cloned, and subjected to DNA sequencing (Fig. 2). Expected frequencies of in frame VDJ junctions in selected and unselected populations are 71.4% and 33%, respectively (42). As expected, $CD44^{+}NK1.1^{+}$ cells of wt mice are highly selected for productive Vβ8DJ rearrangements, and against productive Vβ5DJ rearrangements. In frame Vβ8DJ and in frame Vβ5DJ junctions were indeed detected in $CD44^{+}NK1.1^{+}$ thymocytes of ζ/Lck-dd mice, at frequencies not significantly different from the 33% expected in non-selected populations. Among $CD44^{+}NK1.1^{+}$ thymocytes of TCRα deficient mice, $TCR\beta IC^{-}$ cells are partially depleted of in frame TCRβ joints, consistent with the expression of TCRβ proteins soon after the generation of productive rearrangements. In contrast to mature NKT cells of wt mice, the $TCR\beta IC^{+}$ subpopulation in TCRα deficient mice is positively selected for both Vβ8DJ and Vβ5DJ joints, consistent with indiscriminate expression of all in frame TCRβ VDJ genes in pre-NKT cells. These results suggest that NKT cell development in ζ/Lck-dd mice is arrested at a stage prior to β-selection owing to lack of TCRβ expression. In contrast, NKT cell development in TCRα deficient mice is arrested after general β-expression and before positive selection for TCR Vβ8 family gene products.

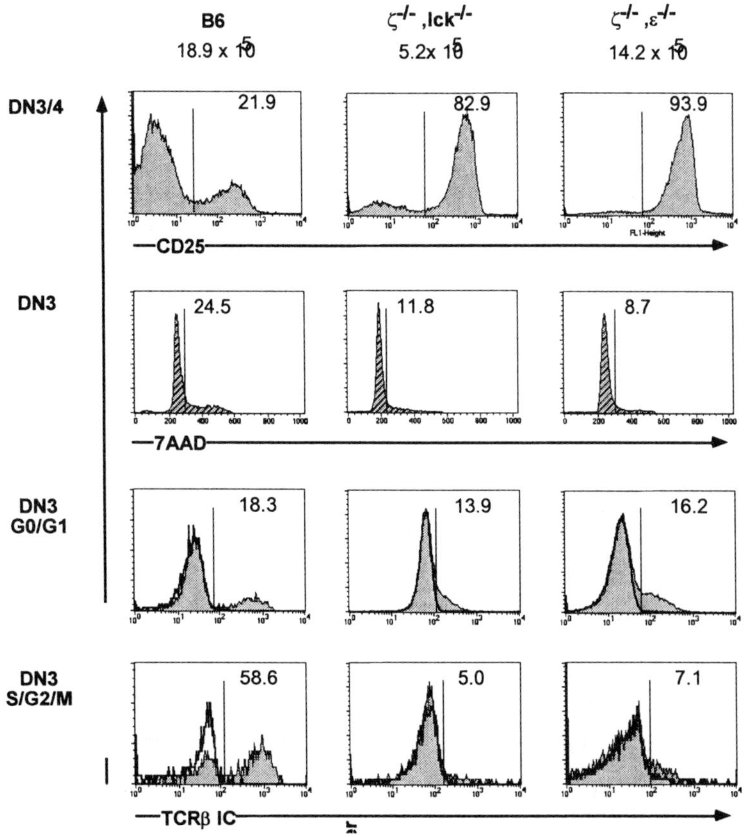

Figure 1.Four color FCM analysis of intracellular (IC) TCRβ expression in DN3 thymocytes in the G0/G1 and the S/G2/M phases of the cell cycle. B6 wt mice, ζ/lck-dd mice, and ζ/ε-dd mice were analysed; results from representative individual mice are shown. DN3/DN4 subpopulations were negatively gated with a pool of mAb as described in the text, all APC labelled. Additional colors were anti-CD25 (biotin+ PerCP), DNA staining with 7AAD, and anti-TCRβIC (PE). The $CD25^+$ (DN3) subsets were gated as shown in the top row. Gating for DN3 cells with diploid (G0/G1) and hyperdiploid (S/G2/M) DNA content is shown in the second row. TCRβIC staining profiles are shaded (third and fourth row); negative controls were done by blocking with an excess of unlabelled anti-TCRβ mAb (superimposed bold profiles). Relative intracellular TCRβ protein levels were estimated by the ratio of the mean fluorescence channel of the positively gated cells over the mean fluorescence channel of the negatively gated cells. In DN3 G0/G1 cells these ratios were: B6, 28; ζ/Lck-dd, 3.1; ζ/ε-dd, 5.2. Percentages of relevant subpopulations are shown in each frame, total numbers of DN3/DN4 cells per mouse are shown on top.

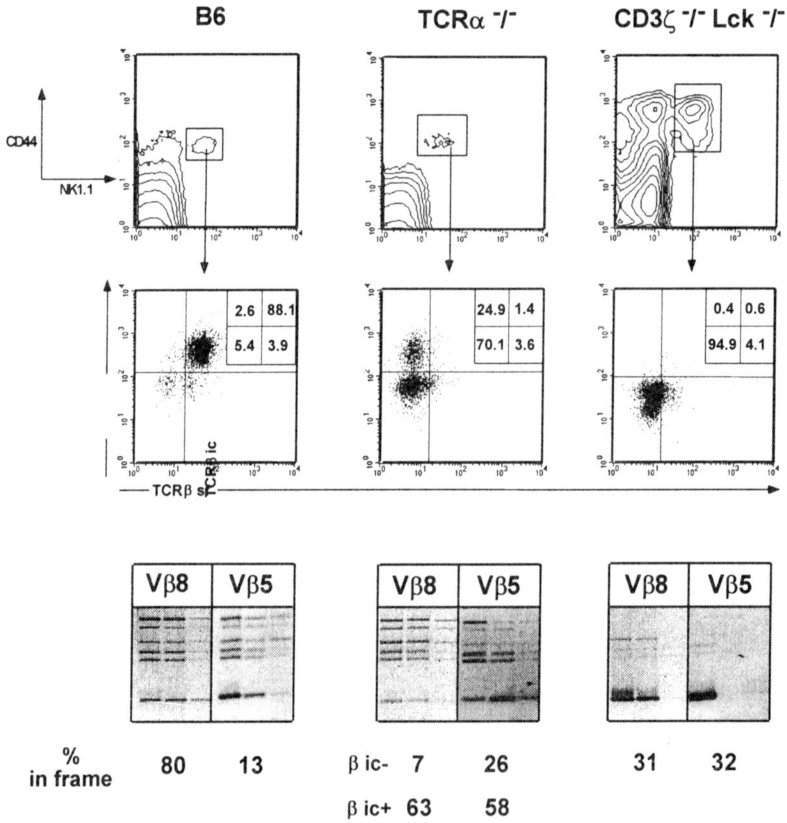

Figure 2. Analyses of intracellular (ic) and surface (sf) TCRβ polypeptide chains and of TCRβ rearrangements in CD44$^+$ NK1.1$^+$ cells of B6 wt mice, TCRα deficient mice, and ζ/Lck-dd mice. Total thymocytes were stained with anti-CD44 (APC), anti-NK1.1 (B+PerCP), and with anti-TCRβ first at the cell surface (FITC) and subsequently by intracellular staining (PE). CD44$^+$NK1.1$^+$ populations were gated (top panels) and analysed for TCRβsf vs TCRβic (middle panels). Data are from individual representative mice. Percentages of subpopulations are given in the insets. CD44$^+$ NK1.1$^+$ thymocytes were purified by preparative flow cytometry. DNA was prepared and adjusted to similar concentrations using spectrophotometric determination and PCR amplification of the insulin gene[13] at 2-fold dilutions (not shown). Vβ8DJβ2 and Vβ5DJβ2 junctions were amplified at at 2-fold dilutions as shown in the bottom panels. PCR products were separated on agarose gels, stained with ethidium bromide, and inversely photographed. Rearranged TCRβ VDJ genes display as 6 bands corresponding to Jβ2.1 to Jβ2.6 from top to bottom. PCR products were randomly cloned, and sequenced. The percentages of in frame rearrangements are given at the bottom.

3. DISCUSSION

In this paper we compare the control of TCRβ expression levels in mainstream pre-αβ T cells and pre-NKT cells by CD3 complex associated signaling. For mainstream pre-αβ T cells the results suggest that CD3 signals upregulate expression of rearranged TCRβ VDJ genes in the DN3 stage 5-10fold above a low constitutive level that is seen in DN3 cells of CD3 signaling-deficient mice. TCRβ levels are upregulated in DN3 cells of wt mice with diploid DNA content. Most of these cells are likely to be still in G0 for the following reasons: The DN3 stage lasts for about 3 days, and TCRβ VDJ rearrangements are likely to occur throughout this period. Most TCRβ VDJ rearrangements will therefore have occurred less than 3 days ago. The onset of proliferation follows the appearance of TCRβ polypeptide chains with a delay of 1-2 days [18]. During most of the DN3 stage, TCRβIC$^+$ cells therefore reside in the interval between expression of TCRβ protein and onset of cell cycle. Thus, CD3 mediated upregulation of TCRβ gene expression takes place in most DN3 cells before they enter the cell cycle. Together, these results suggest that TCRβ gene expression is so far the earliest CD3 regulated event in thymocyte differentiation.

In analogy to mainstream pre-αβT cells we identified an early checkpoint of pre-NKT cells at which surface αβTCR/CD3 expression is undetectable by FCM, whereas rearranged TCRβ VDJ genes are present. Moreover, whereas 80-90% of wt NKT cells showed high levels of TCRβIC staining, the pre-NKT cells of ζ/Lck-dd were essentially negative. As we could not detect TCRβ mRNA by RT-PCR in ζ/Lck-dd pre-NKT cells, we think that little if any TCRβ gene expression takes place in pre-NKT cells of severely CD3 signaling-deficient mice. Nevertheless, pre-NKT cells of ζ/Lck-dd mice contained productive TCRβ VDJ rearrangements, at frequencies suggesting a nonselected population. In contrast, pre-NKT cells of TCRα-deficient mice contain a significant population with high TCRβIC staining. The data therefore strongly suggest that the generation of pre-NKT cells with intracellular TCRβ protein is dependent on CD3 complex associated signals. Of note, nearly all of the NKT cells of TCRα-deficient mice express TCRγδ receptors at the cell surface (not shown), whereas TCRβ does not appear at the cell surface. It is therefore possible that the generation of TCRβIC$^+$ NKT cells in TCRα-deficient mice is induced by surface γδTCR/CD3 signals, consistent with our observation that TCRβ protein expression is induced indiscriminately.

Aifantis et al. [16] recently confirmed our initial observations [13,14,26] that early TCRβ gene expression is regulated by CD3 signals and have claimed that early TCRβ gene expression is controled by the pre-TCR. In contrast, we have previously considered the possibility that initial TCRβ gene expression may be controled by the CD3 complexes (CIC, pro-TCR) expressed on pro-T cells prior to TCRβ rearrangement and expression [13,14,26]. In this context it seems important that the CD3 dependence of TCRβ expression in pre-NKT cells appears to be absolute, in contrast to mainstream pre-αβ T cells that exhibit a low CD3 independent level of TCRβ expression. The low CD3 independent TCRβ expression in mainstream pre-αβ T cells may be compatible with pre-TCR mediated regulation. The absolute dependence of TCRβ expression on CD3 signals in pre-NKT cells is more difficult to reconcile with a control by the pre-TCR, as the formation of a pre-TCR requires the presence of TCRβ protein. Although CIC have so far not been demonstrated on pre-NKT cells, an involvement of an early form of CD3 conplex in the control of TCRβ expression may have to be considered.

ACKNOWLEDGEMENTS

We thank Ingrid Falk and Gabi Nerz for able technical assistance, Andreas Würch for valuable help with PCR techniques and flow cytometry, and Dr. H. Mossmann and the animal house staff of the MPI for competent mouse breeding.

REFERENCES

1. Kisielow, P., and von Boehmer, H., 1995, Development and selection of T cells: facts and puzzles. Adv. Immunol. 58:87.
2. Robey, E., and Fowlkes, B.J., 1994, Selective events in T cell development. Annu. Rev. Immunol. 12:675.
3. Godfrey, D.I., and Zlotnik, A., 1993, Control points in early T cell development. Immunol. Today 14:547.
4. Fehling, H.J., and von Boehmer, H., 1997, Early αβ T cell development in the thymus of normal and genetically altered mice. Curr. Biol. 9:263.
5. Godfrey, D.I., Kennedy, J., Suda, T., and Zlotnik, A., 1993, A developmental pathway involving four phenotypically and functionally distinct subsets of CD3-CD4-CD8- triple-negative adult mouse thymocytes defined by CD44 and CD25 expression. J. Immunol. 150:4244.
6. Godfrey, D.I., Kennedy, J., Mombaerts, P., Tonegawa, S., and Zlotnik, A., 1994. Onset of TCRβ gene rearrangement and role of TCRβ expression during CD3-CD4-CD8- thymocyte differentiation. J. Immunol. 152:4783.
7. Groettrup, M., Ungewiss, K., Azogui, O., Palacios, R., Owen, M.J., Hayday, A.C., and von Boehmer, H., 1993, A novel disulfide-linked heterodimer on pre-T cells consists of the T cell receptor β chain and a 33 kDa glycoprotein. Cell 75:283.
8. Saint-Ruf, C., Ungewiss, K., Groettrup, M., Bruno, L., Fehling, H.J., and von Boehmer, H., 1994, Analysis and expression of a cloned pre-T cell receptor gene. Science 266:208.

9. Wiest, D.L., Kearse, K.P., Shores, E.W., and Singer, A., 1994, Developmentally regulated expression of CD3 components independent of clonotypic T-cell antigen receptor complexes on immature thymocytes. J. Exp. Med. 180:1375.
10. Levelt, C.N., and Eichmann, K., 1995, Receptors and signals in early thymic selection. Immunity 3:667.
11. Zunicka-Pflücker, J.L., and Lenardo, M.J., 1996, Regulation of thymocyte development from immature progenitors. Curr. Opin. Immunol. 8:215.
12. Tanaka, Y., Ardouin, L., Gillet, A., Lin, S.Y., Magnan, A., Malissen, B., and Malissen, M., 1995, Early T cell development in CD3-deficient mice. Immunol. Rev. 148:171.
13. Würch, A., Biro, J., Potocnik, A.J., Falk, I., Mossmann, H., and Eichmann, K., 1998, Requirement of CD3 complex-associated signaling functions for expression of rearranged T cell receptor-β VDJ genes in early thymic development. J. Exp. Med. 188:1669.
14. Biro, J., Würch, A., Potocnik, A.J., Falk, I., Mossmann, H., and Eichmann, K., 1999, Regulation of T cell receptor (TCR) β gene expression by CD3 complex signaling in immature thymocytes: implications for TCRβ allelic exclusion. Proc. Nat. Acad. Sci. USA 96:3882.
15. Malissen, M., Gillet, M., Ardouin, L., Bouvier, G., Trucy, J., Ferrier, P., Vivier, E., and B. Malissen, B., 1995, Altered T cell development in mice with a targeted mutation of the CD3-ε gene. EMBO J. 14: 4641
16. Aifantis, I., Feinberg, J., Fehling, H.J., DiSanto, J. P., and von Boehmer, H., 1999, Early T cell receptor □gene expression is regulated by the pre-T cell receptor-CD3 complex. J. Exp. Med. 190: 141.
17. Hoffman, E.S., Passoni, L., Crompton, T., Leu, T.M.J., Schatz, D.G., Koff, A., Owen, M. J., and Hayday, A.C., 1996, Productive T-cell receptor β-chain gene rearrangement: coincident regulation of cell cycle and clonality during development in vivo. Genes Dev. 10:948.
18. Falk, I., Biro, J., Kohler, H., and Eichmann, K., 1996, Proliferation kinetics associated with T cell receptor-β chain selection of fetal murine thymocytes. J. Exp. Med.184: 2327.
19. Bendelac, A., Rivera, M.N., Park, S.H., and, Roark, J.H., 1997, Mouse CD1-specific NK1 T cells: development, specificity, and function. Annu. Rev. Immunol. 15:535.
20. MacDonald, H.R., 1995, NK1.1+ T cell receptor-α/β+ cells: new clues to their origin, specificity, and function. J. Exp. Med. 182:633.
21. Arase, H., Ono, S., Arase, N., Park, S.Y., Wakizaka, K., Watanabe, H., Ohno, H., and Saito, T., 1995, Developmental arrest of NK1.1+ T cell antigen receptor (TCR)-α/β+ T cells and expansion of NK1.1+ TCR-γ/δ+ T cell development in CD3ζ-deficient mice. J. Exp. Med. 182:891.
22. Eberl, G., Lowin-Kropf, B., and MacDonald, H.R., 1999, Cutting Edge: NKT cell development is selectively impaired in Fyn-deficient mice. J. Immunol. 163:4091.
23. Gadue, P., Morton, N., and Stein, P.L., 1999, The Src family tyrosine kinase fyn regulates natural killer T cell development. J. Exp. Med. 190:1189.
24. Eberl, G., Fehling, H.J., von Boehmer, H., and MacDonald, H.R., 1999, Absolute requirement for the pre-T cell receptor α chain during NK1.1+ TCRαβ cell development. Eur. J. Immunol. 29:1966.
25. Cui, J., Shin, T., Kawano, T., Sato, H., Kondo, E., Toura, I., Kaneko, Y., Koseki, H., Kanno, M., Taniguchi, M., 1997, Requirement for Vα14 NKT cells in IL-12-mediated rejection of tumors. Science 278:1623.
26. Würch, A., Biro, J., Falk, I., Mossmann, H., and Eichmann, K., 1999, Reduced generation but efficient TCRβ-chain selection of CD4+8+ double-positive thymocytes in mice with compromized CD3 complex signaling. J. Immunol. 162:2741.

Molecular characterization of gut T cell precursors in euthymic and athymic mice

FLORENCE LAMBOLEZ and BENEDITA ROCHA
INSERM U.345, Institut Necker, 156 rue de Vaugirard, 75730 PARIS CEDEX 15, France

1. INTRODUCTION

The major compartment of effector T cells in the body lines the epithelium of the murine gut. Intraepithelial T lymphocytes (T-IEL) from this location have large intracytoplasmic storage granules containing perforin and granzyme and express γ-INF mRNA. *Ex vivo*, they secrete this lymphokine and kill target cells immediately[1-3]. The number of these T cells is comparable to that of all T cells present in both spleen and lymph-nodes[4]. T-IEL have different origins in normal mice[5-9]. About half derive from activated T cells migrating from the peripheral lymphoid organs to the gut and have a memory phenotype (TcR-$\alpha\beta^+$ $CD5^+$ $CD28^+$ LFA-1^+ $CD44^+$ CD8$\alpha\beta^+$ or $CD4^+$ thymus-dependent-IEL/TD-IEL). The other half differs from peripheral T cells by phenotype (CD8$\alpha\alpha^+$ $CD5^-$ LFA-1^- $B220^+$) and CD3 complex expression (CD3-ζ chain is associated with a ζ analogue, the FcεRIγ chain[10]). They comprise a large proportion of TcR-$\gamma\delta^+$ cells, and the TcR-$\alpha\beta^+$ cells of this lineage are not deleted by self antigens[4,11,12]. CD8αα T-IELs are thought to develop locally: structures named cryptopatches, disseminated randomly at the base of some gut crypts containing TcR^- $Thy1^+$ c-kit^+ IL-$7R^+$ $CD25^+$ cells[13,14] were assimilated to "local" thymus like structures harboring differentiating precursors[14,15]. Although CD8αα T-IELs are generated in athymic mice, the presence of a thymus increases their number by five-to 10 fold and modifies their composition[5,7,16]. In euthymic mice, TcR-αβ and TcR-γδ T cells are equally represented. In athymic mice about 90-95% of TcR^+ T cells are $\gamma\delta^+$. These differences remain after the injection of peripheral T cells (what reconstitutes TD-IEL), and thus are not due to any role of the TD-IEL on the maturation or expansion of CD8αα T-IEL.

The role of the thymus in CD8αα T-IEL generation could be hormone mediated[17]. Other experiments, however, show that the thymus may be a direct cell source to the CD8αα T-IEL population, as ectopic thymus grafts transplanted into athymic mice repopulate the gut with T cells of graft origin[16,18]. If the thymus seeds the gut wall, it is not known at what stage of T cell maturation these migrants colonize the gut.

To define the pathways of the putative T cell differentiation in the gut, and to identify the origin of gut T cell precursors we studied the $CD3^-$ gut populations in euthymic and athymic mice.

2. RESULTS

To obtain $CD3^-$ cells from euthymic or nude mice, the gut wall was separated from the epithelium. Lymphocytes were recovered either from collagenase digests of the wall (Wall Lymphocytes-WL) or dissociated from epithelial cells (intraepithelial lymphocytes-IEL)[9]. WL and IEL populations were labeled with a mixture of several Abs, recognizing mature heamatopoietic cells (Fig. 1), and Lin^- populations analyzed. In the WL, the the majority of cells were $CD8^-$ and expressed Thy1 at different levels. In the IEL, the majority of IEL were $Thy1^-$ and expressed variable levels of CD8α. These two major subpopulations were enriched to 60-70% purity by a first sorting, and sorted to purity by a second sorting.

We compared the expression of several genes by $CD3^-$ thymocytes and gut cells. We studied GATA-2 expression as this gene was reported to be expressed by differentiating haematopoietic cells, before commitment to the B and T cell lineages[19]. GATA-3, a transcription factor reported to be transcribed by T cell lineage committed cells and required for T cell differentiation[20]; CD3-ε, pre-Tα and Rag-1 expression (Fig. 2A). We found that $CD3^-$ thymocytes expressed both GATA-3 and CD3-ε, but did not express GATA-2 mRNAs. The $Thy1^+$ gut cells transcribed all three genes, suggesting that this population contained both non-committed and T cell-committed precursors. In gut $CD8^+$ populations, we only found the transcription of GATA-3 and CD3-ε mRNA, suggesting that these cells are committed to T cell differentiation. We readily found Rag-1 mRNA expression in $Thy1^+$ cells, but not in $CD8^+$ IEL. To compare the relative frequency of recombinase expressing cells in isolates from different mice, we sorted $Thy1^+$ cells from nude and euthymic mice into multiple individual

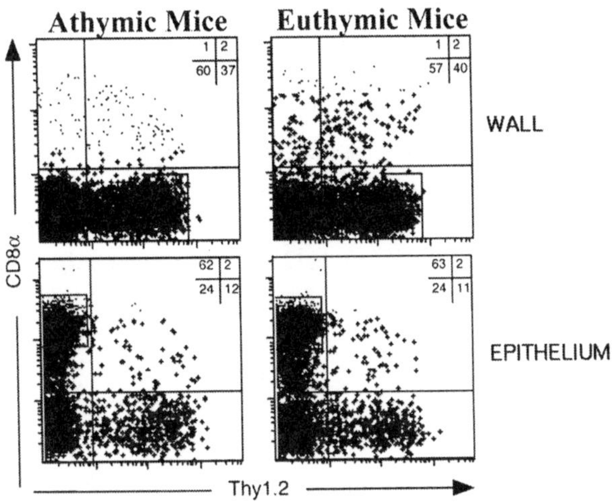

Figure 1. The phenotype of Lineage negative gut cells: cells isolated from the gut wall or the epithelium were labeled with a cocktail of antibodies recognizing T cells, B cells, granulocytes, macrophages and red blood cells. Results show gated Lineage negative (Lin$^-$) cells.

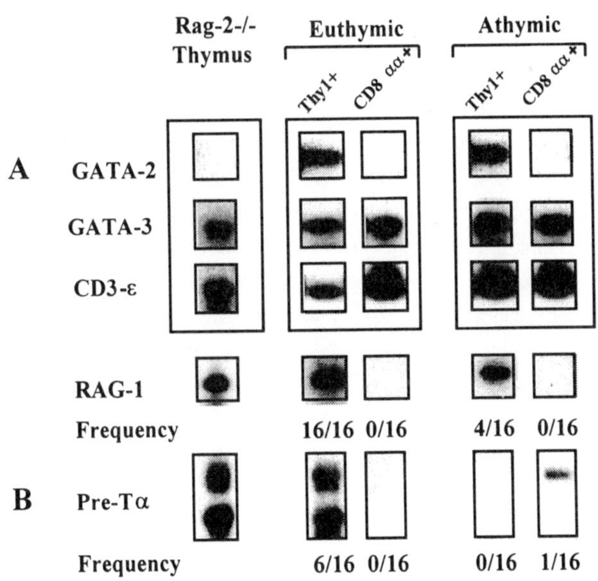

Figure 2. Expression of different genes by gut precursors. Lineage negative cells were sorted and tested for the expression of several genes as described previously[21]. PcR products were blotted and hybridized with specific probes. The primers used[22] do not amplify DNA.

wells containing 1,000 cells each. The conditions of PcR amplification we used are efficient enough to detect Rag-1 mRNA expression by 83% of individual $CD44^-$ $CD25^+$ thymocytes. In nude mice but 1/3 to 1/4 of the wells were detected as containing Rag-1 mRNA. In euthymic mice $Thy1^+$ cells, Rag-1 mRNA was found in all tested samples. These results suggest that lymphocyte receptor rearrangements are more active in euthymic than in athymic mice. To study TcR rearrangements in $CD3^-$ gut populations (Fig. 3) we evaluated: the extension of TcR-β DJ rearrangement by a PcR that allows the identification of both germline Dβ2.1-Jβ2.7 fragment, and all Dβ2.1-Jβ2 rearrangements[23]; TcR-β V(D)J rearrangements by using a mixture of V region primers together with a J region primer[24] and TcR-α VJ rearrangements by using a mixture of V region primers and a J region primer[25]. These assays can detect rearrangements when TcR-$\alpha\beta^+$ cells constitute but 1% of the total DNA pool. With respect to TcR-γ rearrangements, we characterized two that are those differently expressed in the gut versus the thymus-derived TcR-$\gamma\delta^+$: Vγ2, that is a prevalent in the thymus and Vγ5, abundant in the gut TcR-$\gamma\delta^+$ IEL, but rarely expressed in the thymus[26].

In $Thy1^+$ from euthymic mice cells, the DJ germ line band was present, V(D)J rearrangements were pauciclonal and TcR-α rearrangements could not be detected. In $CD8^+$ the DJ germline band was absent, V(D)J rearrangements were abundant, and TcR-α chain rearrangements were readily detected. With respect to TcR-γ chain rearrangements, we were surprised that Vγ2 (prevalent in the thymus) was also the prevalent rearrangement in the gut $Thy1^+$ population. Vγ5 rearrangements were undetected in these cells. In $CD8^+$ IEL, Vγ5 rearrangements were detected but the Vγ2 rearrangements were yet more abundant.

In nude $CD3^-$ cells the types of TcR rearrangements found were very different. In $Thy1^+$ cells, TcR-β chain rearrangements were virtually absent. In $CD8^+$ IEL the germ line DJ band was still detected, V(D)J rearrangements were pauciclonal and we could not identify rearrangements of the TcR-α chain. This reduced TcR-αβ differentiation contrasted with the prevalent expression of the gut abundant Vγ5 rearrangement. This rearrangement was readily detected in $Thy1^+$ cells, and prevailed in $CD8^+$ IEL.

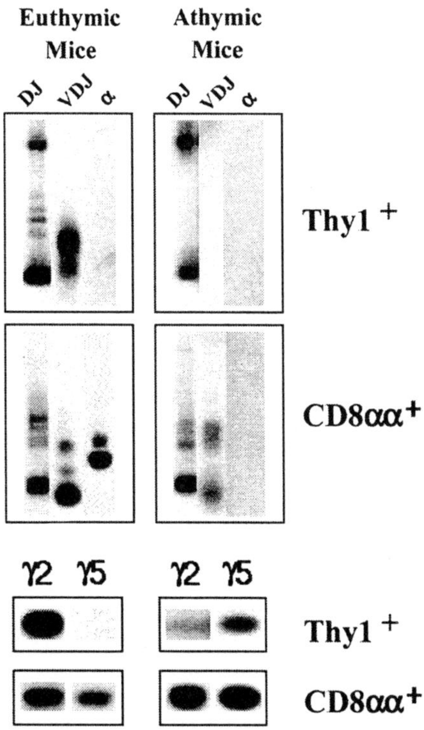

Figure 3. T cell receptor rearrangements in gut precursor cells. TcR-β-DJ[23] and V(D)J rearrangements[24], TcR-α VJ rearrangements[25] were studied using PcR primers, oligonucleotide probes and conditions described previously. The primers and probes used for TcR-γ rearrangements were a gift from P. Pereira. All samples contain the same amount of DNA (as destermined by the amplification of germ-line Cβ gene) corresponding to 10,000 cells.

One of the likely mechanisms to explain the different TcR-$\alpha\beta^+$/TcR-$\gamma\delta^+$ ratio in euthymic and athymic CD8αα T-IEL would implicate the pre-Tα chains. These chains are expressed by $CD3^-$ thymocytes and bind to the TcR-β chains to form the pre-TcR. This pre-TcR plays a fundamental role in TcR-αβ T cell differentiation, driving a considerable expansion of TcR-β^+ $CD25^+$ thymocytes and their maturation into $CD25^-$ $CD4^-$ $CD8^-$ and eventually into $CD4^+$ $CD8^+$ cells[27]. This expansion/maturation process, called β selection, was also reported to play a role in TcR-αβ versus TcR-γδ commitment, by driving the differentiation of immature T cell precursors into the TcR-αβ lineage[28].

In the thymus, the expression of two isoforms of the pre-Tα chain were reported[29]. We studied the expression of the two isoforms of the pre-Tα chain in thymocytes and gut $CD3^-$ populations (Fig. 2B). As reported previously, we found mRNA coding for both forms in immature thymocytes. Similarly, in euthymic mice, $Thy1^+$ cells also expressed both pre-Tα mRNA types. $CD8^+$ IEL did not express pre-Tα mRNA. We found a very different expression in nude mice. The $Thy1^+$ wall nude cells, (that expressed Rag-1 and may thus may undergo TcR rearrangements), did not express pre-Tα mRNA and thus could not form a pre-TcR. We detected pre-Tα mRNA expression on $CD8^+$ IEL, but only the long form was present.

We next compared the frequency of pre-Tα mRNA expression in the thymus and the gut precursors. For this purpose, we sorted gut $CD3^-$ populations into multiple individual wells containing 1,000 cells each. The conditions of PcR amplification we used are efficient enough to detect pre-Tα mRNA expression by 71% of individual $CD44^-$ $CD25^+$ thymocytes. As found in PcRs from mRNA extracted from bulk populations, we only detected pre-Tα mRNA in $Thy1^+$ cells from euthymic mice, and in the $CD8^+$ cells from nude mice. In $Thy1^+$ cells from euthymic mice, we found multiple wells where pre-Tα mRNA was not detected, suggesting a much lower expression rate, as compared to that found in thymus precursors. In the $CD8^+$ nude populations we found that the expression of the long form was indeed very rare.

3. DISCUSSION

The characterization of the two major Lin^- cell types from the gut indicated that the $Thy1^+$ cells were more immature than the $CD8^+$ population. $Thy1^+$ cells expressed mRNA coding for Rag-1 and pre-Tα and harbored cells with incomplete T cell receptor rearrangements. In contrast, the $CD3^-$ $CD8^+$ no longer expressed Rag-1 or the short form of the pre-Tα chain mRNA; TcR rearrangements were more abundant or/and more mature. The progression of TcR rearrangements in between $Thy1^+$ and $CD8\alpha\alpha^+$ cells; associated with the absence of recombinase gene transcription and the acquisition of the phenotype of the mature CD8αα T-IEL is compatible with the notion that the $CD3^-$ $Thy1^+$ more immature precursors may originate $CD3^-$ $CD8\alpha\alpha^+$ cells, that eventually differentiate into CD8αα T-IEL. This hypothesis is also supported by the presence of minor populations with transitional intermediate phenotypes.

The differences in number and composition of CD8αα T-IEL in athymic mice and euthymic mice are well documented[5,7,16]. We found a direct correlation between the mature T cell types recovered from the epithelium, and the local processes of T cell differentiation. In euthymic mice (where TcR-$\alpha\beta^+$ and TcR-$\gamma\delta^+$ cells are equally represented), TcR-β, α and γ rearrangements are detected in $CD3^-$ precursors. In contrast in nude mice, where > 90% of CD8$\alpha\alpha$ T-IEL are TcR-$\gamma\delta^+$ which a large fraction is TcR-V$\gamma 5^+$, the most abundant rearrangement found in $CD3^-$ populations was the Vγ5 rearrangement. Euthymic and athymic gut precursors also differed by their expression of pre-Tα chains. Euthymic Rag-1^+ Thy1^+ cells expressed both isoforms of pre-Tα chain, and V(D)J TcR-β rearrangements. These cells could therefore form the pre-TcR and undergo β selection. It is very unlikely that such process occurs in nude gut T cell differentiation. The Thy1^+ Rag-1^+ nude cells did not express pre-Tα chain. A very small minority of $CD8^+$ T-IEL expressed the long form. Such delayed expression might not play a major role in TcR-$\alpha\beta$ differentiation, as $CD8^+$ nude IEL no longer expressed recombinase genes and thus could not undergo further T cell receptor rearrangements. Moreover, we cannot exclude that the long pre-Tα chain mRNA we detected was expressed by rare dendritic cell precursors contaminants. The absence of β-selection in nude $CD3^-$ cells may contribute to the paucity of the TcR-$\alpha\beta$ generation in the athymic epithelium.

The origin of the gut T cell precursors has been a subject of considerable debate. The deficient TcR-$\alpha\beta$ T cell generation in both nude mice or neonatal thymectomized mice was initially attributed to an insufficient epithelium differentiation by a local impact of the nude mutation, or by the absence of thymic hormones produced during the perinatal period[17]. Reconstitution experiments performed later, however, demonstrated that a normal adult gut epithelium was unable to support the efficient generation of TcR-$\alpha\beta^+$ CD8$\alpha\alpha^+$ IEL in the absence of the thymus[7]. The thymus origin of at least part of gut TcR$^+$ CD8$\alpha\alpha^+$ cells was subsquentially demonstrated[16,18]. It is not yet known if such precursors migrate directly from the thymus to the gut wall, or if they colonize intermediate sites, like the bone-marrow. Our results are compatible with a thymus origin of gut precursors. Thy1^+ wall cells from euthymic mice already differ considerably from nude of the pre-Tα chain isoforms, the extent of TcR-β rearrangements. Moreover, these cells also express abundant TcR-γ2 rearrangements, supporting that these cells might be of thymic origin as these rearrangements prevail in thymus-derived TcR-$\gamma\delta$ cells.

It is tempting to speculate that the thymocyte precursors migrating to the gut originate mainly from Thy1^+ c-kit^{low} IL-7R$^+$ CD25$^{-/low}$ CD44$^+$ thymocytes, or from their immediate precursors. These thymocytes phenotype is similar to that of pre-Tα chain mRNA expression, and the extent of TcR-β and TcR-γ chain rearrangements[30]. These very immature thymocytes also express the FcεRIγ chain (characteristic of CD8$\alpha\alpha$ IEL)[24], that is lost in further stages of thymocyte ontogeny[10]. In such case the thymus might be able to shed committed precursors to the peripheral pools. A similar phenomenon was recently described during bone-marrow B cell generation[31].

4. CONCLUSION

The present work establishes that gut T cell differentiation differs in euthymic and athymic mice.

ACKNOWLEDGMENTS

Florence Lambolez is supported by a grant from the Association Claude Bernard. We thank Delphine Guy-Grand for her help and advice.

REFERENCES

1. Lefrancois, L., and Goodman, T., 1989, In vivo modulation of cytolytic activity and Thy-1 expression in TCR-gamma delta+ intraepithelial lymphocytes. *Science* **243**: 1716-1718.
2. Viney, J.L., Kilshaw, P.J., and MacDonald, T.T., 1990, Cytotoxic alpha/beta+ and gamma/delta+ T cells in murine intestinal epithelium. *European Journal of Immunology* **20**: 1623-1626.
3. Guy-Grand, D., DiSanto, J.P., Henchoz, P., Malassis-Seris, M., and Vassalli, P., 1998, Small bowel enteropathy: role of intraepithelial lymphocytes and of cytokines (IL-12, IFN-gamma, TNF) in the induction of epithelial cell death and renewal. *European Journal of Immunology* **28**: 730-744.
4. Rocha, B., Vassalli, P., and Guy-Grand, D., 1991, The V beta repertoire of mouse gut homodimeric alpha CD8+ intraepithelial T cell receptor alpha/beta + lymphocytes reveals a major extrathymic pathway of T cell differentiation. *Journal of Experimental Medicine* **173**: 483-486.
5. Guy-Grand, D., Cerf-Bensussan, N., Malissen, B., Malassis-Seris, M., Briottet, C., and Vassalli, P., 1991, Two gut intraepithelial CD8+ lymphocyte populations with different T cell receptors: a role for the gut epithelium in T cell differentiation. *Journal of Experimental Medicine* **173**: 471-481.
6. Ohteki, T., and MacDonald, H.R., 1993, Expression of the CD28 costimulatory molecule on subsets of murine intestinal intraepithelial lymphocytes correlates with lineage and responsiveness. *European Journal of Immunology* **23**: 1251-1255.
7. Rocha, B., Vassalli, P., and Guy-Grand, D., 1994, Thymic and extrathymic origins of gut intraepithelial lymphocyte populations in mice. *Journal of Experimental Medicine* **180**: 681-686.
8. Rocha, B., Guy-Grand, D., and Vassalli, P., 1995, Extrathymic T cell differentiation. *Current Opinion in Immunology* **7**: 235-242.
9. Arstila, T., Arstilla, T. P., Calbo, S., Selz, F., Malassis-Seris, M., Vassalli, P., Kourilsky, P., and Guy-Grand, D., 2000, Identical T cell clones are located within the mouse gut epithelium and lamina propia and circulate in the thoracic duct lymph. *Journal of Experimental Medicine* **191**: 823-834.

10. Guy-Grand, D., Rocha, B., Mintz, P., Malassis-Seris, M., Malissen, B., and Vassalli, P., 1994, Different use of T cell receptor transducing modules in two populations of gut intraepithelial lymphocytes are related to distinct pathways of T cell differentiation. *Journal of Experimental Medicine* **180**: 673-679.
11. Rocha, B., von Boehmer, H. and Guy-Grand, D., 1992, Selection of intraepithelial lymphocytes with CD8 alpha/alpha co-receptors by self-antigen in the murine gut. *Proceedings of the National Academy of Sciences of the United States of America* **89**: 5336-5340.
12. Yamada, H. *et al.*, 1998, Positive selection of extrathymically developed T cells by self-antigens. *Journal of Experimental Medicine* **188**: 779-784.
13. Kanamori, Y. *et al.*, 1996, Identification of novel lymphoid tissues in murine intestinal mucosa where clusters of c-kit+ IL-7R+ Thy1+ lympho-hemopoietic progenitors develop [see comments]. *Journal of Experimental Medicine* **184**: 1449-1459.
14. Saito, H. *et al.*,1998, Generation of intestinal T cells from progenitors residing in gut cryptopatches [see comments]. *Science* **280**: 275-278.
15. Suzuki, K. *et al.*, 2000, Gut cryptopatches: direct evidence of extrathymic anatomical sites for intestinal T lymphopoiesis. *Immunity* **13**: 691-702.
16. Lin, T., Matsuzaki, G., Kenai, H., Nakamura, T., and Nomoto, K., 1993, Thymus influences the development of extrathymically derived intestinal intraepithelial lymphocytes. European *Journal of Immunology* **23:** 1968-1974.
17. Wang, J., and Klein, J. R., 1994, Thymus-neuroendocrine interactions in extrathymic T cell development. *Science* **265:** 1860-1862.
18. Lefrancois, L., and Olson, S., 1994, A novel pathway of thymus-directed T lymphocyte maturation. *Journal of Immunology* **153:** 987-995.
19. Tsai, F.Y. *et al.*, 1994, An early haematopoietic defect in mice lacking the transcription factor GATA-2. *Nature* **371**: 221-226.
20. Ting, C.N., Olson, M.C., Barton, K.P. and Leiden, J.M., 1996, Transcription factor GATA-3 is required for development of the T-cell lineage. *Nature* **384**: 474-478.
21. Veiga-Fernandes, H., Walter, U., Bourgeois, C., McLean, A. and B. Rocha., 2000, Response of naïve and memory CD8+ T cells to antigen stimulation *in vivo. Nature Immunology* **1**: 47-53.
22. Lambolez, F., Joret, A-M., Garcia, C., von Boehmer, H. and Rocha, B., Charcterization of T cell development in the mouse gut (submitted).
23. Rodewald, H.R., Kretzschmar, K., Takeda, S., Hohl, C. and Dessing, M., 1994, Identification of pro-thymocytes in murine fetal blood: T lineage commitment can precede thymus colonization. *EMBO Journal* **13**: 4229-4240.
24. Rodewald, H.R. *ett al.*, 1993, Fc gamma RII/III and CD2 expression mark distinct subpopulations of immature CD4-CD8- murine thymocytes: in vivo developmental kinetics and T cell receptor beta chain rearrangement status. *Journal of Experimental Medicine* **177**: 1079-1092.
25. Levin, S. D., Anderson, S. J., Forbush, K. A., and Perlmutter, R. M., 1993, A dominant-negative transgene defines a role for p56lck in thymopoiesis. *EMBO Journal* **12:** 1671-1680.
26. Takagaki, Y., DeCloux, A., Bonneville, M. and Tonegawa, S., 1989, Diversity of gamma delta T-cell receptors on murine intestinal intra-epithelial lymphocytes. *Nature* **339**: 712-714.
27. von Boehmer, H. *et al.*, 1998, Crucial function of the pre-T-cell receptor (TCR) in TCR beta selection, TCR beta allelic exclusion and alpha beta versus gamma delta lineage commitment. *Immunological Reviews* **165**: 111-119.
28. Aifantis, I. *et al.*, 1998, On the role of the pre-T cell receptor in alpha-beta versus gamma-delta T lineage commitment. *Immunity* **9**: 649-655.
29. Barber, D.F., Passoni, L., Wen, L., Geng, L. and Hayday, A.C., 1998, The expression in vivo of a second isoform of pT alpha: implications for the mechanism of pT alpha action. *Journal of Immunology* **161**: 11-16.

30. Wilson, A., de Villartay, J. P., and MacDonald, H. R., 1996, T cell receptor delta gene rearrangement and T early alpha (TEA) expression in immature alpha beta lineage thymocytes: implications for alpha beta/gamma delta lineage commitment. *Immunity* **4**: 37-45.
31. Nagaoka, H., Yu, W., and Nussenzweig MC., 2000, Regulation of RAG expression in developing lymphocytes. Current Opinion *Immunology* **12**: 187-190.

CRTH2: marker for the detection of human Th2 and Tc2 cells

LORENZO COSMI, FRANCESCO ANNUNZIATO, GRAZIA GALLI, ROBERTO MANETTI, ENRICO MAGGI and SERGIO ROMAGNANI
**Department of Internal Medicine, Section of Clinical Immunology, Allergy and Respiratory Diseases, University of Florence, Italy*

1. INTRODUCTION

Th1 and Th2 cells represent two extremely polarized forms of the specific CD4+ Th cell-mediated immune response. Murine Th1 cells secrete interleukin IL-2, TNF-β and IFN-γ, promoting cell-mediated immunity to intracellular pathogens, whereas Th2 cells produce IL-4, IL-5, IL-6, IL-10 and IL-13, which are mainly involved in the humoral immunity to parasites. Although human T-cell clones with similar characteristics exist, a better definition of Th1/Th2 cells may rest on their ability to produce IFN-γ, but not IL-4 (Th1) or IL-4 but not IFN-γ (Th2), respectively[1].

1.1 Surface molecules associated with human Th1 or Th2 cells

In the last few years, some surface molecules have been described, which preferentially associate with human Th1 or Th2 cells, respectively. The Th1-associated molecules include CD26, membrane IFN-γ and lymphocyte activation gene (LAG)-3, whereas CD62L and CD30 have been shown to be preferentially expressed by Th2 cells[2,3]. More recently, it has been reported that chemokine receptors can also associate with human Th1 or Th2 cells. CCR5 and CXCR3 were found to be preferentially associated with Th1 cells.

By contrast, CCR3, CCR4, and CCR8 associated with Th2 cells, whereas CXCR4 was found to be equally distributed on human Th1 or Th2 cells, but it was found to be up-regulated by IL-4 and down-regulated by IFN-γ[4]. However, the association of chemokine receptors with one or the other T-cell population was mainly assessed at mRNA level.

1.2 Chemoattractant recetor-homologous molecule expressed on Th2 cells (CRTH2)

Recently, a novel surface molecule, chemoattractant receptor-homologous molecule expressed on Th2 cells (CRTH2) was described, which appeared to be capable of discriminating between human Th1 and Th2 cells[5]. CRTH2 is an orphan receptor closely related to the N-formyl peptide receptor and the C5a receptor. CRTH2 was found to be expressed not only on Th2 cells, but also on peripheral blood basophils and eosinophils, and cord blood-derived mast cells were identified as the possible producers of CRTH2 ligand(s)[6,7]. Recently it has been shown that prostaglandin D2 induces chemotaxis in Th2 cells, eosinophils and basophils via CRTH2[8].

2. CHARACTERIZATION OF CRTH2-EXPRESSING CELLS

We have assessed the reliability of CRTH2 as a selective marker of circulating human Th2 cells by comparing its expression on the surface of unfractionated or CRTH2-enriched PBMC with that of other Th2-associated molecules, such as CCR3 and CCR4, as well as with the intracellular synthesis at single cell level of IL-4, IL-5, IL-13, and IFN-γ.

Very small percentages of CD3+ PBMC showed expression of CRTH2 or CCR4 and even less of CCR3. While virtually all CCR4+ cells were T cells, variable proportions of CRTH2+ and CCR3+ PBMC from healthy individuals also stained positive for FcεR1, suggesting their basophil nature. In order to determine the relative proportions of T cells and basophils among CCR4+, CRTH2+, and CCR3+ PBMC, each of the three small populations was positively selected by using the MACS system, and assessed for the simultaneous expression of CD3 and FcεR1. The results of these experiments confirmed that virtually all CCR4+ cells were T lymphocytes, whereas a few CRTH2+ cells and about a half of CCR3+ cells were basophils.

The cytokine profile of CRTH2+, CCR3+, and CCR4+ T cells was then assessed by flow cytometry for intracellular synthesis at single cell level. Unfractionated CD4+ and CD8+ T cells contained remarkable proportions of IFN-γ-, but low proportions of IL-4- and IL-13-, and virtually no IL-5-, producing cells. By contrast, the majority, even not all, of CRTH2+ cells in both the CD4+ and the CD8+ subsets produced IL-4 and IL-13, a small proportion of them also produced IL-5, whereas very few CD4+ and CD8+ IFN-γ-producing T cells were observed. The few CCR3+ T cells (both CD4+ and CD8+) were only slightly enriched in cells producing IL-4, IL-5, and IL-13. However, proportions of IFN-γ-producing cells within the CCR3+ T cell subset were not significantly different from those present in unfractionated populations. Both CD4+ and CD8+ T cells selected for CCR4 expression were enriched for cells producing IL-4 alone or IL-4 and IL-13, but not for IL-5-producing cells. However, the proportion of T cells able to produce IFN-γ in the CCR4+ population was not signficantly reduced in comparison with the unfractionated populations (Fig. 1).

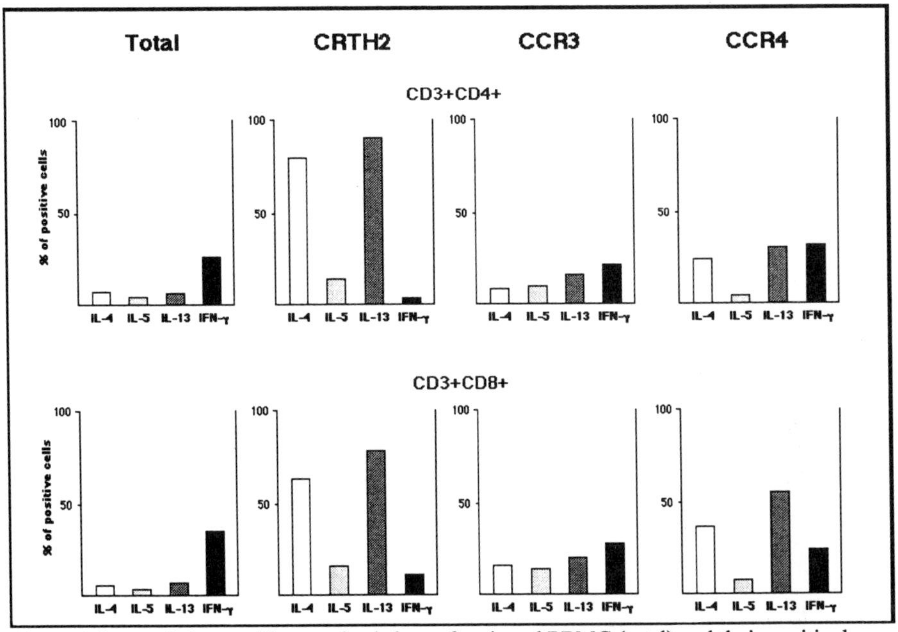

Figure 1. Intracellular cytokine synthesis by unfractioned PBMC (total) and their positively selected subsets.

The expression of CRTH2 by circulating T cells was then compared with the expression of different chemokine receptors. CXCR3 was expressed by high numbers of CD4+ and CD8+, T cells in unfractionated populations, and the number of CXCR3-expressing cells was strongly decreased in positively CRTH2+ cells, but not in CCR3+ cells. The number of CXCR3-expressing cells was also reduced in CD8+, but not in CD4+, T cells positively selected for CCR4 expression. CCR5 expression was higher in CD8+ than in CD4+ T cells from unfractionated populations, and the presence of CCR5-expressing cells was virtually abolished in the CRTH2+ CD4+, and strongly decreased in the CRTH2+ CD8+, T-cell population. By contrast, in CCR3+

populations, the number of CCR5-expressing cells was virtually unchanged at level of both CD4+ and CD8+ T cells, and in the CCR4+ population it was even increased among both CD4+ and CD8+ T cells in comparison with unfractionated populations. The number of CCR4-expressing cells was strongly increased in both CD4+ and CD8+ T cells from CRTH2-selected populations, whereas the number of CCR3-expressing cells was not. By contrast, the numbers of CCR4-expressing cells were not increased in either CD4+ or CD8+ T cells selected for CCR3 expression, whereas the numbers of CRTH2+, but not of CCR3+, cells were strongly increased among both CD4+ and CD8+ T cells positively selected for CCR4 expression.

The possibility to use CRTH2 as a marker for the detection of circulating Th2 and Tc2 cells in disease was then evaluated. Significantly higher values of CRTH2+ (both CD4+ and CD8+) T cells were found in both patients with atopic dermatitis and HIV-infected patients showing values of CD4+ T cells lower than $500/mm^3$, in comparison with healthy individuals. By contrast, no significant differences in the values of CCR3+ or CCR4+ T cells among the three groups of subjects were observed.

3. CONCLUSION

CRTH2 is the only surface marker selectively associated with single circulating T (both CD4+ and CD8+) cells able to produce IL-4 (as well as IL-5 and IL-13), but not IFN-γ. Finally and most importantly, this date provide the first evidence that the proportions of circulating CRTH2+ (both CD4+ and CD8+) T cells are significantly increased in patients affected by atopic dermatitis or advanced HIV infection, thus supporting the existence of a Th2 and Tc2 cell polarization in subjects suffering from these conditions.

REFERENCES

1. Romagnani, S. 1997, The Th1/Th2 paradigm in disease. Springer, Heidelberg/R.G. Landes Company, Austin.
2. Assenmacher, M., Scheffold, A., Schmitz, J., Segura Checa, J.A., Miltenyi, S., Radbruch, A. 1996, Specific expression of surface interferon-γ on interferon-γ-producing T cells from mouse and man. *Eur. J. Immunol.*. **26**: 263-267.
3. Annunziato, F., Manetti, R., Tomasevic, L., Giudizi, M-G., Biagiotti, R., Giannò, V., Germano, P., Mavilia, C., Maggi, E., Romagnani, S. 1996, Expression and release of LAG-3-encoded protein by human CD4+ T cells are associated with IFN-γ production. *FASEB J.* **10**: 769-776.
4. Bonecchi, R., Bianchi, G., Bordignon Panina, P., D'Ambrosio, D., Lang, R., Borsatti, A., Sozzani, S., Allavena, P., Gray, P.A., Mantovani, A., Sinigaglia, F. 1998, Differential

expression of chemokine receptors and chemotactic responsiveness of Th1 and Th2 cells. *J. Exp. Med.*. **187**: 129-134.

5. Nagata, K., Tanaka, K., Ogawa, K., Kemmotsu, K., Imai, T., Yoshie, O., Abe, H., Tada, K., Nakamura, M., Sugamura, K., Takano, S. 1999, Selective expression of a novel surface molecule by human Th2 cells in vivo. *J. Immunol.*. **162**: 1278-1286.
6. Nagata, K., Hirai, H., Tanaka, K., Ogawa, K., Aso, T., Sugamura, K., Nakamura, M., Takano, S. 1999, CRTH2, an orphan receptor of T-helper-2-cells, is expressd on basophils and eosinophils and responds to mast cell-derived factor(s). *FEBS Letters*. **459**: 195-199.
7. Cosmi, L., Annunziato, F., Iwasaki, M, Galli, G., Manetti, R., Maggi, E., Nagata, K., Romagnani, S, 2000, CRTH2 is the most reliable marker for detection of circulating human type 2 Th and type 2 T cytotoxic cells in health and disease. *Eur.J. Immunol.* **2**: 255-261.
8. Hirai, H., Tanaka, K., Yoshie, O, Ogawa, K., Kenmotsu, K., Takamori, Y., Ichimasa, M., Sugamura, K., Nakamura, M., Takano, S. Nagata, K., 2001, prostaglandin D2 selectively induces chemotaxis in T helper type 2 cells, eosinophils and basophils via seven-transmembrane receptor CRTH2. *J. Exp. Med.*. **2**: 255-261.

GILZ, a glucocorticoid hormone induced gene, modulates T lymphocytes activation and death through interaction with NF-kB

CARLO RICCARDI, STEFANO BRUSCOLI, EMIRA AYROLDI, MASSIMILIANO AGOSTINI and GRAZIELLA MIGLIORATI
Department of Clinical and Experimental Medicine, University of Perugia, Via del Giochetto, 06122, Perugia, Italy

1. INTRODUCTION

In the T-cell lineage, several pathways have been identified which regulate apoptosis. In particular, in normal T lymphocytes activation, differentiation and death are under regulation of a number of signals and stimuli that can contribute either to positive or negative selection[1-5].

After Ag/TCR interaction, proliferation and differentiation contribute to generate activated effectors and immune response and, at a later time, most of the activated cells are eliminated to end the immune response, to avoid a continuos clone expansion and the generation of auto-immunity[6-7]. TCR-driven stimulation involves the activation of different transduction signals, including calcineurin/calmodulin and ras/ERK pathways. Moreover, TCR activates the co-ordinated expression of a number of molecules involved in clonal expansion, such as for example IL-2/IL-2R, and in the activation induced cell death (AICD), such as the case of Fas/FasL[7-10]. Moreover, a number of genes coding for transcription factors are involved as regulators of T cell activation and death, such as for example P53, cAMP response element binding proteins (CREB), AP-1, NFAT and NF-kB. In particular, the role of NF-kB as a regulator (either apoptotic or anti-apoptotic) of death in thymocytes, peripheral T cells, and T-cell hybridomas has been evidenced[11-16].

Stimuli, other than Ag/TCR-interaction regulate T-cell activation and death, including cytokines and co-accessory molecules[17-19]. Among different stimuli, Glucocorticoid hormones (GCH) are also critical regulators of T-cell development in that can either induce or inhibit apoptosis[20-25].

In particular, GCH inhibit T lymphocytes activation and death and also counter activation-induced IL-2/IL-2R and Fas/FasL expression[24,26]. The inhibitory effect on T-cell activation and death relates in part to the GCH-induced inhibition of NK-kB activity[17,27]. In fact, it has been reported that GCH antagonise NF-kB activity through augmentation of I-kBα expression, through competition for the co-activator protein CBP/300 and through direct association of GR with NF-kB sub-units[28-33]. Moreover, it has also been reported that dexamethasone (DEX) treatment can down-modulate p65 NF-kB transactivation potential in the absence of any I-kB up-regulation[32].

1.1 Initial Comments

We have previously shown that GCH can modulate T lymphocytes apoptosis in that can either activate or inhibit cell death.

In particular, the protective effect is mRNA and protein synthesis-dependent and may be mediated via the induction of expression of GCH-induced genes including GITR,[34-36] (a membrane receptor of the TNF receptor superfamily, TNFRSF18, cloned in DEX-treated hybridoma cells and also induced, in normal T lymphocytes, by triggering of the TCR/CD3 complex but not by DEX), and GILZ[37,38] (a gene of the leucine zipper family, with a putative transcription suppressor activity, rapidly induced by DEX-treatment in normal T lymphocytes in vitro).

Moreover, we have shown that GILZ over-expression results in inhibition of activation-induced Fas/FasL expression[37].

To further analyse the possible relevance of GILZ in the control of T lymphocytes activation, we performed experiments to evaluate the capability of DEX to induce GILZ expression in vivo in different cells of the lymphohaemopoietic system and the possible interaction of GILZ with the NF-kB transcription factor that has been previously shown to regulate the T-cell activation process including Fas/FasL expression.

2. IN VIVO DEX ADMINISTRATION UP-REGULATES GILZ MRNA AND PROTEIN EXPRESSION IN LYMPHOID TISSUES

Results indicated that GILZ mRNA (Fig 1), evaluated by RPA analysis (Ribonuclease Protection Assay) was clearly increased in isolated thymus (a), spleen (c) and lymph nodes (e) of mice treated with DEX (10mg/Kg ip) at different times. In particular, GILZ mRNA levels increase 3 hours after treatment and return to control levels at 24 hours. We have also investigated, by western blot analysis using a polyclonal anti-GILZ antibody, the GILZ protein expression in the same tissues (Fig 1: b,d,f). Results shown in the figure indicate that the GILZ protein expression correlates with GILZ mRNA.

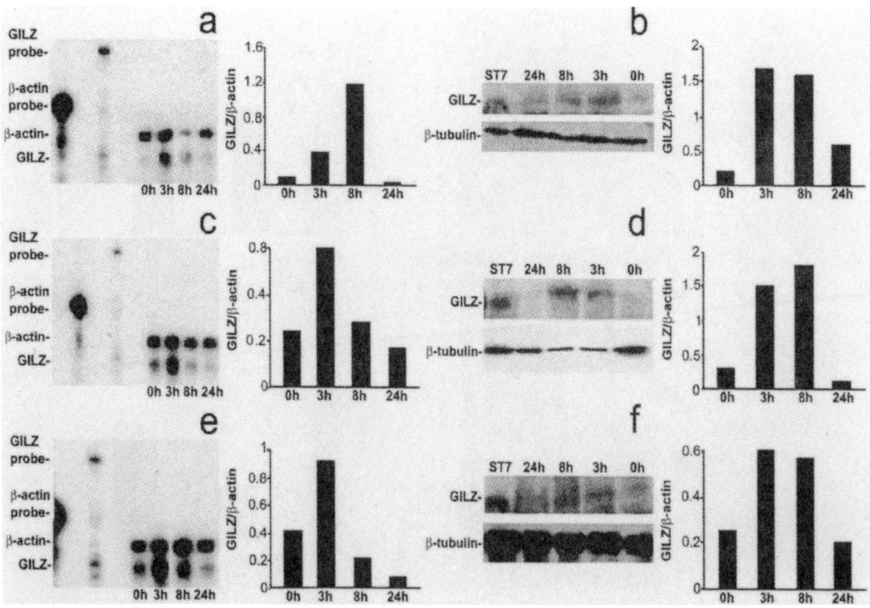

Figure 1. In-vivo DEX administration (10mg/Kg ip) up-regulates GILZ mRNA and protein expression in: thymus (a) GILZ mRNA, (b) GILZ protein; spleen (c) GILZ mRNA, (d) GILZ protein and lymph-nodes (e) GILZ mRNA, (f) GILZ protein. Mice were injected intraperitoneally with DEX or PBS as control.

2.1 Expression of GILZ mRNA in lymphocyte subpopulations and in peritoneal macrophages

We evaluated GILZ mRNA expression in DEX-treated and untreated B cells by RPA analysis. Results indicate that GILZ mRNA is up-regulated 3 hours after DEX-treatment in B cells (Fig 2a).

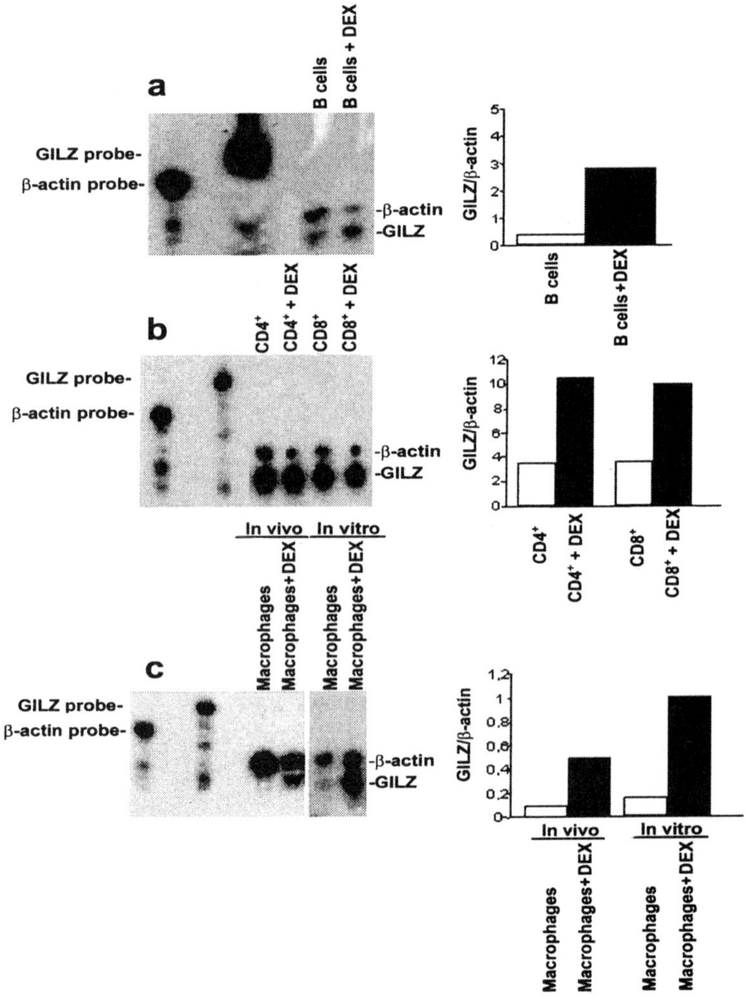

Figure 2. Expression of GILZ mRNA in cells subpopulation before and after in-vitro DEX (10^{-7} M)-treatment for 3 hours. B cells (a), $CD4^+$ or $CD8^+$ T cells (b) were enriched from spleen and lymph-nodes by negative selection using FITC-conjugated anti CD3, B220, CD4 and CD8 respectively, followed by depletion with anti-FITC-conjugated magnetic beads. The purity of cells was usually greater than 90%. (c) Expression of GILZ mRNA in peritoneal macrophages before and after in-vitro o in-vivo DEX-treatment for 3 hours.

We also evaluated GILZ mRNA expression in DEX-treated and untreated $CD4^+$ and $CD8^+$ cells by RPA analysis. Results show that GILZ mRNA is up-regulated after 3 hours of treatment in $CD4^+$ and $CD8^+$ cells (Fig 2b). We have analysed GILZ mRNA levels in DEX-treated or untreated peritoneal macrophages both *in vitro* and *in vivo* by RPA analysis. In figure 2c it is shown that GILZ mRNA is up-regulated by DEX-treatment in peritoneal macrophages both *in vitro* and after *in vivo* administration.

These results indicate that *in vivo* DEX administration rapidly up-regulates GILZ expression in T, B lymphocytes and macrophages further suggesting a possible role in the control of lymph-haematopoietic cells compartment.

2.2 GILZ binds to NF-kB

Previous results indicated that GILZ is able to counter activation induced cell death and through inhibition Fas/fasL up-regulation. A number of transcription factors are involved in the control, of T-cell activation and Fas/FasL expression.

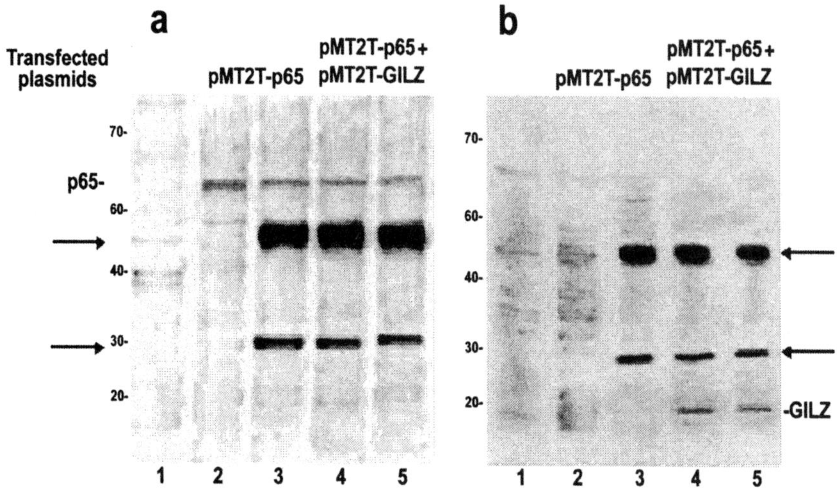

Figure 3. In vivo association of GILZ and p65 in NTera-2 cells. NTera-2 cells were transfected with 3µg of expression vector (pMT2T) for p65 alone or p65 and GILZ, cells extracts were immunoprecipitated with p65 and GILZ antibodies, and analyzed by Western blot with p65 antibodies (a) or GILZ antibodies (b). Lane 1, untransfected and unprecipitated cell extracts; lane 2, extracts of cells transfected with p65 and unprecipitated; lane 3, extracts of cells transfected with p65 and immunoprecipitated with anti-p65; lane 4, extracts of cells transfected with p65 and GILZ and immunoprecipitated with anti-p65; lane 5, extracts of cells transfected with p65 and GILZ and immunoprecipitated with anti-GILZ. Arrows indicate the high and low chain of antibody.

To investigate the possible mechanism responsible of GILZ effect we analysed the in vivo protein-to-protein interaction between GILZ and p65. For that purpose, we performed co-immunoprecipitation experiments in GILZ and p65 co-transfected cells. In particular, NTera-2 cells, which lack the NF-kB complex including I-kB molecules, were co-transfected with expression vectors encoding for GILZ and p65, and immunoprecipitated with antibodies against GILZ or p65. Western blots were performed with anti-p65 or anti-GILZ antibodies.

As shown in figure 3, untransfected NTera-2 cells do not contain detectable p65 (lane 1 of figure a) and GILZ (lane 1 of figure b) protein, while p 65 was evident in cells transfected with p65 as evidenced by western blot (lane 2 of figure a) or immunoprecipitation (lane 3 of figure a) with anti-p65 antibodies. Furthermore, p65 band was also evident in the groups transfected with both p65 and GILZ and immunoprecipitated with anti-p65 (lane 4 of figure a) or anti-GILZ (lane 5 of figure a). This results suggest that p65 interact with GILZ protein, and its was confirmed in the figure 3b, in facts anti-GILZ antibody immunoprecipitated GILZ protein (lane 5 of figure b), and coimmunoprecipitated p65 (lane 4 of figure b).

3. CONCLUSION

The newly identified glucocorticoid-responsive gene, GILZ, is regulated by GCH *in vivo* at the same manner as *in vitro*. In this work we have show that there is an early increased of GILZ induced by DEX-treatment in vivo. In fact after 3 hours of treatment GILZ mRNA expression increased in T-lymphocytes (CD4+ or CD8+), B lymphocytes and macrophages, and return to control levels at 24 hours. Also GILZ protein expression correlates with GILZ mRNA.

Furthermore, GILZ coimmunoprecipitates in vitro with p65, inhibiting its transactivation, and this suggest a possible mechanism responsible for GILZ-mediated biological effects, which could occur also in vivo.

Future studies need to be made to deepen the GILZ molecular mechanisms.

ACKNOWLEDGMENTS

The work from our laboratory was supported by Associazione Italiana Ricerca sul Cancro (AIRC), Milan, and by CNR target project on Biotechnology, Rome, Italy.

REFERENCES

1. Jenkinson, E.J., Kingston, R., Smith, C.A., Williams, G.T., and Owen, J.J., 1989, Antigen-induced apoptosis in developing T cells: a mechanism for negative selection of the T cell receptor repertoire. *Eur. J. Immunol.* 19:2175-2177.
2. MacDonald, H.R., and Lees., R.K., 1990, Programmed death of autoreactive thymocytes. *Nature* 343:642-644.
3. Raff, M.C., 1992, Social controls on cell survival and cell death. *Nature* 356:397-399.
4. Boise, L.H., and Thompson, C.G., 1996, Hierarchical control of lymphocyte survival. *Science* 274:67-68.
5. Backstrom, B.T., Muller, U., Hausmann, B., and Palmer, E., 1998, Positive selection through a motif in the αβ T cell receptor. *Science* 281:835- 838.
6. Webb, S., Morris, C., Sprent, J., 1990, Extrathymic tolerance of mature T cells: Clonal elimination as a consequence of immunity. *Cell* 63:1249-1254.
7. Kabelitz, D., Pohl, T., and Pechhold, K., 1993, Activation-induced cell death (apoptosis) of mature peripheral T lymphocytes. *Immunol. Today* 14:338-339.
8. Ju, S.T., Panka, D.J., Cui, H., Ettiger, R., el-Khatib, M., Sherr, D.H., Stanger, B.Z., and Marshak-rothstein, A., 1995, Fas(CD95)/FasL interactions required for programmed cell death after T-cell activation. *Nature* 373:444-448.
9. Suda, T., Okazaki, T., Naito, Y., Yokota, T., Arai, N., Ozaki, S., Nakao, K., and Nagata, S., 1995, Expression of the Fas ligand in cells of T cell lineage. *J. Immunol.* 154: 3806-3813.
10. Green, D.R., and Ware, C.F., 1997, Fas-ligand: privilege and peril. *Proc. Natl. Acad Sci. USA* 94:5986-5990.
11. Jain, J., Loh, C., and Rao, A, 1995, Transcriptional regulation of the IL-2 gene. *Curr. Opin. Immunol.* 7:333-342.
12. Boothby, M.R., Mora, A.L., Scherer, D.C., Brockman, J.A., and Ballard, D.W., 1997, Perturbation of the T lymphocyte lineage in transgenic mice expressing a constitutive repressor of nuclear factor (NF)-kappaB. *J. Exp. Med.* 185:1897-1907.
13. Kuo, C.T., Veselits, M.L., and Leiden, J.M., 1997, LKLF: a transcriptional regulator of single-positive T cell quiescence and survival. *Science* 277:1886-1990.
14. Magginvar, S.B., Harhaj, E.W., and Sun, S.C., 1997, Regulation of the interleukin-2 CD28 responsive element by NF-Atp and various NF-kappaB/Rel transcription factors. *Mol. Cell. Biol.* 17:2605-2614.
15. Gerondakis, S., Grumont, R., Ropurke, R., and Grossman, M., 1998, The regulation and roles of Rel/NF-kappaB transcription factors during lymphocyte activation. *Curr. Opin. Immunol.* 10:353-359.
16. Lin, B., William-Skipp, C., Tao, Y., Schleicher, M.S., Cano, L.L., Duke, R.C., and Scheinman, R.I., 1999, NF-kB functions as both proapoptotic and antiapoptotic regulatory factor within a single cell type. *Cell Death Differ* 6:570-582.
17. Migliorati, G., Nicoletti, I., Pagliacci M.C., D'Adamio, L., and Riccardi, C., 1993, Interleukin-4 Protects Double-Negative and CD4 Single-Positive Thymocytes from Dexamethasone-Induced Apoptosis *Blood* 81:1352-1358.
18. Ayroldi, E., Zollo O., Cannarile, L., D'Adamio F., Grohmann, U., Delfino, V.D., and Riccardi, C., 1998, Interleukin-6 (IL-6) Prevents Activation-Induced Cell Death: IL-2-Independent Inhibition of Fas/fasL Expression and Cell Death *Blood* 92:4212-4219.
19. Ayroldi, E., Migliorati G., Cannarile, L., Moraca, R., Delfino, D., and Riccardi, C., 1997, CD2 rescues T cells from T-cell receptor/CD3 apoptosis: a role for the Fas/FasL system *Blood* 89 3717-37.

20. Wyllie, A.H., 1972, Glucocorticoid-induced thymocyte apoptosis is associated with endogenous endonuclease activation. *Nature* 284:555-558.
21. Cohen, J.J., and Duke, R.C., 1984, Glucocorticoid activation of a calcium dependent endonuclease in thymocyte nuclei leads to cell death. *J. Immunol.* 132:38-43.
22. Vacchio, M.S., Papadopoulos, V., and Ashwell, J.D., 1994, Steroid production in the thymus: implications for thymocyte selection. *J. Exp. Med.* 179:1835-1846.
23. Chrousos, G.P., 1995, The hypothalamic-pituitary-adrenal axis and immune mediated inflammation. *N. Engl. J. Med.* 332:1351-1362.
24. King, L.B., Vacchio, M.S., Dixon, K., Hunziker, R., Margulies, D.H., and Ashwell, J.D., 1995, A targeted Glucocorticoid receptor antisense transgene increases thymocyte development. *Immunity* 3:647-656.
25. Riccardi, C., Cifone, G., and Migliorati, G., 1999, Glucocorticoid hormone-induced modulation of gene expression and regulation of T-cell death: role of GITR and GILZ, two dexamethasone-induced genes. *Cell Death Differ.* 12:1155-1163.
26. Yang, Y., Mercep, M., Ware C.F., and Ashwell, J.D., 1995, Fas and activation-induced Fas ligand mediate apoptosis of T cell hybridomas: inhibition of Fas ligand expression by retinoic acid and glucocorticoids. *J. Exp. Med.* 181:1673-1682.
27. Ramdas, J., and Harmon, J.M., 1998, Glucocorticoid-Induced Apoptosis and Regulation of NF-kB Activity in Human Leukemic T Cells. *Endocrinology* 139:3813-3821.
28. Ray, A., and Prefontaine, K.E., 1994, Physical association and functional antagonism between the p65 subunit of transcription factor NF-kappaB and the glucocorticoid receptor. *Proc. Natl. Acad. Sci. USA* 91:752-756.
29. Auphan, N., DiDonato, J.A., Rosette, C., Hejmberg, A., and Karin, M., 1995, Immunosuppression by glucocorticoids: inhibition by NF-kB activity through induction of IkB synthesis. *Science* 270:286-290.
30. Caldenhoven, E., Liden, J., Wissink, S., Van de Stolpe, A., Raaijmakers, J., Koenderman, L., Okret, S., Gustafsson, J.A., and Van der Saag, P.T., 1995, Negative cross-talk between RelA and the glucocorticoid receptor: a possible mechanism for the antinflammatory action of glucocorticoids. *Molecular Endocrinology* 9:401-412.
31. Scheinman, R.I., Cogswell, P.C., Lofquist, A.K., and Baldwin Jr., A.S., 1995 Role of transcriptional activation of IkBα in mediation of immunosuppression by glucocorticoids. *Science* 270:283-286.
32. Scheinman, R.I., Gualberto, A., Jewell, C.M., Cidlowski, J.A., and Baldwin Jr, A.S., 1995, Characterization of the Mechanisms Involved in the Transrepression of NF-kB by Activated Glucocorticoid Receptors. *Mol. Cell. Biol.* 15:943-953.
33. De Bosscher, K., Schimtz, M.L., Vanden Berghe, W., Plaisance, S., Fiers, W., and Haegeman, G., 1997, Glucocorticoid-mediated repression of nuclear factor-kappaB-dependent transcription involves direct interference with transactivation. *Proc. Natl. Acad. Sci. USA* 94:13504-13509.
34. Nocentini, G., Giunchi, L., Ronchetti, S., Krausz, L.T., Bartoli, A., Moraca, R., Migliorati, G., and Riccardi, C., 1997, A new member of the tumor necrosis factor/nerve growth factor receptor family inhibits T cell receptor-induced apoptosis. *Proc. Natl. Acad. Sci. USA* 94: 6216-6221.
35. Nocentini, G., Bartoli, A., Ronchetti, S., Giunchi, L., Cupelli, A., Delfino, D., Migliorati, G., and Riccardi, C., 2000 Gene Structure and Chromosomal Assignment of Mouse GITR, a Member of Tumor Necrosis Factor/Nerve Growth Factor Receptor Family *DNA and Cell Biology* 19:205-217.
36. Nocentini, G., Ronchetti, S., Bartoli, A., Spinicelli, S., Delfino, D., Brunetti, L., Migliorati, G., and Riccardi, C., 2000, Identification of three novel mRNA splice variants of GITR *Cell Death and Differentation* 7:408-410.

37. D'Adamio, F., Zollo, O., Moraca, R., Ayroldi, E., Bruscoli, S., Bartoli, A., Cannarile, L., Migliorati, G., and Riccardi, C., 1997, A new Dexamethasone-induced gene of the leucine zipper family protects T lymphocytes from TCR/CD3-activated cell death. *Immunity* 7:803-812.
38. Cannarile, L., Zollo, O., D'Adamio, F., Ayroldi, E., Marchetti, C., Tabilio, A., bruscoli, S., and Riccardi, C., 2001, Cloning, chromosomal assignment and tissue distribution of human GILZ, a glucocorticoid hormone-induced gene *Cell Death and Differentation* Plenum Press.

Tyrosine phosphorylation of PICOT and its translocation to the nucleus in response of human T cells to oxidative stress

YAEL BABICHEV AND NOAH ISAKOV
Department of Microbiology and Immunology, Faculty of Health Sciences, and the Cancer Research Center, Ben-Gurion University, Beer Sheva, Israel

1. INTRODUCTION

Protein kinase C θ (PKCθ) is a Ca^{2+}-independent isoform expressed in T but not B lymphocytes, and is therefore suggested as being linked to the T cell antigen receptor (TCR) function (1, 2). PKCθ was shown to function as an upstream regulator of critical transcription factors, such as AP-1 and NF-κB, in activated T lymphocytes (3). More recent studies demonstrated that PKCθ colocalizes with the TCR at the core of the supramolecular activation complex (SMAC) formed at the contact region between antigen-responding T cells and antigen-presenting cells (APC) (4). Finally, PKCθ–deficient mice were found to be impaired in T cell-mediated immune responses, apparently, due to inability of their antigen triggered T cells to activate the AP-1 and NF-κB transcription factors (5).

2. PKCθ-BINDING PROTEINS

Although studies have established the critical role of PKCθ in T cell activation, its exact mechanism of action during the T cell activation response is yet unresolved. For example, the function of PKCθ in the TCR-linked signal transduction pathway is not clear, neither are the mechanisms

Progress in Basic and Clinical Immunology, Edited by Mackiewicz *et al.*
Kluwer Academic/Plenum Publishers, New York, 2001

by which PKCθ translocates to the plasma membrane, recruits to the SMAC region, and becomes coupled to the TCR signaling machinery.

It has been postulated that distribution of PKC isoenzymes within the cell, and regulation of their enzymatic activity, are regulated in part, by the direct physical interaction with specific anchoring proteins (6). It has also been suggested that individual PKC isoforms interact with distinct anchoring proteins, and that two sets of anchoring proteins may alternate in binding to the active and inactive PKC isoenzymes (6).

In a search for PKCθ anchoring proteins, Meller *et al.* have found that PKCθ interact with the cytosolic protein 14-3-3τ in resting T cells (7). Upon expression of a genetically modified membrane targeted form of 14-3-3τ, a large fraction of the cellular pool of PKCθ is translocated to the plasma membrane of resting T cells. In addition, physical interaction of PKCθ with 14-3-3τ downregulated PKCθ enzymatic activity.

Studies in HIV infected T cells demonstrated that PKCθ associate with the HIV negative factor (Nef) protein, suggesting that altered regulation of PKCθ by Nef may contribute to the T cell impairments in HIV infected individuals (8). In addition, PKCθ in activated T cells was shown to interact with Fyn, a member of the Src family of protein tyrosine kinases (9). It has been indicated that the TCR-associated Fyn may account for the relocalization of PKCθ to the SMAC region of activated T cells.

3. PICOT

To test whether PKCθ is regulated by additional hitherto unknown interacting proteins, Witte *et al.* have used the yeast two-hybrid system in order to identify new putative PKCθ-interacting proteins (10). These studies led to the identification of a new gene product, termed PICOT (GenBank accession no. AAF28844), which consists of 335 amino acids and possesses a molecular mass of ~38-kDa on a SDS-PAGE. PICOT displays an N-terminal thioredoxin-homology domain, which lacks a critical cysteine residue at the putative catalytic center. In contrast, the C-terminal region of PICOT is made up of two tandem repeats of a conserved motif, which includes 84 amino acids. This novel sequence, termed PICOT homology domain (PICOT-HD) (alignment number: ds44360, at the EMBL database (<http://www3.ebi.ac.uk/Services/align/listali.html>), was found to be evolutionary conserved from bacteria to mammals (11).

4. T CELL TREATMENT WITH HYDOROGEN PEROXIDE AFFECTS PICOT TYROSINE PHOSPHORYLATION LEVELS AND SUBCELLULAR LOCALIZATION

Antigen-induced T cell stimulation results in the activation of tyrosine kinases and increased phosphorylation of multiple effector molecules that mediate the activation response. Many of these effects can be mimicked by reactive oxygen intermediates (ROS), such as hydrogen peroxide, that is likely to represent a physiological second messenger during the activation response (12). The fact that PICOT associates with PKCθ, which is found in the SMAC of activated T cells (4), and the potential involvement of PICOT in redox-regulated biochemical pathways, encouraged us to test whether PICOT may serve as a target for tyrosine kinases in hydrogen peroxide-treated T cells.

We found that treatment of Jurkat T cells with hydrogen peroxide induces tyrosine phosphorylation of PICOT in a dose response manner. Cotransfection of cells with PICOT and a constitutively activated form of Lck (LCK Y505F) also induced tyrosine phosphorylation of PICOT. The results indicated that tyrosine phosphorylation of PICOT may be directly or indirectly dependent upon Lck, an assumption, which is further substantiated by the fact that Lck undergoes activation by hydrogen peroxide.

Lck is constitutively associated with the cytoplasmic tail of CD4 or CD8 on the surface of T cells. Upon engagement of the TCR, it is recruited into the SMAC region at the contact site of the responding T cell with the APC (4). The directed inclusion of Lck in SMACs reflects the spatially regulated temporal association of CD4 or CD8, with antigen presenting MHC class II or class I molecules, respectively, on the surface of the APC. Staining of activated T cells demonstrated that PKCθ undergoes recruitment into the SMAC region, via a mechanism, which is yet unclear (4). However, if PICOT molecules associate with SMAC-residing PKCθ in antigen-responding T cells, they are likely to be in the vicinity of Lck, and therefore undergo phosphorylation in a similar manner to that of the TCR subunit cytoplasmic tails and the ζ-chain associated protein (ZAP) –70. We assume therefore that PICOT may play a role in cell activation-dependent signaling pathways, or in cellular responses to stress signals, which are mediated predominantly by reactive oxygen intermediate.

5. CONCLUSIONS

While the biological function of PICOT-HD-containing proteins is unknown, the high degree of sequence conservation of PICOT-HDs in proteins from different species, which are extremely remote from each other in evolutionary terms, suggest that PICOT-HD-containing proteins and their overall conformation and function are critical for the conservation of the species. We found that PICOT is expressed in a wide range of cell lines and organs and resides predominantly in the cell cytosol. Overexpression of PICOT in Jurkat T cells followed by stimulation with hydrogen peroxide resulted in phosphorylation of PICOT on tyrosine residues. We suggest that PICOT plays a role in cell activation-dependent signal transduction pathways and/or cellular responses to stress signals mediated by reactive oxygen intermediates.

ACKNOWLEDGEMENTS

Research at our laboratory is supported, in part, by grants from the Israel Science Foundation, the United States-Israel Binational Science Foundation, the Chief Scientist of the Ministry of Health, the Israel Cancer Research Association, and the Israel Cancer Research Fund.

REFERENCES

1. Baier, G., D. Telford, L. Giampa, K. M. Coggeshall, G. Baier-Bitterlich, N. Isakov, and A. Altman, 1993, Molecular cloning and characterization of PKC θ, a novel member of the protein kinase C (PKC) gene family expressed predominantly in hematopoietic cells. *J. Biol. Chem.* **268**:4997-5004.
2. Meller, N., Y. Elitzur, and N. Isakov, 1999, Protein kinase C-θ (PKCθ) distribution analysis in hematopoietic cells. Proliferating T cells exhibit high proportions of PKCθ in the particulate fraction. *Cell. Immunol.* **193**:185-193.
3. Altman, A., N. Isakov, and G. Baier, 2000, Protein kinase C-θ: a new essential superstar on the T cell stage. *Immunol. Today.* **21**:567-573.
4. Monks, C. R. F., B. A. Freiberg, H. Kupfer, N. Sciaky, and A. Kupfer, 1998, Tree-dimensional segragation of supramolecular activation clusters in T cells. *Nature* **395**:82-86.
5. Sun, Z., C. W. Arendt, W. Allmeier, E. M. Schaeffer, M. J. Sunshine, L. Gandhi, J. Annes, D. Petrzilka, A. Kupfer, P. L. Schwartzberg, and D. R. Littman, 2000, PKC-θ is required for TCR-induced NF-κB activation in mature but not immature T lymphocytes. *Nature* **404**:402-407.

6. Mochly-Rosen, D., and A. S. Gordon, 1998, Anchoring proteins for protein kinase C: a means for isozyme selectivity. *FASEB J.* **12**:35-42.
7. Meller, N., Y. C. Liu, T. L. Collins, N. Bonnefoy Berard, G. Baier, N. Isakov, and A. Altman, 1996, Direct interaction between protein kinase C θ (PKCθ) and 14-3-3τ in T cells: 14-3-3 overexpression results in inhibition of PKC θ translocation and function. *Mol. Cell. Biol.* **16**:5782-5791.
8. Smith, B. L., B. W. Krushelnycky, D. Mochly-Rosen, and P. Berg, 1996, The HIV Nef protein associates with protein kinase C θ. *J. Biol. Chem.* **271**:16753-16757.
9. Ron, D., E. W. Napolitano, A. Voronova, N. J. Vasquez, D. N. Roberts, B. L. Calio, R. H. Caothien, S. M. Pettiford, S. Wellik, J. B. Mandac, and L. M. Kauvar, 1999, Direct interaction in T-cells between θPKC and the tyrosine kinase p59fyn. *J. Biol. Chem.* **274**:19003-19010.
10. Witte, S., M. Villalba, K. Bi, Y. Liu, N. Isakov, and A. Altman, 2000, Inhibition of the c-Jun N-terminal kinase/AP-1 and NF-κB pathways by PICOT, a novel protein kinase C-interacting protein with a thioredoxin-homology domain. *J. Biol. Chem.* **275**:1902-1909.
11. Isakov, N., S. Witte, and A. Altman, 2000, PICOT-HD, a highly conserved protein domain that is often associated with thioredoxin and glutaredoxin modules. *Trends Biochem. Sci.* **25**:537-539.
12. Meier, B., H. H. Radeke, S. Selle, M. Younes, H. Sies, K. Resch, and G. G. Habermehl, 1989, Human fibroblasts release reactive oxygen species in response to interleukin-1 or tumour necrosis factor-alpha. *Biochem. J.* **263**:539-545.

IMMUNE RECEPTORS

The molecular specificity of IgG-Fc interactions with Fcγ receptors

YUSUKE MIMURA, RODOLFO GHIRLANDO*, PETER SONDERMANN+, JOHN LUND, AND ROY JEFFERIS
Division of Immunity and Infection, The Medical School, Birmingham B15 2TT, UK
**LMB-NIDDK-NIH, 5 Centre Drive MSC 0540, Bethesda MD 20892-0540, USA; +Max-Planck Institute, D-82152, Martinsried, Germany.*

The molecular specificity and mechanisms for the interaction of immunoglobulins with Fc binding ligands has been a subject of intensive investigation for many years. Significant information has been gained for human IgG-Fc from x-ray crystallographic analysis of IgG-Fc and IgG-Fc/ligand complexes. The crystal complexes of IgG-Fc with FcRn, SpA, SpG and rheumatoid factor autoantibody ligands revealed binding sites at the C_H2/C_H3 interface and an IgG-Fc:ligand stoichiometry of 1:2; reflecting the two fold symmetry of the IgG molecule [1]. For FcγR and C1q monomeric IgG must necessarily be functionally monovalent since IgG, FcγR bearing cells and C1 co-exist in the blood, in the absence of activation and the consequent inflammatory reactions.

The IgG-Fc region is a homodimer comprised of inter-chain disulphide bonded hinge regions, glycosylated C_H2 domains, bearing N-linked oligosaccharide at asparagine 297 and non-covalently paired C_H3 domains. Effector mechanisms mediated through FcγRI, FcγRII, FcγRIII and C1q are severely compromised for aglycosylated or deglycosylated forms of IgG [1]. The triggering of FcγR and C1 effector functions results from the multivalent array of IgG-Fcs presented by immune complexes. Crystal structures for soluble recombinant FcγRIIa and FcγRIIb have been published and interpreted to propose interaction sites for IgG-Fc [2,3]. The FcγRIIa molecule was seen to form a dimer that was proposed to generate a univalent binding site for a hinge proximal interaction site on IgG-Fc [1]. A NMR study observed interaction between IgG-Fc and FcγRII and also mapped the interaction site to the hinge proximal region [4]. The FcγRIIb structure was interpreted to propose an interaction site at the C_H2/C_H3 interface of IgG-Fc; such that the IgG would be divalent for FcγR with a 2:1 stoichiometry [3].

More recently a crystal structure, at 3.2A° resolution, for the complex of IgG1-Fc with soluble, recombinant FcγRIII has been published [5]. This shows that the interaction site on IgG-Fc is localised to the hinge proximal region of the C_H2 domain and includes the lower hinge region. The site is asymmetrical with both heavy chains making contact with a single FcγRIII molecule – thus accounting for the mono-valency of monomeric IgG. It was proposed that this model might serve as a paradigm for other Ig-FcR interactions. A similar conclusion was drawn from the crystal structure of IgE-Fc in complex with soluble, recombinant alpha chain of the high affinity epsilon receptor [6].

The influence of glycosylation on FcγR recognition has been extensively investigated through a study of the contribution of a series of truncated IgG-Fc glycoforms to IgG-Fc stability and effector function activity [7]. Differential scanning microcalorimetry was used to compare the stabilities of the homogeneous glycoforms of IgG1-Fc. The native IgG-Fc yields a thermogram with transition temperatures (Tm) of 71° C and 82° C for the C_H2 and C_H3 domains, respectively. For the truncated glycoforms the Tm of the C_H2 domain is progressively lowered whilst that of the C_H3 domain is not affected. This correlates with attenuation of FcγR binding and activation. The results show that all truncated oligosaccharides confer a degree of functional activity and thermodynamic stability to the IgG1-Fc, in comparison with deglycosylated IgG1-Fc [7]. The same truncated glycoforms of an intact IgG1 anti-MHC Class II antibody were shown to exhibit differential functional activity for FcγRI and C1 ligands, relative to deglycosylated IgG1. The minimal glycoform investigated had a trisaccharide attached to each heavy chain and can be expected to influence protein structure primarily in the hinge proximal region of the C_H2 domain, implicated as a binding site for multiple effector ligands [1]. This is consistent with the observation that recombinant FcγRIII makes a crystal contact with the primary N-acetylglucosamine residue [5]. These data provide a thermodynamic rationale for the modulation of antibody effector functions by different glycoforms.

These studies have been extended to a determination of the influence of the tertiary/quaternary structure on IgG-Fc glycosylation and FcγRI activation [8]. A series of truncated, humanised IgG1 antibodies was expressed in Chinese hamster ovary cells, to evaluate the contribution of structural components to glycosylation and function. The series includes L243 IgG1 (α-MHC Class II) lacking a C_H3 domain pair (ΔC_H3-IgG1), single chain Fv fusion proteins with Fc (scFvFc) or a hinge-C_H2 domain (scFvhC_H2), Fc with/out a hinge, and a single C_H2 domain. Fluorescence HPLC analysis of released pyridylaminated oligosaccharides indicates that intact IgG1 and scFvFc antibodies are galactosylated and sialylated to levels similar to those observed previously for normal human IgG1. The truncated forms express increased levels of digalactosylated (30-83%) or sialylated (9-21%) oligosaccharide chains with the highest levels observed for the single C_H2 domain. These data show which architectural components influence IgG glycosylation processing and that the $(C_H3)_2$ pair is particularly influential.

When MHC Class II bearing (JY) cells were sensitised with L243 ΔC_H3-IgG1, scFvFc, or scFvhC_H2 they elicited superoxide production, through FcγRI on U937 cells, at levels of 35-45% relative to that obtained for intact L243 IgG1 (100%). Mild reduction and alkylation of the hinge disulphide bonds of scFvhC_H2 greatly decreased its capacity to trigger superoxide production. Thus, the L243 scFvhC_H2 homo-dimer constitutes the minimal truncated form that binds the MHC Class II molecule antigen and triggers superoxide production through FcγRI.

Isothermal titration calorimetry (ITC) has been used to analyse interactions between human IgG1-Fc and a soluble form of FcγRIIb (Mimura, Sondermann, Jefferis et al., manuscript in preparation). A 1:1 stoichiometry was observed irrespective of whether the IgG1-Fc was titrated into sFcγRIIb or sFcγRIIb into IgG1-Fc. The values of the thermodynamic parameters at 30° C were identical for each titration: Ka, 1.2×10^6 M^{-1}; ΔH, -6.2 kcal mol^{-1}; ΔG, -8.4 kcal mol^{-1}; TΔS, 2.2 kcal mol^{-1}. The same 1:1 stoichiometry and thermodynamics were obtained when sFcγRIIb was titrated into intact native IgG1. When sFcγRIIb was titrated into deglycosylated IgG1-Fc there was no evidence of an interaction (*i.e.* Ka $< 10^5$ M^{-1}). These data confirm a 1:1 stoichiometry for the interaction of IgG1 with sFcγRIIb.

From present and previous studies [1, 7, 8] the influence of glycosylation on IgG-Fc structure and function may be summarized as followings:

•i) reciprocal interactions between the protein and the oligosaccharide influence the conformation of each.

•ii) "core" oligosaccharide is essential for FcγRI, FcγRII and FcγRIII recognition and C1 activation.

•iii) outer arm sugar residues can influence interactions at the C_H2-C_H3 interface, e.g. FcRn, SpA, SpG etc.

•iv) radical replacements of amino acid side chains contacting "core" oligosaccharide can modulate Fc effector functions.

•v) The same replacements can influence outer arm sugar addition.

•vi) conservative amino acid side chain replacements in C_H2 can influence outer arm sugar addition.

•vii) The quaternary structure of the IgG molecule influences effector ligand activation and the glycosylation profile.

•viii) The oligosaccharide can function as a structural *"rheostat"* through which effector functions can be modulated.

These studies contribute to a molecular understanding of IgG-Fc/ FcγR interactions and further the possibility of designing small molecules that might selectively inhibit IgG-Fc/ FcγR interactions.

Two recent papers have reported peptides having inhibitory activity for FcγR. One was an IgG-Fc mimetic that was presumed to bind to FcγRI [9], and, the other a peptide that binds to IgG-Fc [10]. Improved x-ray crystallographic resolution and analysis of IgG-Fc and/or sFcγR complexes with such small peptides should provide for the development of a new generation of customized inhibitors of IgG-Fc/FcγR interactions having therapeutic potential.

REFERENCES

1. IgG-Fc mediated effector functions: molecular definition of interaction sites for effector ligands and the role of glycosylation. Jefferis R., Lund J. and Pound JD. 1998. Immunol.Rev. 1998,163:59-76.
2. Crystal structure of the human leucocyte Fc receptor, FcγRIIa Maxwell K., Powell M., Hogarth M. et al. Nature Structural Biology, 1999, 6:437-442.
3. Crystal structure of the soluble form of the human FcγgRIIb: a new member of the Ig superfamily at 1.7A resolution. Sondermann P., Huber R., Jacob U. The EMBO J. 1999, 18:1095-1103.
4. Structural basis of the interaction between IgG and Fcγ receptors Kato K., Sautes-Fridman C. et al. J.Mol.Biol. 2000, 295:213-224.
5. The 3.2-Å Crystal Structure of the Human IgG1 Fc Fragment–FcγRIII Complex. Sondermann P.; Huber R.; Oosthuizen, V.; Jacob U. Nature, 2000, 406:267-273.
6. Structure of the Fc fragment of human IgE bound to its high-affinity receptor FcεRI Garman S., Wurzburg B., Tarchevskaya S., Kinet J-P., Jardetzsky T. Nature 2000, 406:359-266.
7. The influence of glycosylation on the thermal stability and effector function expression of human IgG1-Fc. Mimura Y., Church S., Ghirlando R., Dong S., Goodall M., Lund J., Jefferis R. Molecular Immunology. In press.
8. Expression and characterisation of truncated glycoforms of humanised L243 IgG1: architectural features can influence synthesis of its oligosaccharide chains and affect superoxide production triggered through human FcγRI. Lund J., Takahashi N., Popplewell A., Goodall M., Pound J., Tyler R., King D and Jefferis R. Eur.J.Biochemistry. 2000; 267:7246-7257.
9. Solid-phase synthesis and cyclization of a large branched peptide from IgG-Fc with affinity for FcγRI. Sheridan J., Hayes G., Austen B. J.Peptide Sci., 1999, 5:555-562.

10. Prevention of systemic lupus erythematosus by administration of an immunoglobulin binding peptide. Marino M., Ruvo M., de Falco S., Fassina G. Nature biotechnology, 2000, 18:735-739.

Regulation of myeloid cell proliferation and survival by p75/AIRM1 and CD33 surface receptors

MARIA CRISTINA MINGARI[1,2], CHIARA VITALE[3], CHIARA ROMAGNANI[2], MICHELA FALCO[3,4] AND LORENZO MORETTA[3,4]
[1]*Istituto Nazionale per la Ricerca sul Cancro c/o Centro Biotecnologie Avanzate, Genova;* [2]*Dipartimento di Oncologia, Biologia e Genetica, Università degli Studi di Genova,* [3]*Dipartimento di Medicina Sperimentale, Università degli Studi di Genova;* [4]*Istituto Giannina Gaslini, Genova, ITALY*

1. INTRODUCTION

Major progresses have recently been made toward a better understanding of the molecular mechanisms regulating the NK cell function. This is primarily the result of the discovery of a number of receptors which regulate the NK cell function. Thus, the identification of various MHC-class I-specific inhibitory NK receptors (iNKR) revealed a sophisticated capability of discriminating between normal and tumor (or virally-infected) cells (1-4). All iNKR are characterized by the presence of an immunoreceptor tyrosine-based inhibition motif (ITIM) in their cytoplasmic tail (3-6). The surface expression of iNKR that inhibit the NK-cell function, explains why NK cells lyse only those target cells that have lost or express insufficient amounts of MHC class I molecules, a phenomenon that frequently occurs in tumors and virus-infected cells. Each inhibitory receptor is expressed only by a fraction of NK cells. In addition, each NK cell expresses at least one receptor specific for self-MHC alleles. As a consequence, the whole NK cell pool can sense the loss of even single MHC-class I alleles on self cells. NK cells also express surface receptors responsible for the activation during the process of natural cytotoxicity. These recently identified receptors include NKp46 (7,8), NKp30 (9) and NKp44 (10,11), collectively referred to as natural

Progress in Basic and Clinical Immunology, Edited by Mackiewicz *et al.*
Kluwer Academic/Plenum Publishers, New York, 2001

cytotoxicity receptors (NCR) (12). Another receptor which plays a complementary role with NCR in the processo of NK cell activation is NKG2D (13,14), while additional triggering surface molecules expressed by human NK cells, including 2B4 and NKp80, appear to play a role as coreceptors rather than as true receptors (15,16).

A general interest in NK receptors was consequent to the finding that various inhibitory receptors, originally identified in NK cells, may also be expressed by other leukocyte populations, thus suggesting that they may play a more general role in the control of leukocyte function. Thus, iNKR are expressed by certain memory CTLs in which they can inhibit TCR-mediated cell function (17-19). Additional inhibitory NK receptors of still undefined specificity including p75/AIRM1 (20), p40/LAIR1 (21,22) and IRp60 (23), are also expressed by myeloid cells, including monocytes, dendritic cells (DC) and granulocytes, in which they may mediate inhibition of cell function or proliferation. Here we will briefly discuss on p75/AIRM1 and its homologue CD33 in view of their role in regulation of proliferation and survival of normal and leukemic myeloid cells.

2. P75/AIRM1, A NOVEL MEMBER OF THE SIALOADHESIN FAMILY HOMOLOGUE TO CD33

Studies that led to the discovery of p75/AIRM1 were aimed at the identification of novel receptors, possibly involved in the negative regulation of NK cell function. We selected mAbs specific for a novel inhibitory surface molecule of ~75 kD (p75) also termed adhesion receptor molecule 1 (AIRM1). Molecular cloning revealed a novel member of the sialoadhesin family characterized by one IgV and two IgC2-type Ig-like domains in the extracellular portion. It displays maximal similarity with CD33, i.e. an important marker of both normal differentiation and leukemic cell typing (20,24-26).

Similar to other sialoadhesins, p75/AIRM1 binds erythrocytes and this binding could be inhibited by mAbs to p75/AIRM1 or by pretreating the erythrocytes with neuraminidase. This suggests that p75/AIRM1 may function as a receptor which recognizes its ligand(s) in a sialic acid-dependent fashion. The homology between p75/AIRM1 and CD33, including the presence of an ITIM sequence in the cytoplasmic tail led us to reinvestigate the role of CD33, especially with respect to a possible inhibitory effect on myeloid cell function or proliferation (see below) (27-29).

The homology between CD33 and p75/AIRM1 molecules prompted us to analyze whether the latter was also expressed by cells of the myeloid lineage. FACS analysis of cells isolated (on Ficoll-hypaque gradients) from cord blood and gated on myeloid populations revealed that p75/AIRM1 is expressed by most $CD33^+$ cells and by the majority of $CD14^+$ cells. Analysis of mature granulocytes revealed a dim staining with anti-p75/AIRM1 (but not with anti-CD33). Fresh $CD34^+$ cells isolated from cord blood did not express p75/AIRM1 or CD33. In $CD34^+$ cells cultured with suitable growth factors (SCF and GM-CSF), an early expression of CD33 (but not of p75/AIRM1) occurred in a fraction of cells (30). After 3-4 days of culture, a high proportion of cells expressed CD33 while only a minor fraction expressed p75/AIRM1. At later culture intervals, most cells expressed both CD33 and p75/AIRM1. Thus, although CD33 and p75/AIRM1 were expressed by virtually the same cells in fresh cord blood, their time of appearance during myeloid differentiation was different, the expression of CD33 preceding that of p75/AIRM1 (30).

3. MAB-MEDIATED CROSSLINKING OF P75/AIRM1- OR CD33 INHIBITS PROLIFERATION AND DIFFERENTIATION OF NORMAL IMMATURE MYELOID CELLS

We investigated whether p75/AIRM1, beside the inhibitory effect on NK cell cytotoxicity, could also induce inhibition of myeloid cell functions as well. A similar effect could also be envisaged for CD33 in view of its homology with p75/AIRM1. $CD34^+$ cells were cultured with SCF and GM-CSF to induce cell differentiation towards the myelomonocytic cell lineage. The cell recovery at day 6 revealed a sharp inhibition in cultures containing either anti-p75/AIRM1 or anti-CD33 mAb. Thus, while no information was available on the possible function of CD33, our data suggest that it may actually play a regulatory role on normal hemopoiesis. A similar function could be hypotized for p75/AIRM1.

4. ANTI-P75/AIRM1 AND ANTI-CD33 MABS INHIBIT THE *IN VITRO* PROLIFERATION OF MYELOID LEUKEMIC CELLS

Leukemic cells from chemotherapy-free patients affected by CML were analyzed for the surface expression of p75/AIRM1 and the potential capability of anti-p75/AIRM1 or anti-CD33 mAbs to inhibit cell proliferation. While leukemic cells from different patients expressed variable proportions of p75/AIRM1. Leukemic cells, cultured in the presence of GM-CSF underwent variable degrees of proliferation, as assessed by evaluating the cell recovery at different culture intervals or by measuring the uptake of [3H] thymidine. Analysis of the effect of the addition of mAbs directed against p75/AIRM1 or CD33, revealed 80-40% inhibition of the proliferation of CMLs expressing the corresponding surface antigen.

In view of this inhibitory effect exerted by mAbs specific for p75/AIRM1 or CD33 on the proliferation of CML cells, we analyzed their surface expression on acute myeloid leukemias (AML) that are characterized by a particularly severe prognosis. AML are usually subdivided on the basis of the french-american-british (FAB) classification. The analysis of a panel of AML samples belonging to different FAB subtypes revealed that p75/AIRM1 was selectively expressed by M4 and M5 subtypes but not by M1, M2 and M3 (31). As p75/AIRM1 is not expressed by normal or leukemic T or B lymphocytes, it may represent an additional marker for identifying M4 and M5 AML.

AML cells isolated at diagnosis from chemotherapy-free patients, were cultured for 4 d in the presence or in the absence of GM-CSF. Under these conditions, upon addition of anti-CD33 mAb, virtually no viable cells could be detected after 4 d of culture in all cases analyzed. p75/AIRM1 exerted a variable effect. Thus, AML cells displaying a high degree of *in vitro* proliferation were inhibited, while no substantial effect could be detected on cell survival. Therefore, it appears that anti-CD33 mAb may affect AML cell proliferation by acting on cell survival, while anti-p75/AIRM1 mAb may simply inhibit cell proliferation.

5. CD33-MEDIATED APOPTOSIS OF AML CELLS

Since the engagement of CD33 affected cell survival, we investigated the mechanism(s) responsible for cell death. Different experimental evidences indicated that anti-CD33 mAb could induce apoptosis. Indeed, treatment of AML cells with anti-CD33 led to binding of annexin V and to oligonucleosomal DNA fragmentation. No such events occurred in cultures containing anti-p75/AIRM1 mAb: it is possible that the engagement of p75/AIRM1 may affect the cell cycle progression and that only cells characterized by a high proliferation rate may be susceptible to the p75/AIRM1-mediated inhibitory effect (31).

Experiments in which anti-CD33 was used in combination with etoposide (ETP) revealed an additional and even a synergistic effect. Thus, a suboptimal dosage of ETP that, when used alone, did not induce binding of annexin V over the control values, displayed a marked effect when used in combination with anti-CD33 mAb.

Remarkably, anti-CD33 mAb has also been shown to induce apoptotic death of macrophages and to prevent their development into DC (32). Again, this data may have important implications for a novel therapeutic approach to counteract the macrophage survival and function as well as to modulate excessive immune reactions. This may be particularly relevant in autoimmune diseases or in infectious diseases characterized by overwelming macrophage responses.

ACKNOWLEDGMENTS

This work was supported by grants awarded by Associazione Italiana per la Ricerca sul Cancro (A.I.R.C.), Istituto Superiore di Sanità (I.S.S.), Ministero della Sanità, and Ministero dell'Università e della Ricerca Scientifica e Tecnologica (M.U.R.S.T.), MURST 5%–CNR Biotechnology program 95/95 and Consiglio Nazionale delle Ricerche, Progetto Finalizzato Biotecnologie.

REFERENCES

1. Trinchieri G.Biology of natural killer cells. Adv. Immunol. 1989; 47: 176-187
2. Ljunggren HG and Karre K. In search of the "missing self". MHC molecules and NK cell recognition. Immunol. Today 1990; 11:237-244
3. Moretta A, Bottino C, Vitale M, Pende D, Biassoni R, Mingari MC and Moretta L.. Receptors for HLA-class I molecules in human Natural Killer cells. Annu. Rev. Immunol. 1996; 14 : 619-648
4. Lanier LL. NK cell receptors. Annu. Rev. Immunol. 1998; 16:359-393
5. Long EO. Regulation of immune responses through inhibitory receptors. Annu. Rev. Immunol. 1999; 17: 875-804
6. Bolland S, Ravetch JV. Inhibitory pathways triggered by ITIM containing receptors. Adv Immunol. 1999; 72: 149-177
7. Sivori S et al. NKp46, a novel Natural Killer cell-specific surface molecule which mediates cell activation. J.Exp. Med. 1997; 186: 1129-1136
8. Pessino A et al. Molecular cloning of NKp46: a novel member of the immunoglobulin superfamily involved in triggering of natural cytotoxicity. J. Exp. Med. 1998. 188: 953-960

9. Pende D et al. Identification and molecular characterization of NKp30, a novel triggering receptor involved in natural cytotoxicity mediated by human natural killer cells. J. Exp. Med. 1999; 190 : 1505-1516
10. Vitale M et al. NKp44, a novel triggering surface molecule specifically expressed by activated Natural Killer cells is involved in non-MHC restricted tumor cell lysis. J. Exp. Med. 1998; 187: 2065-2072.
11. Cantoni C et al. NKp44, a triggering receptor involved in tumor cell lysis by activated human Natural Killer cells, is a novel member of the immunoglobulin superfamily. J. Exp. Med. 1999; 189:787-796
12. Bauer S, Groh V, Wu J, Steinle A, Phillips JH, Lanier LL, Spies T. Activation of NK cells and T cells by NKG2D, a receptor for stress-inducible MICA. Science 1999; 285:727-729.
13. Pende D et al. Role of NKG2D in tumor cell lysis mediated by human NK cells: cooperation with natural cytotoxicity receptors and capability of recognizing tumors of nonepithelial origin. Eur. J. Immunol. 2001; 31 (in press)
14. Sivori S et al. 2B4 functions as a co-receptor in human natural killer cell activation. Eur. J. Immunol. 2000; 30: 787-793
15. Moretta A, Biassoni R, Bottino C, Mingari MC, and Moretta L.. Natural Cytotoxicity Receptors that trigger human NK-mediated cytolysis. Immunol. Today 2000; 21:228-234.
16. Vitale M et al. Identification of NKp80 a novel triggering molecule expressed by human Natural Killer cells. Eur. J. Immunol. 2001; 31: 233-242
17. Mingari, MC, Vitale C, Cambiaggi A , Schiavetti F, Melioli G, Ferrini S, Poggi, A. Cytolytic T lymphocytes displaying Natural Killer (NK)-like activity. Expression of NK-related functional receptors for HLA class I molecules (p58 and CD94) and inhibitory effect on the TCR-mediated target cell lysis or lymphokine production. Int Immunol. 1995; 7:697-703
18. Mingari MC et al. Human CD8+ T lymphocyte subsets that express HLA class I-specific inhibitory receptors represent oligoclonally or monoclonally expanded cell populations. Proc. Natl. Acad. Sci. USA. 1996; 93:12433-12438
19. Mingari MC, Moretta A, Moretta L. Regulation of KIR expression in human T lymphocytes. A safety mechanism which may impair protective T cell responses. Immunol. Today 1998; 19:153-157
20. Falco M et al. Identification and molecular cloning of p75/AIRM1, a novel member of the sialoadhesin family which functions as an inhibitory receptor in human natural killer cells. J. Exp. Med. 1999; 190:793-802
21. Poggi A et al. p40, a novel surface molecule involved in the regulation of the non-MHC restricted cytolytic activity in humans. Eur. J. Immunol. 1995; 25:369-376
22. Meyaard L, Adema GJ, Chang C, Woollatt E, Sutherland GR, Lanier LL, Phillips JH. LAIR-1, a novel inhibitory receptor expressed on human mononuclear leukocytes. Immunity 1997; 7 :283-290
23. Cantoni C et al. Molecular and functional characterization of IRp60, a member of the immunoglobulin superfamily that functions as an inhibitory receptor in human natural killer cells. Eur. J. Immunol. 1999; 29 :3148-3159
24. Peiper SC, Ashmun RA, Look AT. Molecular cloning , expression, and chromosomal localization of a human gene encodong the CD33 myeloid differentiation antigen. Blood 1988; 72:314-321
25. Freeman SD, Kelm S, Barber KE, and Crocker PR. Characterization of CD33 as a new member of the sialoadhesin family of cellular interaction molecules. Blood 1995; 85: 2005-2012.

26. Caron PC et al. Murine and humanized constructs of monoclonal antibody M195 (anti-CD33) for the therapy of acute myelogenous leukemia. Cancer 1994; 73: 1049-1056
27. Taylor VC, Buckley CD, Douglas M, Cody AJ, Simmons DL, and Freeman SD .The myeloid-specific sialic acid binding receptor, CD33, associates with the protein-tyrosine phosphatases,SHP-1 and SHP-2. J.Biol.Chem. 1999; 274 : 11505-11512.
28. Ulyanova T, Blasioli J, Woodford-Thomas TA, and Thomas ML. The sialoadhesin CD33 is a myeloid-specific inhibitory receptor. Eur. J. Immunol. 1999; 29: 3440-3449.
29. Sujatha PP, Taylor LS, Stransbury EK, and McVicar DV. Myeloid specific human CD33 is an inhibitory receptor with differential ITIM function in recruiting the phosphatases SHP-1 and SHP-2. Blood 2000; 96, 483-490.
30. Vitale C et al. Engagement of p75/AIRM1 or CD33 inhibits the proliferation of normal or leukemic myeloid cells. Proc. Natl. Acad. Sci. USA 1999; 96: 15091-15096.
31. Vitale C et al. Surface Expression and function of p75/AIRM-1 or CD33 in acute myeloid leukemias. Engagement of CD33 induces apoptosis of leukemic cells. Proc.Natl.Acad.Sci. USA. 2001 ; in press.
32. Ferlazzo, G , Spaggiari GM , Semino C , Melioli G , and Moretta L. Engagement of CD33 surface molecules prevents the generation of dendritic cells from both monocytes and CD34+ myeloid precursors. Eur. J. Immunol. 2000; 30: 827-833.

X-linked lymphoproliferative disease: the dark side of 2b4 function

CRISTINA BOTTINO[1], SILVIA PAROLINI[2], ROBERTO BIASSONI[1], MICHELA FALCO[3], LUIGI NOTARANGELO[4] and ALESSANDRO MORETTA[3]
[1]Istituto Nazionale per la Ricerca sul Cancro, 16132 Genova, Italy; [2]Dipartimento di Scienze Biomediche e Biotecnologie, Università di Brescia, 25123 Italy; [3]Dipartimento di Medicina Sperimentale, Università di Genova, 16132 Italy. [4]Istituto di Medicina Molecolare Angelo Nocivelli, Clinica pediatrica, Università di Brescia, 25123 Italy.

1. INTRODUCTION

A series of different receptor/ligand interactions are responsible for HLA class I-independent NK cell activation in humans. In this context, three NK-specific triggering receptors termed NKp46 (1,2), NKp44 (3,4) and NKp30 (5) have been identified, and termed Natural Cytotoxicity Receptors (NCR)(6). These receptors play a predominant role in NK cell activation in the process of natural cytotoxicity. Importantly, heterogeneity exists among different NK cells in their surface density of NCR. Thus, NCR^{bright} and NCR^{dull} NK cells were shown to display sharp differences in the ability to kill a panel of NK susceptible target cells. In particular, the strong cytolytic activity correlates with the expression of the NCR^{bright} phenotype whereas the expression of the NCR^{dull} phenotype is invariably associated with a low cytolytic activity of NK cells (7).

Additional receptors co-operate with NCR to induce NK cell triggering; among these the 2B4 molecule has been shown, both in mouse (8) and in humans (9,10), to activate NK cell cytotoxicity upon mAb-mediated cross-linking. Moreover, CD48 has been shown to represent the major

Progress in Basic and Clinical Immunology, Edited by Mackiewicz *et al.*
Kluwer Academic/Plenum Publishers, New York, 2001

physiological ligand of 2B4 (11-14) thus suggesting a role of 2B4 in non-MHC-restricted cytotoxicity

2. 2B4 IS A CO-RECEPTOR INVOLVED IN HUMAN NK CELL TRIGGERING

We previously showed that the stimulatory ability of 2B4 might differ in different NK cells when analyzed in redirected killing assays against murine target cells (9). Indeed, only a fraction of the human NK cell clones analyzed were responsive to anti-2B4 mAb-mediated stimulation. More recently, we demonstrated that NK clones responding to anti-2B4 mAb, in redirected killing express high levels of NKp46 surface molecules ($NKp46^{bright}$) (7). On the other hand, in NK clones characterized by the $NKp46^{dull}$ phenotype no responses to anti-2B4 could be observed. This suggested that a strict correlation existed between the surface density of NKp46 and the ability to respond to 2B4-mediated stimulation in a redirected killing assay. Previous experimental evidence indicated that the ligand of NKp46 was expressed on murine cells (3). Thus, it was conceivable that in cytolytic assays against murine target cells, the stimulating ability of anti-2B4 mAb could be dictated by the extent of cross-linking of NKp46 molecules mediated by its ligand (s) expressed on target cells. Along this line, mAb-induced modulation of NKp46 surface molecules in $NKp46^{bright}$ cells resulted in complete unresponsiveness to anti-2B4 mediated stimulation (although the surface expression of 2B4 was not affected). Therefore, the finding that NK cell clones are heterogeneous in their ability to respond to anti-2B4 mAb, reflects the fact that 2B4 may function as a co-receptor for NKp46 (9). Since the NKp46 ligand is expressed on most types of human target cells (3,7), it is likely that under physiological conditions, the co-receptor function of 2B4 would primarily depend on the expression of the 2B4 ligand (CD48) on target cells. In this context, it is important to note that expression of CD48 is up-regulated in Epstein Barr virus (EBV)-infected cells. These cells are highly susceptible to NK-mediated lysis indicating that the appropriate ligands are available for the interaction with NCR or their co-receptor(s). Previous data indicated that the major NCR implied in killing of EBV-infected B cells is represented by NKp46 (7). Thus, killing of these cells could be partially inhibited by mAb-mediated masking of this receptor. Notably, the simultaneous masking of 2B4 by appropriate mAb is able to increment the inhibitory effect observed in the presence of anti-NKp46 mAb thus suggesting that the 2B4/CD48 interaction is required for optimal recognition and killing of EBV-infected cells. The role of 2B4 in the recognition of CD48 molecules expressed in EBV cells can also be appreciated in a tumor NK cell line termed NK92. This cell line although expressing low levels of NKp46, is able to kill EBV cells such as the HLA class I-negative LCL 721.221. The NK92-mediated killing is partially inhibited by mAb-mediated masking of 2B4 while no effects can be observed with anti-NKp46 mAb. This suggests that, in this particular case, another receptor involved in the recognition of EBV-infected cells could co-operate with 2B4. Recently, in our laboratory we were able to identify this novel triggering molecule that was termed NTB-A (manuscript in preparation). Indeed, the combined masking of both 2B4 and NTB-A is able to abrogate NK92-mediated killing of EBV-infected cells (LCL 721.221).

3. SIGNALING VIA 2B4 IN HUMAN NK CELLS

2B4 is a member of the CD2 sub-family of the Immunoglobulin superfamily (Ig-SF) which also includes CD48, CD58, CD84, CD150 (also termed SLAM) and Ly9 (11-14). Is characterized in the extracellular portion by a, membrane-distal, IgV domain and a, membrane-proximal, IgC2 domain. The transmembrane portion lacks charged amino acids and, according to this, 2B4 does not associate with signaling polypeptides such as DAP12, CD3ζ, FcεRIγ and DAP10. The cytoplasmic tail does not contain classical ITAM consensus sequences however it is characterized by the presence of four TxYxxI/V motifs. Importantly, cell triggering with an anti-2B4 mAb was shown to induce tyrosine phosphorylation of 2B4 in normal NK cells (15). This results in the recruitment of a small a (15kD) intracytoplasmic protein characterized by a single SH2 domain termed Src homology 2 domain-containing protein (SH2D1A) or alternatively, SLAM-associated protein (SAP) (15). 2B4 also associate with SH2-containing phosphatases (SHP); however is still debated whether this SHP is represented by SHP-1, as detected in normal cells, (15) or by SHP-2 as shown in cell transfectants (16). The finding that the amounts of SHP-1 associated to 2B4 appear to be reduced upon tyrosine phosphorylation and SH2D1A-binding support the hypothesis that, in normal NK cells, SH2D1A participates to the triggering cascade by competing with SHP-1 for binding to 2B4 (15,16).

A recent study (17) provided evidence for a constitutive association between 2B4 molecules and the Linker for Activation of T cells (LAT) (18) in human NK cells. Moreover, upon specific engagement of 2B4, LAT becomes Tyrosine phosphorylated and recruits downstream elements such as PLCγ and Grb2 (17). In this context, it is of note that 2B4 is characterized by a CxC/+ motif (i.e. a CxC sequence surrounded by positive-charged residues) in the transmembrane/cytoplasmic portion. This may mediate its association with LAT that, in turn, displays a "CxxC/-" motif (i.e. a CxxC sequence followed by negative-charged amino acids) in the transmembrane/cytoplasmic portion. Altogether, these data suggests that LAT may participate to the 2B4-dependent activation of human NK cells. Interestingly, it was shown that NK cell triggering induced by interaction with NK-sensitive targets, such as C1R and 721.221 LCL, resulted in increased Tyrosine phosphorylation of LAT molecules (19). A possible explanation for these data is that Tyrosine phosphorylation of LAT may result from the interaction between 2B4 and CD48 molecules expressed on EBV-positive target cells.

4. 2B4 DYSFUNCTION IN NK CELLS DERIVED FROM PATIENTS AFFECTED BY X-LINKED LYMPHOPROLIFERATIVE DISEASE (XLP)

XLP is a severe inherited immune deficiency that is characterized by abnormal immune responses to the Epstein Barr virus (EBV) (20,21). After exposure to EBV, XLP males often succumb to fulminant infectious mononucleosis or develop lymphoma. The gene defective in XLP is located at Xq25 (22-24) and, in normal individuals, codes for SH2D1A (see above). Different mutations of the SH2D1A gene have been identified the result of which is either the absence of SH2D1A or the presence of truncated non-functional products. Thus, the genetic basis of XLP, i.e. mutations in SH2D1A encoding gene (22-24), was known, however the molecular events responsible for this disease remained undefined until recently. The absence of SH2D1A suggested that, in XLP patients, 2B4 molecules could be non-functional. Thus the function of 2B4 molecules in NK cells derived from XLP patients was analyzed in detail. While different triggering receptors including CD16 and NCR displayed a normal function, the signaling pathway initiated by 2B4 was dramatically altered. Indeed, engagement of 2B4 (by specific mAbs or its ligand CD48) resulted in the generation of inhibitory rather than activating signals (15). Importantly, this blocked not only the spontaneous NK cytotoxicity, but also the target-cell lysis induced via CD16 or NCR. As a consequence, XLP NK cells can efficiently kill $CD48^-$ but not $CD48^+$ target cells. Indeed, XLP-NK cells are unable to kill EBV^+ B cell lines (such as LCL 721.221 and Daudi) and their cytolytic activity can be restored by mAb-mediated disruption of the 2B4/CD48 interactions. As expected in XLP-NK cells the 2B4 co-receptor does not associate with SH2D1A while it associates with SHP-1 phosphatase. Notably, different from normal NK cells, in XLP-NK cells the amount of

2B4-associated SHP-1 is not reduced upon tyrosine phosphorylation of 2B4 (15). This suggests that, in the absence of SH2D1A, 2B4-engagement and phosphorylation does not result in SHP-1 dislocation from 2B4. The stable association of this phosphatase may be responsible for the 2B4-mediated down-regulation of cytolytic activity (25).

In conclusion, in XLP patients, clearance of EBV-infected cells would be impaired because of the occurrence of inhibitory rather than activating interactions between 2B4 and CD48. Thus, it appears conceivable that the altered 2B4 function may contribute to the inefficient control of EBV^+ B cells in XLP-patients.

ACKNOWLEDGEMENTS

This work was supported by grants awarded by Associazione Italiana per la Ricerca sul Cancro (A.I.R.C.), Istituto Superiore di Sanità (I.S.S.), Ministero della Sanità, and Ministero dell'Università e della Ricerca Scientifica e Tecnologica (M.U.R.S.T.) and Consiglio Nazionale delle Ricerche, Progetto Finalizzato Biotecnologie. The financial support of Telethon-Italy (grant no.E.0892 and grant no.E.668) is gratefully acknowledged.

REFERENCES

1. Sivori, S., M. Vitale, L. Morelli, L. Sanseverino, R. Augugliaro, C. Bottino, L. Moretta, and A. Moretta. 1997. p46, a novel Natural Killer cell-specific surface molecule which mediates cell activation. J.Exp.Med. 186: 1129-1136.
2. Pessino, A., S. Sivori, C. Bottino, A. Malaspina, L. Morelli, L. Moretta, R. Biassoni, and A. Moretta. 1998. Molecular cloning of NKp46: a novel member of the immunoglobulin superfamily involved in triggering of natural cytotoxicity. J.Exp.Med. 188: 953-960.
3. Vitale, M., C. Bottino, S. Sivori, L. Sanseverino, R. Castriconi, E. Marcenaro, R. Augugliaro, L. Moretta, and A. Moretta. 1998. NKp44, a novel triggering surface molecule specifically expressed by activated Natural Killer cells is involved in non-MHC restricted tumor cell lysis. J.Exp.Med. 187: 2065-2072.
4. Cantoni, C., C. Bottino, M. Vitale, A. Pessino, R. Augugliaro, A. Malaspina, S. Parolini, L. Moretta, A. Moretta, and R. Biassoni. 1999. NKp44, a triggering receptor involved in tumor cell lysis by activated human Natural Killer cells, is a novel member of the immunoglobulin superfamily. J.Exp.Med. 189: 787-796.
5. Pende, D., S. Parolini, A. Pessino, S. Sivori, R. Augugliaro, L. Morelli, E. Marcenaro, L. Accame, A. Malaspina, R. Biassoni, C. Bottino, L. Moretta, and A. Moretta. 1999. Identification and molecular characterization of NKp30, a novel triggering receptor involved in natural cytotoxicity mediated by human natural killer cells. J.Exp.Med. 190: 1505-1516.

ANTIGEN PRESENTATION/ DENDRITIC CELLS

Role of tapasin in MHC class I antigen presentation *in vivo*

NATALIO GARBI, PAMELA TAN, FRANK MOMBURG, GÜNTER J. HÄMMERLING

Department of Molecular Immunology, German Cancer Research Center, Heidelberg, Germany

1. INTRODUCTION

Antigen presentation on MHC class I molecules is a key event for $CD8^+$ T cell development as well as initiation and maintenance of immunological responses against intracellular microorganisms. For a cellular immune response to be initiated, peptides derived from invading pathogens need to be generated, loaded onto MHC class I molecules in the endoplasmic reticulum (ER) and displayed at the cell surface for $CD8^+$ T cell recognition[1,2]. The generation of antigenic peptides is usually achieved by proteolytic degradation in the cytosol by the proteasome. Peptides are then selectively transported into the ER lumen by the transporter associated with antigen presentation (TAP) and loaded onto "peptide-receptive" class I molecules in a process assisted by several molecular chaperones and accessory proteins.

2. HOUSE-KEEPING AND SPECIALISED MOLECULES FACILITATE FOLDING AND PEPTIDE LOADING OF MHC CLASS I

The folding and assembly of proteins in the ER is facilitated by molecular chaperones. The house-keeping chaperones calnexin and ER60[3]

Progress in Basic and Clinical Immunology, Edited by Mackiewicz *et al.*
Kluwer Academic/Plenum Publishers, New York, 2001

bind to newly synthesised MHC class I heavy chains (HC) ensuring proper folding and disulphide bond formation. This process is then continued with the recruitment of MHC class I light chain β_2-microglobulin (β_2m), the exchange of calnexin by calreticulin and the bridging to TAP by the class I-specific accessory protein tapasin to form the "loading complex"[1,2] (Figure 1). The loading complex allows for the existence of "empty" and otherwise unstable conformations of HC and facilitates the loading of peptides brought into the ER lumen via TAP transporters that consist of TAP1 and TAP2 subunits. Loading of peptides with sufficient stability causes the release of trimeric HC-β_2m-peptide complexes from the loading complex, probably via conformational changes of the MHC class I molecules, and their export to the cell surface.

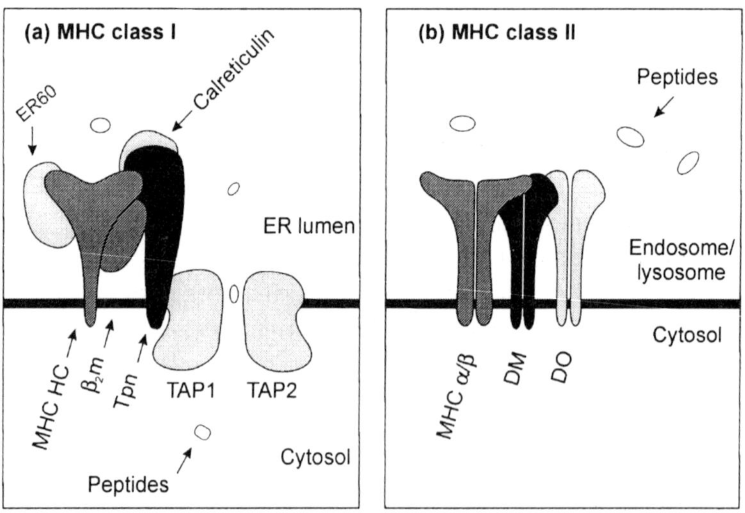

Figure 1. Accessory molecules stabilise empty MHC class I (a) or class II (b) molecules (dark grey) for optimal peptide binding. Tapasin and DM (black) directly associate with their respective MHC molecule facilitating peptide loading and allowing stable MHC-peptide complexes to be displayed on the cell surface for T cell recognition. Adapted from ref. 4.

The role of the loading complex and the relative importance of its different components for antigen presentation has been the subject of extensive research based on mice and cell lines deficient in individual components. Tapasin, a recently identified[5] 48–kD ER-resident transmembrane glycoprotein belonging to the immunoglobulin superfamily, is emerging as an essential class I-specialised molecule with different functions in the loading complex. Firstly, tapasin stabilises peptide-receptive HC molecules until peptide binding occurs[6,7,8]. Secondly, TAP expression is stabilised by tapasin resulting in an increased peptide translocation into the

ER[8,9]. Finally, tapasin appears to lead to an increased half-life of class I-peptide complexes, although recent evidence suggests that the mass spectrometric peptide profiles are very similar in the presence and absence of tapasin[10,11]. However, research on tapasin has focused on the mutant human B cell line 721.220, which is defective for full-length tapasin although it expresses residual amounts of a trunacated tapasin form, and on an insect cell line transfected with different components of the class I antigen presentation machinery. Therefore we generated mice with a targeted tapasin gene disruption to study its role in T cell development and antigen presentation *in vivo*[12].

3. QUANTITATIVE DIFFERENCES IN ANTIGEN PRESENTATION INDUCED BY TAPASIN

3.1 Reduced MHC class I expression and $CD8^+$ T cell frequency in tapasin-deficient mice

Lymphocytes and bone marrow-derived dendritic cells (BMDC) from tapasin-deficient ($Tpn^{-/-}$) mice have a reduction in surface $H2\text{-}K^b$ and $H2\text{-}D^b$ expression of about 90%[12]. This reduction is, however, not as profound as that in cells from $\beta_2m^{-/-}$ or $TAP1^{-/-}$ mice[13,14]. Presumably due to low class I expression in the thymus, positive selection of $CD8^+CD4^-$ T cells in $Tpn^{-/-}$ mice is reduced by an approximate two-fold factor. In the periphery, $CD8^+$ T cell frequency is reduced about four-fold. In agreement with class I expression, more profound defects in $CD8^+CD4^-$ T cell positive selection are observed in $\beta_2m^{-/-}$ or $TAP1^{-/-}$ than in $Tpn^{-/-}$ mice.

3.2 Decreased antigen presentation and reduced viral CTL response in tapasin-deficient mice

Presentation of influenza virus and ovalbumin has been investigated to elucidate the role of tapasin for loading antigenic peptides onto class I molecules. Ovalbumin crosspresentation by $Tpn^{-/-}$ BMDC and splenic dendritic cells is abolished as indicated by the K^b:OVA reactive T cell hybridoma B3Z[12]. Similarly, introduction of ovalbumin into the cytosol of $Tpn^{-/-}$ spleen cells by electroporation does not result in activation of B3Z. These results are comparable to those obtained with $TAP1^{-/-}$ cells and in sharp contrast with wild-type cells. However, $Tpn^{-/-}$ BMDC are able to present influenza viral antigens and are killed by wild-type-derived anti-influenza CTL, albeit to a significantly lower extent than infected wild-type BMDC. Thus, tapasin does not exert an all-or-nothing but rather a quantitative effect on peptide loading onto MHC class I molecules. Generation of anti-influenza CTL *in vivo* is accordingly affected in $Tpn^{-/-}$ mice as assessed by a reduced capacity to kill H-2^b target cells loaded with influenza virus nucleoprotein (NP) 366-374[12]. However, in another study the CTL response against vaccinia virus and LCMV was not reduced in the absence of tapasin[15]. Therefore the presentation of more epitopes should be investigated to ascertain the importance of tapasin in the generation of CTL responses against a diversity of pathogens.

The lowered anti-influenza CTL activity in $Tpn^{-/-}$ mice may be due to two non-exclusive factors. First, $Tpn^{-/-}$ cells are less able to present antigen than cells from wild-type mice, as observed in dendritic cells pulsed with ovalbumin or infected with influenza virus; second, the $CD8^+$ T cell frequency is drastically reduced in $Tpn^{-/-}$ mice. Although the percentage of $CD8^+$ T cells in $Tpn^{-/-}$ mice is reduced, these mice are able to generate a strong primary allogeneic CTL response which is comparable to that of wild-type mice after restimulation with alloantigen *in vitro*. This demonstrates a fully functional $CD8^+$ T cell repertoire in $Tpn^{-/-}$ mice that is expandable in the presence of antigen.

4. QUALITATIVE DIFFERENCES IN ANTIGEN PRESENTATION IN $TPN^{-/-}$ MICE

4.1 $Tpn^{-/-}$ mice present a less stable class I-peptide repertoire but are tolerant to wild-type MHC class I antigens

As discussed above, tapasin plays a quantitative role in antigen presentation. However, it was not clear if tapasin has also a qualitative effect by modulating the selection of peptides to be presented on class I molecules *in vivo*. The stability of surface class I-peptide molecules is dependent on the affinity of the peptides for class I molecules. Therefore the half life ($t_{1/2}$) of surface class I molecules provides an indication of the affinity of the peptide repertoire selected in the absence of tapasin. After blocking *de novo* transport of class I molecules to the surface with brefeldin A, the half-life of surface class I molecules (K^b and D^b) in $Tpn^{-/-}$ splenocytes is strongly reduced[12] ($t_{1/2}$ K^b 2h in $Tpn^{-/-}$ *vs* 10h in $Tpn^{+/+}$, D^b 4h in $Tpn^{-/-}$ *vs* 11h in $Tpn^{+/+}$) as indicated by staining with the conformation-dependent antibodies

K10-56 and B22-249. The reduced class I-peptide stability is not merely due to an increased presence of empty surface class I molecules in $Tpn^{-/-}$ cells, as suggested in transfected insect cells[6], since surface class I-peptide $t_{1/2}$ is similarly reduced in cells whose proteasome was blocked with lactacystin to prevent the generation of most class I epitopes but not treated with brefeldin A. Therefore, most class I molecules in $Tpn^{-/-}$ cells recognised by the above mentioned antibodies are peptide occupied but less stable than those on wild-type cells, suggesting an impaired peptide selection in $Tpn^{-/-}$ mice.

It is known that $CD8^+$ T cells from $\beta_2m^{-/-}$ and $TAP1^{-/-}$ mice are not tolerant to wild-type MHC class I antigens[16,17], possibly due to an altered class I-peptide repertoire in these mice. $Tpn^{-/-}$ mice, however, failed to mount a secondary syngeneic CTL response against wild-type cells. This suggests that although the peptide repertoire is altered in these mice, some overlap with that of wild-type mice exists and the generation of syngeneic CTL responses is thus prevented.

4.2 Altered NK cell repertoire in tapasin knockout mice

Tapasin-deficient mice have normal numbers of natural killer (NK) cells, as assessed by the pan-NK antibody DX5 and they are able to kill YAC-1 targets as efficiently as wild-type NK cells[12]. However, wild-type NK cells readily kill $Tpn^{-/-}$ targets whereas $Tpn^{-/-}$ NK cells do not, indicating that tapasin-deficient mice have an NK cell repertoire with altered specificity. These results are similar to those observed in $TAP1^{-/-}$ mice[18].

5. TAPASIN AND HLA-DM: SIMILAR MECHANISMS IN DIFFERENT ANTIGEN PRESENTATION PATHWAYS ENSURING STABLE MHC-PEPTIDE COMPLEXES?

Antigen presentation on MHC class I and II molecules, although different in many aspects, have common fundamental features. Apart from differences in molecular structure, peptide loading onto class I and II molecules takes place in different compartments reflecting the diverse localisation of antigens they present. Class II molecules are loaded in endosomal/lysosomal compartments with peptides derived from antigens that have access to this compartment, e.g. many endogenous antigens and extracellular bacteria after being internalised. On the other hand, class I molecules are loaded in the ER with peptides derived from cytosolic antigens usually synthesised within the APC such as viral antigens or brought into the cytosol by the still unknown croos-presentation mechanism. However, antigen presentation alerts T cells of invading pathogens and evolution has provided both pathways with different mechanisms yet the same purpose: selection of optimal peptide binders resulting in an improved MHC-peptide stability at the cell surface for T cell recognition. In the class I pathway several factors have been shown to contribute to peptide selection leading to the binding of an optimum repertoire onto class I molecules:

- *Proteasome*. The actual class I-binding ligand or slightly longer peptides are cleaved out of protein antigens by abundant multisubunit proteases in the cytosol, the proteasomes[19].
- *TAP*. Both the length and carboxyl terminus of the peptide are important features for transport efficiency by TAP[20]. The optimal length for transport is about 8-12 amino acids and the preferred carboxyl termini for transport are those also preferred for binding to class I molecules.
- *MHC heavy chain*. Due to structural limitations of the peptide binding groove, HC preferentially binds 8-11mer peptides. Furthermore, binding of peptides that contain class I allele-specific motifs (the so-called peptide anchor residues) results in a stronger interaction with the binding groove and thus higher complex stability[21].
- *Tapasin*. As discussed here, tapasin stabilises empty class I molecules in the loading complex and selects for a more stable class I-peptide repertoire to be presented at the cell surface.
- *Amino-terminal trimming of peptides*. Cytosolic and ER trimming of peptides resulting in best-fitting epitopes has been shown in model peptides[22,23]. However, the extent to which N-terminal trimming is a generalised process remains unknown.

A strikingly common feature in the two antigen presentation pathways is the function of tapasin and HLA-DM (H-2M in mice) in stabilising MHC molecules and selecting a more stable peptide repertoire (Figure 1). DM has been shown to associate to class II molecules in the loading compartment and catalyse the exchange of peptides by others that result in a higher stability of the class II-peptide complex[24]. DM is also able to act as a chaperone stabilising empty class II molecules until peptide binding occurs[25]. The following are similarities between tapasin and DM in their respective antigen presentation pathways:

- Both associate with their respective MHC molecules in their peptide loading compartments.
- Both stabilise empty MHC molecules.

- Both allow for the existence of loading complexes with highly peptide-receptive MHC molecules. A significant proportion of MHC class I and II molecules in the respective loading complexes are peptide-receptive and can be rapidly loaded with peptide. Stabilisation of peptide-receptive MHC molecules may be an important factor during early infection for a rapid presentation of pathogen epitopes.
- Both modulate peptide binding resulting in a stable MHC-peptide repertoire on the cell surface. DM selects and edits the peptides that bind to class II molecules until a high stability class II-peptide is formed. Although tapasin selects for binding of higher affinity peptides, its editing function remains unknown.

ACKNOWLEDGEMENTS

This work was supported by the EC project ERB-4061-PL-95-1079 (G.J.H.).

REFERENCES

1. Cresswell, P., Bangia, N., Dick, T. and Diedrich, G., 1999, The nature of the MHC class I peptide loading complex. Immunol. Rev. **172**: 21-28.
2. Solheim, J. C., 1999, Class I MHC molecules: assembly and antigen presentation. Immunol. Rev. **172**: 11-19.
3. Lindquist, J. A., Jensen, O. N., Mann, M. and Hämmerling, G. J., 1998, ER-60, a chaperone with thiol-dependent reductase activity involved in MHC class I assembly. Embo J. **17**: 2186-2195.
4. Vogt, B. A., Hämmerling, G. J. and Kropshofer, H, 1998, HLA-DM and HLA-DO: A chaperone and its modulator inflzuencing the peptide repertoire seen by T cells. The immunologist **6/5**:186-193.
5. Sadasivan, B., Lehner, P. J., Ortmann, B., Spies, T. and Cresswell, P., 1996, Roles for calreticulin and a novel glycoprotein, tapasin, in the interaction of MHC class I molecules with TAP. Immunity **5**: 103-114.
6. Schoenhals, G. J., Krishna, R. M., Grandea, A. G. 3rd, Spies, T., Peterson, P. A., Yang, Y. and Fruh, K., 1999, Retention of empty MHC class I molecules by tapasin is essential to reconstitute antigen presentation in invertebrate cells. Embo J. **18**: 743-753.
7. Suh, W. K., Derby, M. A., Cohen-Doyle, M. F., Schoenhals, G. J., Fruh, K., Berzofsky, J. A. and Williams, D. B., 1999, Interaction of murine MHC class I molecules with tapasin and TAP enhances peptide loading and involves the heavy chain alpha3 domain. J. Immunol. **162**: 1530-1540.
8. Li, S., Paulsson, K. M., Chen, S., Sjogren, H. O. and Wang, P., 2000, Tapasin is required for efficient peptide binding to transporter associated with antigen processing. J. Biol. Chem. **275**: 1581-1586.

9. Lehner, P. J., Surman, M. J. and Cresswell, P., 1998, Soluble tapasin restores MHC class I expression and function in the tapasin-negative cell line .220. Immunity **8**: 221-231.
10. Barnden, M. J., Purcell, A. W., Gorman, J. J. and McCluskey, J., 2000, Tapasin-Mediated Retention and Optimization of Peptide Ligands During the Assembly of Class I Molecules. J. Immunol **165**: 322-330.
11. Purcell, A. W., Gorman, J. J., Garcia-Peydro, M., Paradela, A., Burrows, S. R., Talbo, G. H., Laham, N., Peh, C. A., Reynolds, E. C., Lopez De Castro, J. A.andMcCluskey, J., 2001, Quantitative and Qualitative Influences of Tapasin on the Class I Peptide Repertoire. J. Immunol. **166**: 1016-1027.
12. Garbi, N., Tan, P., Diehl, A. D., Chambers, B. J., Ljunggren, H.-G., Momburg, F. and Hammerling, G. J., 2000, Impaired immune responses and altered peptide repertoire in tapasin-deficient mice. Nature Immunol. **1**: 234-238.
13. Zijlstra, M., Bix, M., Simister, N. E., Loring, J. M., Raulet, D. H. and Jaenisch, R., 1990, β_2-microglobulin deficient mice lack $CD4^-8^+$ cytolytic T cells. Nature **344**: 742-746.
14. Van Kaer, L., Ashton Rickardt, P. G., Ploegh, H. L. and Tonegawa, S., 1992, TAP1 mutant mice are deficient in antigen presentation, surface class I molecules, and $CD4^-8^+$ T cells. Cell **71**: 1205-1214.
15. Grandea III, A. G., Golovina, T. N., Hamilton, S. E., Sriram, V., Spies, T., Brutkiewicz, R., harty, J. T., Eisenlohr, L. C. and Van Kaer, L., 2000, Impaired assembly yet normal trafficking of MHC class I molecules in tapasin mutant mice. Immunity **13**: 213-222.
16. Glas, R., Ohlen, C., Hoglund, P. and Karre, K., 1994, The $CD8^+$ T cell repertoire in β2-microglobulin-deficient mice is biased towards reactivity against self-major histocompatibility class I. J. Exp. Med. **179**: 661-672.
17. Aldrich, C. J., Ljunggren, H. G., Van Kaer, L., Ashton Rickardt, P. G., Tonegawa, S. and Forman, J., 1994, Positive selection of self- and alloreactive $CD8^+$ T cells in Tap-1 mutant mice. Proc. Natl. Acad. Sci. USA **91**: 6525-6528.
18. Ljunggren, H. G., Van Kaer, L., Ploegh, H. L. and Tonegawa, S., 1994, Altered natural killer cell repertoire in Tap-1 mutant mice. Proc. Natl. Acad. Sci. USA **91**: 6520-6524.
19. Niedermann, G., Geier, E., Lucchiari-Hartz, M., Hitziger, N., Ramsperger, A. and Eichmann, K., 1999, The specificity of proteasomes: impact on MHC class I processing and presentation of antigens. Immunol. Rev. **172**: 29-48.
20. Momburg, F. and Hammerling, G. J., 1998, Generation and TAP-mediated transport of peptides for major histocompatibility complex class I molecules. Adv. Immunol. **68**: 191-256.
21. Rammensee, H. G., Falk, K. and Rotzschke, O., 1993, Peptides naturally presented by MHC class I molecules. Annu. Rev. Immunol. **11**: 213-44.
22. Stoltze, L., Schirle, M., Schwarz, G., Schröter, C., Thompson, M. W., Hersh, L. B., Kalbacher, H., Stevanovic, S., H -G Rammensee, H.-G. and Schild, H., 2000, Two new proteases in the MHC class I processing pathway. Nature Immunol. **1**: 413-418.
23. Paz, P., Brouwenstijn, N., Perry, R. and Shastri, N., 1999, Discrete proteolytic intermediates in the MHC class I antigen processing pathway and MHC I-dependent peptide trimming in the ER. Immunity **11**: 241-251.
24. Kropshofer, H., Hämmerling, G. J. and Vogt, A. B., 1997, How HLA-DM edits the MHC class II peptide repertoire: survival of the fittest? Immunol. Today **18**: 77-82.
25. Kropshofer, H., Arndt, S. O., Moldenhauer, G., Hämmerling, G. J. and Vogt, A. B., 1997, HLA-DM acts as a molecular chaperone and rescues empty HLA-DR molecules at lysosomal pH. Immunity **6**: 293-302.

Regulation of transporters associated with antigen processing (TAPs) by nucleotide binding to, and hydrolysis by, Walker consensus sequences

LOREDANA SAVEANU and PETER M. VAN ENDERT
Institut National de la Santé et de la Recherche Médicale Unité 25, 161 rue de Sèvres, 75743 Paris Cedex 15, France

1. INTRODUCTION

The TAP transporters (TAP1/TAP2) belong to the large family of ATP-binding-cassette (ABC) transporters which translocate a variety of solutes across cellular membranes in an ATP-dependent fashion. ABC transporters are regulated by nucleotide triphosphate binding to, and hydrolysis by, several conserved sequence elements termed Walker A and B motifs which are located in the two hydrophilic ABC domains found in all members of the family. Nucleotide binding and hydrolysis are thought to be associated with sequential conformational changes that together constitute a transport cycle which starts with a high affinity substrate binding site on one side of the membrane and ends with a low affinity site on the other side (1).

Little is known about nucleotide control of TAP function. TAP fulfils an essential function in antigen presentation by providing peptides to nascent MHC class I molecules. We have previously shown that human wild type TAP complexes undergo a dramatic conformational change upon incubation at 37°C in the absence of nucleotides; this change is associated with loss of peptide binding and transport capacity and can be prevented by addition of nucleotide di- or triphosphates (2). Subsequently, Knittler et al. showed that TAP complexes with mutant Walker A sequences unable to bind nucleotides do not bind or transport peptide. Moreover, such complexes did not release

Progress in Basic and Clinical Immunology, Edited by Mackiewicz *et al.*
Kluwer Academic/Plenum Publishers, New York, 2001

peptide-loaded class I molecules, suggesting conformational changes affecting the class I/TAP interface (3).

We sought to understand regulation of TAP function by nucleotides by producing human TAP proteins with various mutations in the Walker motifs. Some of these were designed to abolish nucleotide binding, while others were expected to affect nucleotide hydrolysis only. Mutant proteins were expressed in the baculovirus/insect cell system, and the effect of mutations analysed in peptide binding and transport assays at various temperatures.

2. RESULTS

TAP1 and TAP2 possess identical 9-residue Walker A sequences, with a critical Gly residue in position 1, and a Lys in 7. These were substituted by Gln and Ala residues, respectively, in mutants T1G538Q and T1544A/T2K509A. Other mutations included deletions of the Walker A sequence (T1Del, T2Del), or its complete replacement (T1Rep, T2Rep) by 9-residue linkers composed mainly of Ala and Ser. Both types of mutation were expected to eliminate nucleotide interaction with the altered TAP subunit. In the case of TAP1, we also introduced a mutation into the Walker B sequence (T1R659Q) that had previously been described in a class I-deficient tumor cell line.

In a Western blot analysis of complete insect cell lysates, all mutant proteins were expressed at similar levels. However, when TAP proteins were solubilised with NP-40 for immuno-precipitation, very low levels of mutant T1Del and T1G538Q were recovered which were assembled correctly with TAP2; all other mutants were solubilised and co-precipitated with complementary wild type subunits efficiently. This suggested that deletion of the TAP1 Walker A sequence, and substitution of Gly538 affected TAP1 folding and induced its aggregation, while the equivalent mutation in TAP2, and all other mutations did not affect folding.

2.1 Peptide transport by mutant TAP proteins

Two methods were used to study transport function: accumulation of glycosylated peptides in purified microsomes expressing mutant subunits together with wild type complementary subunits, and expression of HLA-B27 proteins on the surface of insect cells expressing such complexes. We have previously shown that the latter parameter reflects TAP-dependent peptide loading. Equivalent results were obtained with the two methods. All TAP complexes with mutations in a Walker A sequence of one subunit could not accumulate peptides and provide them to HLA-B27. Surprisingly, mutant T1R659Q, reported to abolish class I expression by a tumour line, reduced TAP transport by 50 percent only. Considering structural models of ABC proteins, this mutation is likely to affect nucleotide hydrolysis but not binding. Therefore, either reduced nucleotide hydrolysis by TAP1 is sufficient to eliminate class I expression by non-lymphoid cells, or the Walker B mutation induces additional alterations without effect in our readout systems, for example by changing TAP interaction with components of class I loading complexes.

2.2 Peptide binding to mutant TAP complexes

Peptide binding to TAP precedes its transport and can be measured at low temperature. When microsomes are studied, peptide binding to TAP at temperatures between 0 and 27°C is not affected by nucleotides, while TAP conformation and peptide binding capacity at 37°C are nucleotide-dependent. In peptide binding assays at low temperature, most mutants had little or no effect on the efficiency of peptide binding. Peptide binding capacity of T1Del/T2wt complexes was reduced to 10 – 20% relative to wild type complexes, reflecting the strongly reduced amount of correctly folded and assembled TAP proteins. In contrast, reduced peptide binding to normally folded and assembled T1wt/T2Del complexes suggested that the TAP2 Walker A sequence, and hence possibly nucleotide binding to TAP2, was important for peptide binding.

When microsomes were incubated at 37°C in the absence of nucleotides prior to binding assays, all mutant TAP complexes lost peptide-binding capacity. However, addition of ATP or ADP prevented loss of binding capacity not only of wild type complexes, but also of those containing mutant TAP1 subunits including T1Rep. Since ADP was as efficient as ATP, nucleotide binding and not hydrolysis preserved TAP peptide binding capacity. In contrast, ATP and ADP did not preserve peptide binding by complexes containing equivalent mutations in TAP2. Thus, nucleotide binding to TAP2 was required to maintain TAP peptide binding capacity at 37°C, while nucleotide binding to TAP1 was not.

In the case of wild type TAP complexes, we had previously shown that loss of peptide binding capacity is associated with conformational changes leading to reduced recognition by several antibodies. When we immuno-precipitated mutant TAP complexes incubated at 37° with these antibodies, we found an unchanged relationship between TAP conformation and peptide binding: complexes with TAP2 Walker A mutations changed conformation, while those with mutations in TAP1 did not. Since other experiments showed that the mutant TAP1 proteins themselves could not bind nucleotides, we conclude that nucleotide binding to TAP2 stabilises TAP1 and TAP2 conformation and peptide binding capacity.

3. CONCLUSIONS

This study demonstrates, first, that the ABC cassettes of both TAP subunits, and probably ATP hydrolysis by both, are required for peptide transport. However, the Walker B substitution studied here represents to our knowledge the only mutation likely to affect only nucleotide hydrolysis (but not binding). Experimental evidence for a requirement for ATP hydrolysis by TAP2 remains therefore to be provided.

Our results also clearly demonstrate that the TAP1 and TAP2 ABC domains have distinct functions. While two mutations of the TAP1 Walker A sequence affect overall TAP folding and assembly, nucleotide interaction with TAP2 only is required and sufficient for maintaining TAP in a conformation with high peptide affinity at physiological temperature. Thus, different from some other well-studied ABC transporters, TAP uses nucleotide binding and hydrolysis by its two subunits at distinct points in its transport cycle.

REFERENCES

1. Schneider, E., and Hunke, S. (1998). ATP-binding-cassette (ABC) transport systems: functional and structural aspects of the ATP-hydrolyzing subunits/domains, *FEMS Microbiol. Rev.* **22**, 1-20.
2. van Endert, P. M. (1999). Role of nucleotides and peptide substrate for stability and functional state of the human ABC family transporters associated with antigen processing, *J. Biol. Chem.* **274**, 14632-8.
3. Knittler, M. R., Alberts, P., Deverson, E. V., and Howard, J. C. (1999). Nucleotide binding by TAP mediates association with peptide and release of assembled MHC class I molecules, *Curr. Biol.* **9**, 999-1008.

The *AIR-1* encoded class II transactivator (CIITA): the master coordinator of MHC class II gene expression and ..more

ROBERTO S. ACCOLLA
Department of Clinical and Biological Sciences, Chair of General Pathology and Immunology, School of Medicine, University of Insubria, Varese; and Istituto Nazionale per la Ricerca sul Cancro (IST), Advanced Biotechnology Center, Genova, ITALY

1. INTRODUCTION

MHC class II genes encode highly polymorphic cell surface glycoprotein heterodimers that play a key role for the homeostasis of the immune response. Class II molecules expressed in appropriate antigen presenting cells (APC) act as receptors for antigenic peptides that only under this form can be presented to regulatory CD4+ T cells (TH) and trigger the cascade of events leading to both humoral and cellular immune effector functions (reviewed in 1).

In order to accomplish this function a series of genetic and biochemical constrains have to be respected. First, class II polymorphism dictates the restriction of T cell recognition, in that only T cells sharing the same allelic specificity of antigen presenting MHC class II molecules can recognize the peptide antigen and be triggered. Second, a sufficient amount of class II molecules should be present on APCs to guarantee an efficient stimulation of CD4 T cells. In this respect reduced or anomalous expression of MHC class II molecules can be at the basis of serious immune disfunctions such as immunodeficiency and autoimmunity, respectively.

Progress in Basic and Clinical Immunology, Edited by Mackiewicz *et al.*
Kluwer Academic/Plenum Publishers, New York, 2001

2. THE REGULATION OF EXPRESSION OF MHC CLASS II GENES.

2.1 Structural anatomy of MHC class II promoter

For the reasons sexpressed above much attention has been devoted to the mechanisms controlling class II gene expression. Biochemical and genetic analysis has clearly demonstrated the crucial role of the highly conserved upstream region of class II genes. Within 300 bases 5' to the transcription initiation site are contained the necessary and sufficient promoter sequences for both constitutive and inducible class II gene expression (see Figure 1). Mutations or deletions in either three of the conserved boxes, Y, X and S/W of the promoter region profoundly decrease or even abolish the transcription of class II genes. Specific transcription factors have been identified and cloned which bind particularly to the X and Y box (reviewed in 2). However these factors are ubiquitously expressed and thus could not explain the exquisite and restricted cell type specific expression of the class II genes.

2.2 The discovery of the master regulator of MHC class II gene expression: the *AIR-1* gene and its product

In 1983 our laboratory isolated a B cell variant from the Burkitt lymphoma line Raji, designated RJ2.2.5, which after mutagenesis and immunoselection had lost the expression of the entire repertoire of class II genes (3). Subsequent genetic and molecular studies identified a locus, *AIR-1* (for Activator of Immune Response genes, number 1), encoding a trans-acting activator, whose function was conserved across species barriers and could complement the defect of RJ 2.2.5 (4,5). Interestingly, the expression of this locus was suppressed in the terminally differentiated B cell, the plasmacell, that do not express MHC class II genes (6). It became clear that the *AIR-1* locus was indeed the major physiological and specific regulator of MHC class II gene expression. Ten years after the original description of RJ2.2.5, the product of the *AIR-1* locus was cloned and designated CIITA (7). Most of, if not all, the genetic regulatory functions previously assigned to the *AIR-1* locus by somatic cell genetics could then be confirmed with the cloned product by molecular complementation studies and by gene knock out in the experimental mouse model (8-11). An historical background of the discovery of the *AIR-1* locus and of its product is summarized in Table 1.

Table 1. Historical background of the discovery of the *AIR-1* locus and of the function of its product.

1983 Mutagenesis and immunoselection identify somatic cell mutants (RJ2.2.5) lacking the constitutive expression of the entire HLA class II gene repertoire (Accolla, J. Exp. Med. 1983, 157:1053).
1985-1986 Trans-species complementation demonstrates the existence of a class II transcriptional activator. The locus encoding the transcriptional activator is mapped to mouse chromosome 16 and designated Air-1 (for Activator of immune response genes number 1) (Accolla et al., J. Exp. Med. 1985, 162:1117; Accolla et al., J. Exp. Med. 1986, 164:369)
1988 The HLA class II negative phenotype in plasma cells is due to active suppression of the human AIR-1 locus function (Latron et al., PNAS 1988, 85:2229)
1989-1991 The AIR-1 locus is the target of the genetic defect occurring in a subgroup of severe combined immunodeficiencies designated Bare Lymphocyte Syndrome (BLS) deficiencies (Hume and Lee, Hum. Immunol., 1989, 26:288; Benichou and Strominger, PNAS 1991, 75:135)
1993 The product of the AIR-1 locus, the class II transcriptional activator (CIITA), is cloned (Steimle et al., Cell 1993, 75:135)
1994-1996 The AIR-1 locus product is the major regulator of both constitutive and IFNγ-induced HLA class II gene transcription in cell lines (Steimle et al., Science 1994, 265:106), in normal thymic epithelial cells (Rigaud et al., J. Immunol. 1996, 156:4254), and in gene knock-out mice (Chang et al., Immunity 1996, 4:167)

An intense investigation started both on the physiological role of the *AIR-1* locus product and on the possible involvement of it in immune-related diseases. Molecular studies have confirmed that CIITA is a transcriptional activator whose expression (as the genes that it regulates) is developmentally controlled. However studies aimed at clarifying the intimate molecular mechanism of CIITA are still elusive. It is recognized that CIITA is not a DNA binding protein; rather, it may function through the interaction with one or more DNA binding factors and in so doing may work as a stabilizer of the appropriate chromatin conformation within and/or around the promoter region (reviewed in 12). Recent data suggest that CIITA is crucial in favouring the enhanceosome formation (13). This may explain the various interactions of the transactivator not only with important elements of the class II promoter but also with basal transcription factors (14), proteins with histone acethyltransferase activity (p300/CBP)(15) , and elongation factors as the the pTEFb complex (Cyclin T1-CDK9) (16) (Figure 1). Furthermore, reciprocal interactions between CIITA and the above transcriptional regulators may be enhanced by homodimer formation of the transactivator.

The AIR-1 gene product CIITA is the MHC class II transcriptional controller

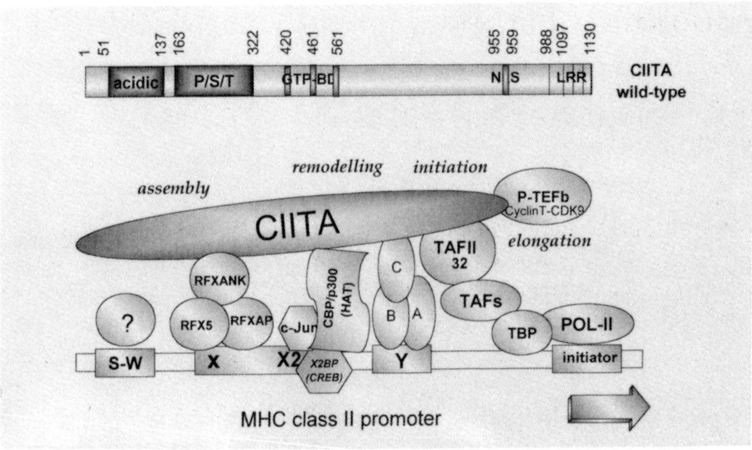

Figure 1. Schematic representation of protein domain organization for the *AIR-1* gene product CIITA (upper part). Numbering corresponds to the B cell form of CIITA. The first 322 amino acids contain both an acidic domain and a Proline/Serine/Treonine domain. Between aa 420 and 561 three GTP binding regions are present. Between aa 955-959 a nuclear localization signal (NLS) is present followed by a C-terminal region with several Leucine-rich motifs. In the lower part of the figure is depicted an hypothetical view of the integrator function of the *AIR-1* gene product. The class II promoter region contains several highly conserved motifs: S-W, X-X2 and Y boxes. These motifs bind transcription factors which are ubiquitously expressed as the RFX complex (RFX5, RFXAP and RFX-ANK) which binds to the X box, CREB and c-Jun that bind to the X2 motif, and the A, B and C subunits of the NFY complex that bind to the Y box. It is still unclear the biochemical nature of the S-W box binding factors. CIITA has been shown to bind to RFX complex, favouring the assembly of the promoter binding factors; CIITA also binds to CBP/p300 which display histone acethyl transferase activity and in so doing probably partecipates to the chromatin remodelling; CIITA binds to basal transcription components, and interestingly, to the P-TEFb complex which is important for phosphorylating the CTD of RNA pol-II that can then elongate primary transcripts. Thus, CIITA can partecipate to both initiation and elongation of transcription.

3. MODULATIONS AND ALTERATIONS OF AIR-1 GENE EXPRESSION: IMPLICATIONS IN THE PHYSIOPATHOLOGY OF THE IMMUNE SYSTEM

The *AIR-1* locus and its product are also clearly involved in human pathology. A subgroup of Bare Lymphocyte Syndrome, a rare syndrome characterized by lack of both constitutive and IFN-γ inducible expression of MHC class II genes , is due to recessive homozygous mutations and/or deletions in the *AIR-1* gene leading to non functional CIITA protein (17,18). These patients have defects in both humoral and cellular immune responses leading to a severe combined immunodeficiency characterized by acute recurrent infections often fatal within the first 2-3 years of life (reviewed in 2).

Recently we become interested in interaction between infectious agents and their cellular hosts. Two model system are currently investigated in our laboratory: phagocytosis of gram-negative bacteria and mycobacteria, and retrovirus infections.

Our studies on phagocytosis have demonstrated that both *E.coli* and *mycobacteria* can transiently downregulate MHC class II, but not class I, expression in the macrophage cell line THP1 (19) and, more importantly, in normal perypheral blood-derived macrophages. The effect is specific for bacterial phagocytosis and cannot be reproduced by phagocytosis of inert particles or by treatment with LPS. In THP1 cell line this effect is mainly due to a block of the export to the cell membrane of newly synthesized class II molecules, although a partial reduction in the IFN-γ induced class II biosynthesis is also observed (19). On the contrary the latter effect dominates in normal perypheral blood macrophages and, interestingly, is due to reduced expression of CIITA-specific mRNA. Of particular importance is the fact that in normal macrophages treated with IFN-γ and undergoing bacterial phagocytosis the reduction of CIITA expression and, consequently, of class II gene transcription is a rather late event taking place after 24-48 hours from treatment, whereas at 6 hours CIITA induction by IFN-γ in bacterial treated cells is as high as in mock treated cells, suggesting that late metabolites either from bacteria or from phagocytes influence the IFN-γ-induced transcription of the *AIR-1* gene. We are presently investigating the molecular correlate of this phenomenon. It is interesting to note that the *AIR-1* gene promoter is a rather complex functional unit including sequences that are sensitive to IFN-γ (promoter IV) or that are constitutively active in B cells (promoter III) or in dendritic cells (promoter I) (20). Whatever the mechanism, this event is of biological importance as the phagocytes cannot adeguately present peptide antigens to T cells (De Lerma et al., submitted for publication). It appears, therefore, that during the first days from bacterial phagocytosis, APC can be refractory to efficient antigen presentation unless other factors relieve the partial block of *AIR-1* gene expression. The equilibrium between expression of CIITA and its inhibitory mediators may play an important role in those pathological states characterized by recurrent bacterial infections.

Viruses have developed several strategies to elude the immune response. Among these strategies reduction of MHC class I expression is of major relevance as class I molecules are the structures that present viral peptides to cytolitic T cells (CTL). For human CMV, EBV, HSV and HIV-1, many viral proteins have been described which influence, cumulatively, almost every step of the biosynthesis of class I molecules (reviewed in 21). Less is known about viral impact on MHC class II expression although some important cases have been described. For example CMV can downregulate expression of CIITA by altering the IFN-γ signal pathway (22).

At present our attention is focussed on retrovirus infections, particularly HIV-1 and HTLV-II. In contrast to previously published observations, we and others found that the major transactivator of HIV-1 viral expression, the Tat protein, does not downregulate class I expression. Interestingly some Tat mutants that are envisaged as possible vaccine components, but not wild-type Tat, profoundly down-regulate the expression of class II genes both in macrophages and in activated T cells, the cellular targets of HIV-1 infection (23). Kanazawa et al. have found that wild type Tat, instead, may downregulates class II gene expression (16). The apparent discrepancy between the results of two laboratories may rely in the different cellular systems and transfectants used, and particularly in the relative amount of Tat protein required to detect the downmodulation effect. However, in both reports no effect on CIITA transcription was observed. As Tat recruits and utilizes P-TEFb for elongating viral transcripts (24) and CIITA binds P-TEFb (16), it is possible that Tat and CIITA may compete for this factor and, depending upon the relative concentration and/or the relative affinities for P-TEFb, may influence each other transactivating function. Within this frame, one possibility is that our Tat mutants may display an "heteroclitic" activity for P-TEFb by binding it with stronger affinity than wild-type Tat, and in so doing reducing the CIITA transactivating function on class II gene transcription. We have recently developed an experimental system that allows to study Tat transactivation function on HIV-1 LTR in a quantitative fashion. HeLa cells (HL3T1) stably transfected with an HIV-1 LTR-CAT plasmid are incubated with synthetic highly purified Tat protein that enters the cells and transactivates the promoter generating CAT protein that can be quantitatively monitored by ELISA. A dose-response curve can be generated depending upon the Tat protein added to the culture and exogenous Tat function can be specifically inhibited by anti-Tat monoclonal antibodies (25). HL3T1 have been stably transfected with CIITA. Addition of Tat protein to HL3T1/CIITA cells cannot longer transactivate the HIV-1 LTR promoter, indicating that CIITA inhibits Tat function. We are investigating whether this finding has functional relevance in influencing, for example, the capacity of susceptible cellular targets to be infected by HIV-1. That *AIR-1* gene expression may influence the capacity of a retrovirus to replicate in its cellular host is strongly suggested by our recent findings that HTLV-II productive infection in permissive T and B cells is reduced, if not inhibited, by the presence of a functional CIITA.

Taken together, the findings summarized in this report open new scenarios for a better understanding of the interactions between bacterial and viral pathogens and their cellular hosts,and call into play the MHC class II regulator not only as a target (whose function on genes for antigen presenting molecules can be inhibited by the pathogen), but also as an actor which, unexpectedly, by itself can inhibit vital pathogen functions.

ACKNOWLEDGEMENTS

This work was supported by the following grants : Istituto Superiore di Sanità (I.S.S.) National Research Project on A.I.D.S. n° 40.B.1; MURST National Project "Meccanismi di resistenza alle neoplasie"; MURST "Structural basis and functional consequences of cell surface recognition processes"; Consiglio Nazionale delle Ricerche (CNR) Target Project on "Biotechnology"; European Vaccine Effort against AIDS (EUROVAC), a European Research Consortium, contract n°QLK2-CT-1999-01321.

REFERENCES

1. Germain, R.N., and Margulies, D.H., The biochemistry and cellular biology of antigen processing and presentation. *Annu. Rev. Immunol.* 1993. 11: 403-450.
2. Mach B, Steimle, V., Martinez-Soria, E., and Reith, W., Regulation of MHC class II genes: lessons from a disease. *Annu. Rev. Immunol.* 1996. 14:301-331.
3. Accolla, R.S. 1983. Human B cell variants immunoselected against a single Ia subset Have lost expression of several Ia antigen subsets. *J.Exp.Med* 1983. 157: 1053-1058.
4. Accolla, R.S., Jotterand-Bellomo, M., Scarpellino, L., Maffei, A., Carra, G., and Guardiola, J., aIr-1, a newly found locus on mouse chromosome 16 encoding a trans-acting activator factor for MHC class II gene expression. *J.Exp. Med.* 1986. 164 : 369-374.

5. Accolla R. S., Scarpellino L., Carra G., Guardiola J., Trans-acting element(s) operating across species barriers positively regulate the expression of major histocompatibility complex class II genes, *J.Exp.Med.* 1985. 162: 1117-1133.
6. Latron F, Jotterand-Bellomo M., Maffei A., Scarpellino L., Bernard M., Strominger J.L., Accolla R.S., Active suppression of major histocompatibility complex class II gene expression during differentiation from B cells to plasma cells, *Proc. Natl. Acad. Sci. USA* 1988. 85: 2229-2233.
7. Steimle, V., Otten, L.A., Zufferey, M., and Mach, B., Complementation cloning of an MHC class II transactivator mutated in hereditary MHC class II deficiency (or Bare Lymphocyte Syndrome). *Cell* 1993. 75:135-146.
8. Steimle V., Siegrist C.A., Mottet A., Lisowska-Grospierre B., Mach B., Regulation of MHC class II expression by interferon-γ mediated by the transactivator gene CIITA, *Science* 1994. 265:106-109.
9. Rigaud G., De Lerma Barbaro A, Nicolis M., Cestari T., Ramarli D., Riviera A.P., Accolla R.S., Induction of CIITA and modification of *in vivo* HLA-DR promoter occupancy in normal thymic epithelial cells treated with IFN-γ, *J.Immunol.* 1996. 156: 4254-4258.
10. Chang C.H, Guerder S., Hong S.C., van Ewijk W., Flavell R.A., Mice lacking the MHC class II transactivator (CIITA) show tissue-specific impairment of MHC class II expression, *Immunity* 1996. 4:167-178.
11. Accolla, R.S., Tosi, G. Sartoris, S. and De Lerma Barbaro, A., MHC class II gene regulation: some considerations on a still ontogenetic and phylogenetic puzzle. *Microbes and Infection* 1999. *1*: 871-877.
12. Harton, J.A., and Ting, J.P.Y., Class II transactivator: mastering the art of major histocompatibility complex expression. *Mol. Cell. Biol.* 2000. 20:6185-6194.
13. Masternack, K., Muhlethaler-Mottet, A., Villard, J., Zufferey, M., Steimle, V., and Reith, W., CIITA is a transcriptional coactivator that is recruited to MHC class Iipromoters by multiple synergistic interactions with an enhanceosome complex. *Gen. & Develop.*, 2000. 14:1156-1166.
14. Fontes, J.D., Jiang, B, and Peterlin, M.B., The class II transactivator CIITA interacts with TBP-associated factor TAFII32. *Nucleic Acid Res.*, 1997. 25:2522-2528.
15. Kretsovali, A., Agalioti, T., Spilianakis, C., Tzortzakaki, E., Merika, M., and Papamatheakis, J., Involvement of CREB binding protein in expression of major histocompatibility complex class II genes via interaction with the class II transactivator. *Mol. Cell. Biol.* 1998. 18: 6777-6783.
16. Kanazawa, S., Okamoto, T., and Peterlin B.M., Tat competes with CIITA for the binding to P-TEFb and blocks the expression of MHC class II genes in HIV infection. *Immunity.* 2000, 12:61-70.
17. Hume, C.R., and. Lee J.S., Congenital immunodeficiencies associated with absence of HLA class II antigens on lymphocytes result from distinct mutations in trans-acting factors. *Human Immunoloy* 1989. 26:288-293.
18. Benichou B., Strominger J.L., Class II-antigen-negative patient and mutant B cell lines represent three, and probably four, distinct genetic defects defined by complementation analysis, *Proc. Natl. Acad. Sci. USA* 1991. 88:4285-4288.
19. De Lerma Barbaro, A., Tosi, G., Valle, M-T., Megiovanni, A.M., Sartoris, S., D'Agostino, A., Soro, O., Mingari, M.C., Canonica, G.W., Manca, F., and Accolla R.S., Distinct Regulation of HLA class II and class I cell surface expression in THP-1 macrophage cell line after bacterial phagocytosis. *Eur. J. Immunol.* 1999. 29: 499-511.

20. Muhlethaler-Mottet, A., Otten, L.A., Steimle, V., and Mach, B., Expression of MHC class Ii molecules in different cellular and functional compartments is controlled by differential usage of multiple promoters of the transactivator CIITA. *EMBO J.* 1997. 16:2851-2860.
21. Tortorella, D., Gewurz, B.E., Furman, M.H., Schust, D.J., and Ploegh, H.L., Viral subversion of the immune system. *Ann. Rev. Immunol.* 2000. 18: 861-926.
22. Miller, D.M., Rahill, B.M., Boss, J.M., Lairmore, M.D., Durbin, J.E., Waldman, J.W., and Sedmak, D.D., Human cytomegalovirus inhibits major histocompatibility complex class Ii expression by disruption of the Jak/Stat path. *J. Exp. Med.* 1998. 187: 675-683.
23. Tosi, G., A. De Lerma Barbaro, A. D'Agostino, M.T. Valle, A.M Megiovanni, F. Manca, A.Caputo, G. Barbanti Brodano, and R.S. Accolla. HIV Tat mutants in the cysteine-rich region down-regulate HLA class II expression in T lymphocytic and macrophage cell lines. *Eur. J. Immunol.* 2000. 30:19-28
24. Wei, P., Gerber, M.E. Fang, S.M. Fisher, W.H. and Jones, K.A., A novel CDK9-associated C-type cyclin interacts directly with HIV-1 Tat and mediates its high-affinity, loop-specific binding to TAR RNA. *Cell* 1998. 92:451-462.
25. Tosi, G., Meazza, R., De Lerma Barbaro, A., D'Agostino, A., Mazza, S., Corradin, G., Albini, A., Noonan, D. M., Ferrini, S., and Accolla R.S., Highly stable oligomerization forms of HIV-1 tat detected by monoclonal antibodies and requirement of monomeric forms for the transactivating function on the HIV-1 LTR. *Eur. J. Immunol.* 2000. 30:1120-1126.

Major histocompatibility complex class II (MHC II) expression during development of human fetal brain and haemopoietic organs

TERESA WIERZBA-BOBROWICZ, ELŻBIETA KOSNO-KRUSZEWSKA, ELIZA LEWANDOWSKA, WALDEMAR LECHOWICZ, BOGNA SCHMIDT-SIDOR
Department of Neuropathology, Institute of Psychiatry and Neurology, Al. Sobieskiego 1/9, Warsaw, Poland

1. INTRODUCTION

Proteins of the major histocopatibility complex class II molecules (MHC II, HLA II, Ia) are surface glycoproteins of cellular membrans. They are products of HLA-DP, HLA-DQ and HLA-DR genes, encoded on at least 100 genes. Molecules of MHC II antigen belong to the most polymorphic proteins among those recognized to date[1-3]. Polymorphism of both genes and MHC proteins, resulting from the evolution process, ensures that many different peptides are bound, hence the organisms are capable to specific immune response. The molecules of this system are responsible for the binding, transport, and presentation of a forein antigen to helper T lymphocytes (Th, CD4). They also stimulate the multiplication of specific B lymphocytes and determine the type of antibodies produced[4-6]. Another important feature of their responsibility is participation in the selection, leading to differentiation of immature into mature lymphocytes. In adult, MHC II molecules are expressed on the surface of cells identified as antigen-presenting cells (APCs); macrophages, B lymphocytes, microglial and dendritic cells. In developing organisms, MHC II expression is also observed on other types of cells: on vascular endothelium, thymic epithelial cells[7-9].

Progress in Basic and Clinical Immunology, Edited by Mackiewicz *et al.*
Kluwer Academic/Plenum Publishers, New York, 2001

Although the discussion about the origin of microglia has been continued for above 100 years, the issue has not yet been resolved[10,11]. The majority of researches[12-15], is convinced that microglial cells originate from mesodermal lineage, monocytic/macrophages lineage, or from blood precursive cells, similarly as dendritic cells (Fig 1).

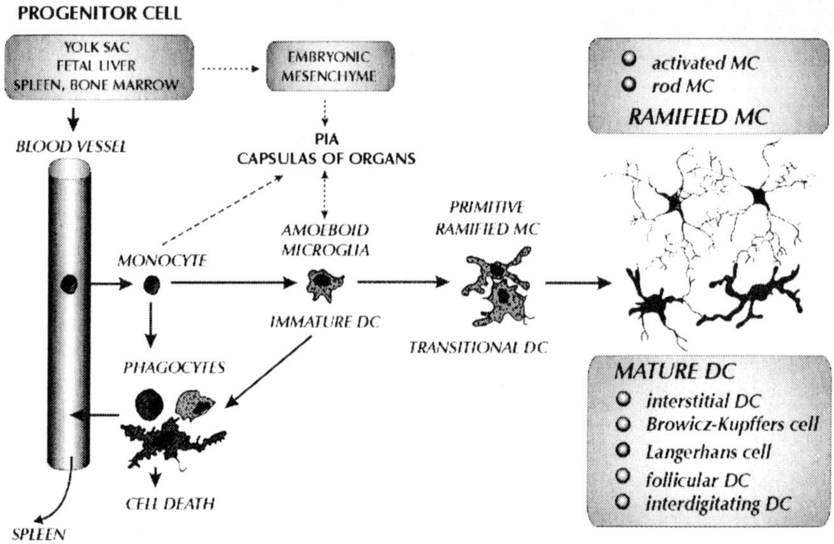

Figure 1. Life cycle of a dendritic cell (DC) / microglia cell (MC)

Until quite recently, it was thought that the fetal development of immunity begins with the development of the lymphatic system. Meanwhile, evidence has been provided that the production of T-cell receptors (TCRs) is fortuitous regardless of the type of peptides present in the organism. Only contact between immature lymphocytes T precursors and thymic cells decides about lymphocyte CD4 survival[12]. It is assumed that the mode of TCRs interaction with MHC II molecules determines the mechanism responsible for the maturation of thymic lymphocytes.

The identification of cells on which MHC II molecules are expressed in the central nervous system (CNS) and haematopoietic organs, during the fetal development, may indicate the fetal age when immunity of a given organs is already matured, as well as evidence for the involvement of cells from this organ in morphogenesis and histogenesis.

2. MATERIAL AND METHODS

Observation were made on the frontal, temporal and occipital lobes, cerebellum and thymus, speen and liver of 30 normal human fetuses, between 11 and 22 week of gestation (GW). Intact brains and other organs were fixed in 4% buffered formalin, embedded in parafin and cut serially at 8 μm. in a frontal sections. H&E was used for routine staining.

Major histocompatibility complex, class II molecules were visualized via immunoreaction using biotin-streptavidin complex. Slides were incubated for 24 h with primary anti-human HLA-DP, DQ, DR (clone DK22, CR3/43, DAKO 1:50). For visualisation of microglial and dendritic cells were used lectin *Ricinus communis* agglutinin (RCA-1, Vector Laboratories, 2.5 μg/ml) and antibodies: HAM 56 (DAKO 1:50), CD68 (clone PG-M1, DAKO 1:100), CD14 (clone TK4, DAKO 1:20), S-100 (Novocastra 1:400). The outcome of the reaction was visualized using diaminobenzidine (DAB, Sigma).

The ultrastructure evaluation was performed on sections fixed in 2% glutaraldehyde, and embedded in epon. Ultrathin sections were stained with uranyl and lead acetate and examined under a transmission electron microscope (Opton Turbo DPS 109).

3. RESULTS

In the whole studied brain (frontal, temporal and occipital lobes and cerebellum), MHC II molecules were observed during the whole period between GW 11 and 22. MHC II molecules were seen on the surface of

round, oval cells in the meninges, choroid plexus, nearby blood vessels and ventricles, as well as in single cells with processes in deeper layers of cortex and white mater (or in an intermediate zone), and in the vicinity the matrix (Fig 2a-c and 3a-c). Morphologicaly, oval and round cells looked like ameboid microglia (AM) cells/macrophages, whereas cells with processes like ramified microglia (RM) (Fig 4 a, b).

The ultrastructural examination revealed AM containing oval or U-shaped nucleus, chromatin accumulated under nuclear membrane, ample cytoplasm with numerous cellular organells. RM had an irregular nucleus surrounded by a wide belt of 'amebic' cytoplasm (Fig 5 a) similarly as the dendritic cell (Fig 5 b).

In the others organs (thymus, spleen and liver), MHC II molecules were observed on the cellular surface during the whole time of gestation under study (between 11 and 22 GW). In the thymic parenchyma, MHC II molecules were expressed on cells with long processes penetrating thymic lobules in the cortex and medulla (Fig 6 a). Morphologically, cells within thymic lobe corresponded with dendritic and epithelial cells (Fig 6 b, c).

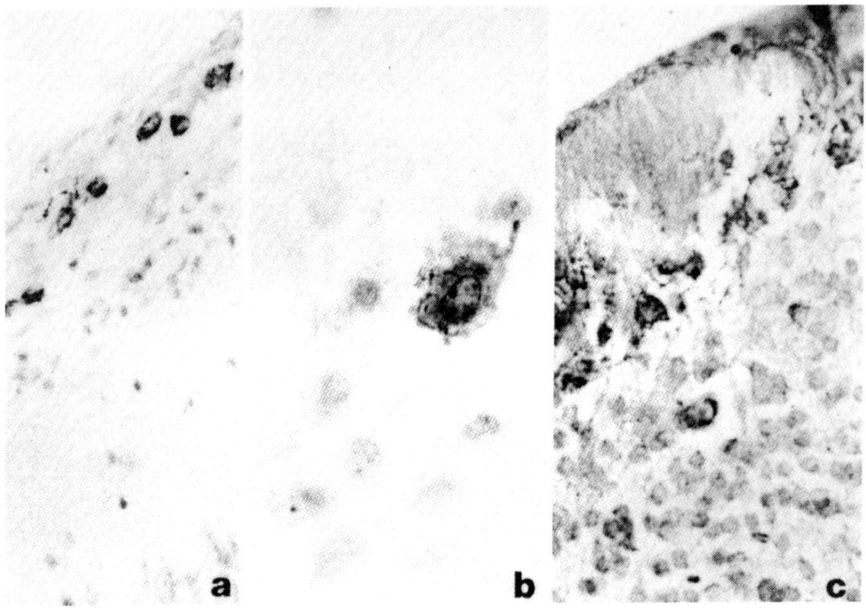

Figure 2. Positive reaction with MHC II molecules of ameboid microglial cells (AM) – (a) cerebral meninges above temporal lobe, 16 GW, x 200; (b) AM nearby blood vessel in cerebellum, 22 GW, x 1000; (c) AM under the layer of germinal cells in occipital lobe, 11 GW, x 400

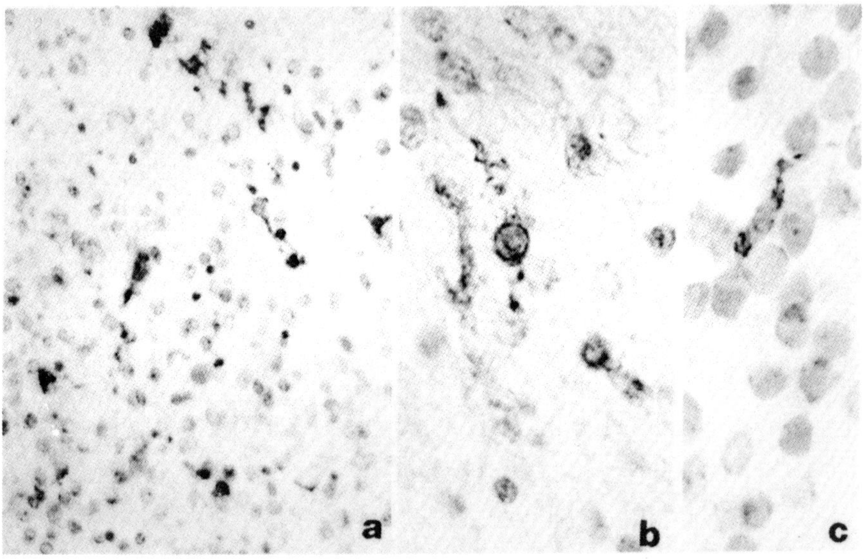

Figure 3. Positive reaction with MHC II molecules of ramified microglial cells in (a) temporal lobe, 22 GW, x 200; (b) frontal lobe, 19 GW, x 1000; (c) cerebellum, 15 GW, x 1000

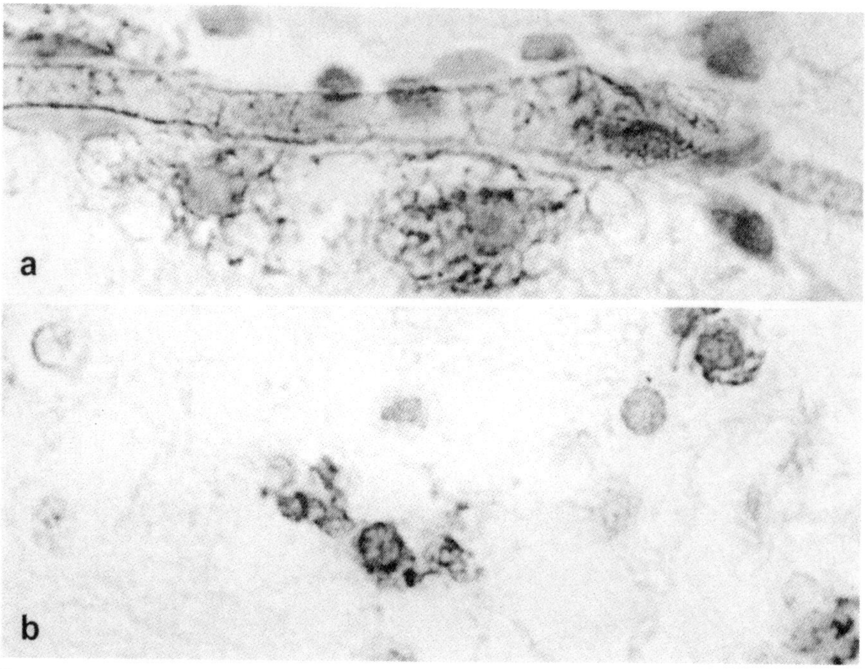

Figure 4. Positive reaction with lectin RCA-1: (a) ameboid microglia in cerebellum, 11 GW, x 1000; (b) ramified microglia in temporal lobe, 15 GW, x 1000

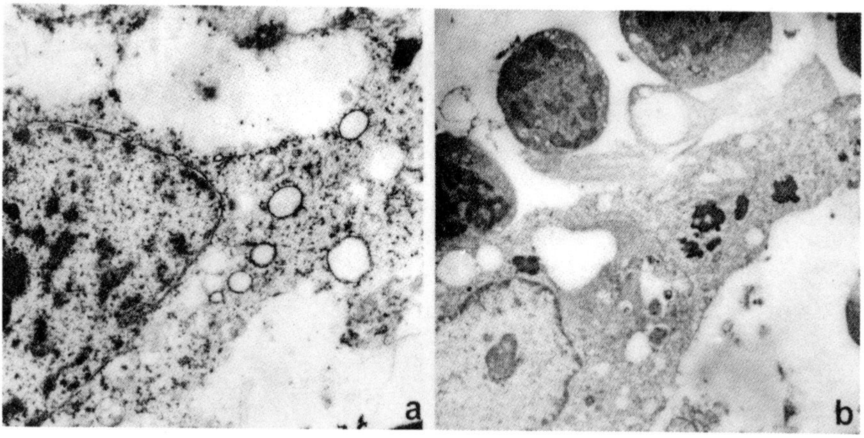

Figure 5. Electronograms of: (a) ramified microglial cell in cerebellum, 18 GW, x 5400, (b) dendritic cell in thymus, 19 GW, x 8000

In the spleen MHC II expression was detected on cells in the spleenic capsula and stroma (Fig 7 a, b). Morphologically, they looked like macrophages or dendritic cells (Fig 7 c, d).

In the liver lobes, the expression of MHC II molecules was found in macrophages located in the capsula, as well as on large cells within the liver lobules (Fig 8 a, b). Morphologically, these cells resembled the Browicz-Kupffer's cells (Fig 8 c).

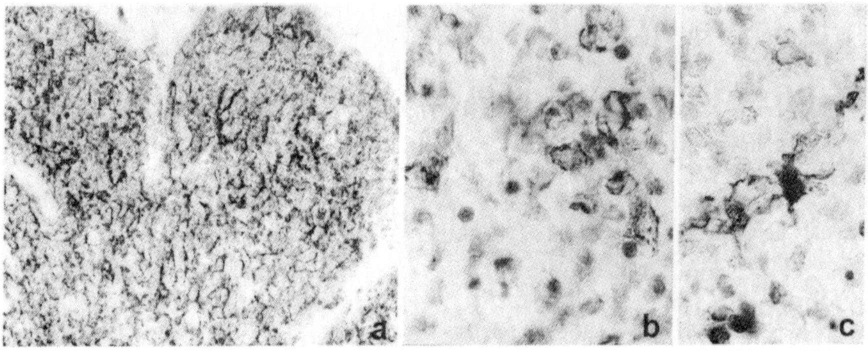

Figure 6. Positive reaction of cells with MHC class II in thymus (a) 16 GW, x 400 and positive reaction of dendritic cells in thymus with (b) antibody CD68, 16 GW, x 1000; (c) antibody S-100, 16 GW, x 1000

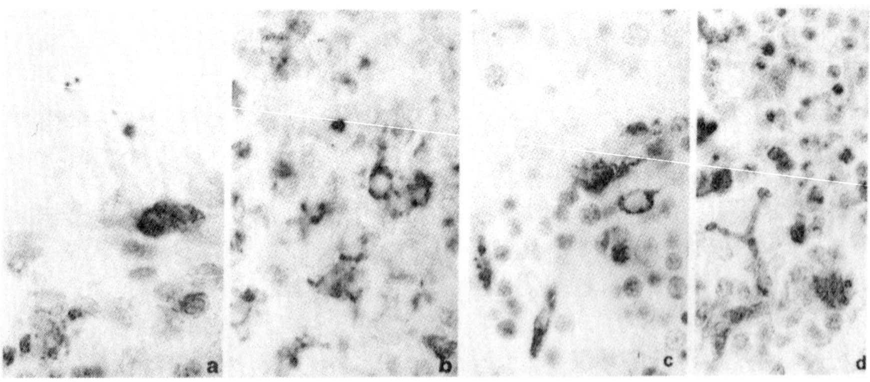

Figure 7. Positive reaction of cells with MHC class II in spleen (a) capsula, 14 GW, x 1000; (b) stroma, 15 GW, x 1000; and positive reaction of dendritic cells in spleen with (c) HAM 56, 16 GW, x 1000; (d) S-100, 16 GW, x 1000

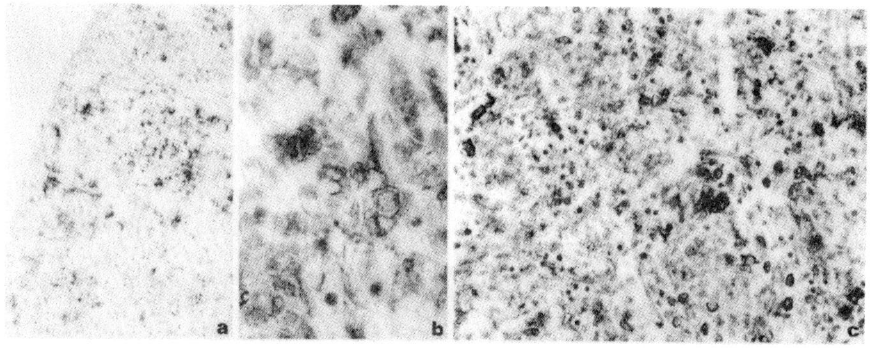

Figure 8. Positive reaction of cells with MHC class II in liver (a) 18 GW, x 100; (b) 18 GW, x 1000; and positive reaction of dendritic cells in liver with (c) CD68, 18 GW, x 200

4. DISCUSSION

In the brain, MHC II molecules were detected at the all intervals on macrophages/AM, in meninges, ventricular choroid plexus and nearby blood vessels, matrix and ventricles. The single RM cells, which expressed MHC II molecules were found in deeper layer of the cortex and white matter. The expresion of MHC II molecules on RM and macrophages/AM cells near the matrix, in the cortex, the white matter, and surrouding of the vessels was most likely related to appoptosis and potential invasion of foreign antigen[11,16].

In the thymus immunocytochemical localization of MHC II molecules were demostrated on macrophages in the organs capsula and on numerous epithelial and dendritic cells in the cortex and medulla at all intervals. The presence of cells with expression of MHC II molecules in the thymus, already at 11 gestation week, may evidence that this expression is influenced during the fetal development by up-regulation. It may be associated with very intensive selection of lymphocytes during the fetal development[17-19]. MHC II expression was also detected on the cells of the liver and spleen that performs a number of functions during the spleen that development, such as production of lymphocytes, monocytes and other blood cells, accumulation of blood cells, phagocytosis of dead erythrocytes, leukocytes and differentiation of immature lymphocytes into effector lymphocytes[5].

The expression of MHC II molecules on the surface of macrophages/AM, RM and DCs, as well as on cells other than APCs in the brain, thymus, spleen and liver, between 11 and 22 GW, provides evidence for potential immune maturity of these organs. Presentation of MHC class II molecules on such a large population of cells, during an early period of the fetal development, may indicate an active involvement of these cells in histogenesis and morphogenesis of the studied organs rather than their reaction to a foreign antigens[20,21].

REFERENCES

1. Blaszczyk, R., Wehling, J., Kubens, B., Hahn, U., Huhn, D., Salama, A. 1995, A novel HLA-A-24 allele (A 2405) identified by single –strand conformation polymorphism analysis and confirmed by solid-phase sequencing and isoelectric focusing. *Tissue Antigens* **46**: 54-58.
2. Castellino, F., Zhong, G., Germain, R.N. 1997, Antigen presentation by MHC class II molecules: invariant chain function, protein trafficking and the molecular basis of diverse determinant capture. *Hum Immunol* **54**: 159-69.
3. Engering, A.J., Richters, C.D., Fluitsma, D.M., et al., 1998, MHC II class II and invariant chain biosynthesis and transport during maturation of human precursor dendritic cells. *Int Immunol* **10**: 1713-1723.
4. Gehrmann, J., Matsumoto, Y., Kreutzberg, G.W., 1995, Microglia: intrinsic immunoneffector cell of the brain. *Brain Res* 20: 269-287.
5. Mc Menamin, P.G., Holthouse, I., Holt, P.G., 1992, Class II major histocompatibility complex (Ia) antigen bearing dendritic cells in the iris and ciliary of the rat eye: distribution, phenotype and relation to retinal microglia. *Immunology* **77**: 385-393.
6. Petranyi, G.G., 1995, The regulation of expression of histocompatibility antigens on the cell surface; molecular genetic basis. *Folia Biol* **41**: 163-177.
7. Keller, R., Joller, P., Keist, R., Binz, H., van der Meide, P.H., 1998, Modulation of major histocompatibility complex (MHC) expression by interferons and microbial agens. *Scand J Immunol* **28**: 113-121.
8. Pujol-Borrell, R., Todd, I., Doshi, M. et al., 1987, HLA class II induction in human island cells by interferon-γ plus tumor necrosis factor or lymphotoxin. *Nature* **326**: 304-306.
9. Wang, C.C., Wu, C.H., Shieh, J.Y., Wen, C.Y., Ling, E.A., 1996, Immunohistochemical study of amoeboid microglial cells in fetal rat brain. *J Anat* **189**: 567-574.
10. Banati, R.B., Hoppe, D., Gottmann, K., Kreutzberg, G.W., Kettenmann, H., 1991, A subpopulation of bone marrow- derived macrophage-like cells shares a unique oin channel pattern with microglia. *J Neurosci Res* **30**: 593-600.
11. Wierzba-Bobrowicz, T., Kosno-Kruszewska, E., Gwiazda, E., Lechowicz, W., 1998, The comparison of microglia maturation in different structures of the human nervous system. *Folia Neuropath* **36**: 152-160.
12. Brocker, T., Riedinger, M., Karjalainen, U., 1997, Targeted expression of major histocompatibility complex (MHC) class II molecules demonstrates that dendriric cells can induce negative but not positive selection of thymocytes in vivo. *J Exp Med* **185**: 541-550.
13. Cuadros, M.A., Martin, C., Coltay, P., Almedros, A., Navascues, J., 1993, First appesrance, distribution, and origin of macrophages in the early development of the avian central nervous system. *J Comp Neurol* 330: 113-129.
14. Giulian, D., Li, J., Bartel, S., Broker, J., Li, X., Kirkpatrick, J.B., 1995, Cell surface morphology identifies microglia as a distinct class of mononuclear phagocyte. *J Neurosci* **15**: 7712-7726.

15. Ling, E.A., 1979, Transformation of monocytes into amoeboid microglia and into microglia in the corpus callosum of postnatal rats, as shown by labelling monocytes by carbon particles. *J Anat* **128**: 847-858.
16. Wierzba-Bobrowicz, T., Schmidt-Sidor, B., Gwiazda, E., Lechowicz, W., Kosno-Kruszewska, E., 2000, Major histocompatibility complex class II expression in the frontal and temporal lobes in the human fetus during development. *Folia Neuropath* **38**: 73-77.
17. Ashwell, K., 1991, The distribution of microglia and cell death in the fetal rat forebrain. *Dev Brain Res* **58**: 1-12.
18. Rescigno, M., Martino, M., Sutherland, C.L., Gold, M.R., Ricciardi-Castagnoli, P., 1998, Dendritic cell survival and maturation are regulated by different singnaling pathway. *J Exp Med* **188**: 2175-80.
19. Tan, M.C., Mommaas, A.M., Drijfhout, J.W. et al., 1997, Mannose receptor-mediated uptake of antigens strongly enhances HLA class II restricted antigen presentation by cultured dendritic cells. *Eur J Immunol* **27**: 2426-2435.
20. Hanau, D., Sandrais, C., Haegel-Kronenberger, H., Bohbot, A., De la Salle, H., Salamero, J., 1999, Fate of class MHC II molecules in human dendritic cells. *Eur J Dermatol* **9**: 7-12.
21. Medzhitov, R., Janeway, C.A., Jr., 1997, Innate immunity:the virtues of a nonclonal system of a nonclonal system of recognition. *Cell* **91**: 295-298.

Interactions between dendritic cells

STELLA C. KNIGHT, FIONA BURKE and PENELOPE A. BEDFORD
Antigen Presentation Research Group, Imperial College School of Medicine, Northwick Park Institute for Medical Research, Watford Road, Harrow, HA1 3UJ, UK.

1. INTRODUCTION

Dendritic cells (DC) of multiple lineages and with functions varying from primary stimulation of different types of B and T cell responses to generation of tolerance are being described. A common property for the identification of DC includes expression of MHC class II molecules and co-stimulatory molecules together with a functional capacity to stimulate primary immune responses. However, such cells may be cells efficient at transferring both MHC and other antigens – including acquired exogenous antigens - to other cells which, in turn, utilise these antigens to stimulate primary immune responses [1;2]. These observations raise questions about the true nature of the cells that directly stimulate primary lymphocyte responses. All so-called 'DC' may be efficient at producing transferable processed antigenic materials but only a proportion may have the property of stimulating lymphocytes directly.

1.1 Background

One of the earliest functional properties of dendritic cells described was the capacity of these cells to stimulate primary allogeneic mixed leucocyte reactions (MLR) [3;4]. The capacity to stimulate an MLR is still considered the functional hallmark of dendritic cells. However, early papers on MLR hinted that some sort of antigen presenting cell of responder type in addition to the allogeneic stimulator cells may be involved in the efficient stimulation of

Progress in Basic and Clinical Immunology, Edited by Mackiewicz *et al.*
Kluwer Academic/Plenum Publishers, New York, 2001

allogeneic T cells [5;6]. Our own recent paper provides evidence that a major stimulus for an MLR is derived from the histocompatibility antigens acquired from allogeneic DC by DC syngeneic with responder lymphocytes [2]. Such an indirect presentation of alloantigens fits more closely with the known properties of MHC restriction and with *in vivo* allograft data showing that the major route of antigen presentation is secondary presentation by DC of the recipient [7;8]. The reason that DC are potent in the stimulation of the allogeneic responses is now becoming apparent. DC shed a high proportion of their MHC molecules in the form of exosomes or 'dendrosomes' [9;10]. It is likely that this material is acquired by other DC which then present these antigens. A similar picture emerges for the stimulation of primary immune responses to exogenous antigens presented by DC to syngeneic lymphocytes. DC pulsed with antigens secrete materials – again possibly in the form of dendrosomes – that have the capacity to stimulate primary immune responses but only in the presence of DC that have not been directly exposed to the antigens. Our studies show that this effective transfer of antigen between DC may be essential for the primary stimulation of T cell responses. These observations have implications for the identification of DC as cells that directly stimulate primary lymphocyte responses; many cell populations that we term 'dendritic cells' may have the major property of secreting or supplying MHC and/or other antigens for acquisition by other cells that directly stimulate lymphocytes. How many of the multiplicity of so-called 'dendritic cells' now being described are efficient at releasing processed antigens and how many have the genuine capacity directly to stimulate lymphocytes? This question is currently being addressed in our laboratory. In this article we will examine further the requirement for DC with and without antigen for the production of primary immune responses.

2. PRESENTATION OF ALLOANTIGENS

Populations of DC isolated from mouse lymph nodes or spleen contain cells which both donate antigens and acquire antigens for the presentation of primary immune responses. DC used in these experiments were separated on metrizamide gradients directly from freshly prepared lymph node cell suspensions or from splenic cells allowed to mature in flasks without added cytokines for 24 hours. Mixing allogeneic spleen DC resulted in transfer of MHC molecules between the allogeneic DC. Figure 1 shows an experiment of this type in which spleen DC from CBA and BALB/c were mixed together. They were then labelled with anti-1-A^k and anti-I-A^d antibodies. A high proportion of DC became double labelled even within 2 hours of mixing. In these particular experiments, the DC mixed included DC that were CD11c$^+$, CD8α^- and cells that were CD11c$^+$, CD8α^+ and the contribution of these two types of DC are currently being assessed. Our published work shows a role for this type of transfer of alloantigen to see optimal proliferation in a mixed leukocyte reaction[2].

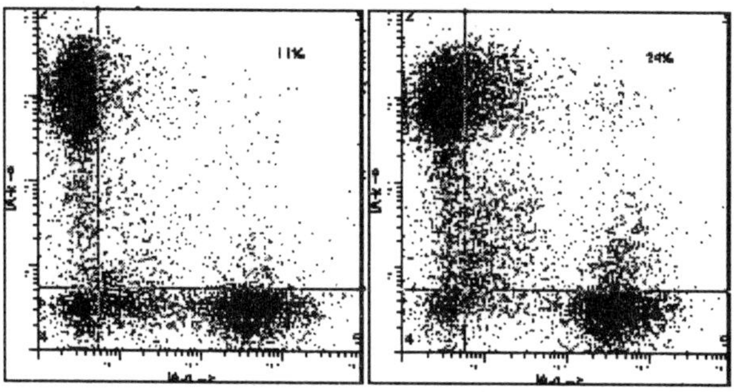

Figure 1. Transfer of class II molecules between allogeneic DC. Splenic DC (Balb/c) enriched on metrizamide gradients were co-cultured for two hours with allogeneic DC (CBA) at 37^{0}C or on ice. The cells were labelled with antibody to class II molecules and labelling measured by flow cytometry. Compared with the staining in the individual cell suspensions, cells mixed at 0 degrees showed 11% of cells double-labelling with evidence of acquisition of 1-A^k 1-A^{d+} cells and vice versa. At 37^{0}C this transfer was more marked with 24% of the cells becoming double-labelled.

In addition to the published work on mouse DC, we have also conducted preliminary experiments on human peripheral blood DC to see whether there is a requirement for both allogeneic DC and DC syngeneic with responder T cells in order to produce a maximum mixed leucocyte reaction. Figure 2 shows an MLC between peripheral blood leucocytes. In this study, DC were isolated from blood mononuclear cells using a metrizamide gradient and used to stimulate primary T cell responses in 20 μl hanging drop cultures. The responder T cell population was also physically depleted of DC through a metrizamide gradient and then depleted of the remaining MHC class II bearing cells using antibody to HLA-DR and complement. Depletion of DC was confirmed by the total loss of a response to the mitogen concanavalin A (1 μg/ml). No proliferation was seen as assessed by tritiated thymidine uptake (2-hr pulse with 1 μg/ml of thymidine at 2 Ci/mM on day 3 added to 10^4 lymphocytes in 20 μl hanging drop cultures). The addition of 200-4000 DC to these cultures restored a full response to concanavalin A with counts per minute in the DC-depleted cells exposed to the mitogen being <50 and those with the DC >3000 counts. In these responder cells deliberately depleted of DC, the addition of either syngeneic or allogeneic DC caused little T cell stimulation (Figure 2). However, a mixture of allogeneic and syngeneic DC caused a normal primary mixed leukocyte reaction. This data provides supporting evidence that both stimulator and responder type DC are also involved in the primary stimulation of human lymphocytes. Antigen transfer as shown formally in the mouse system (figure 1) is likely to underlie this effect. Again, the nature of the 'DC' that supply the alloantigens and those that actually acquire and present it to the T lymphocytes, need to be identified.

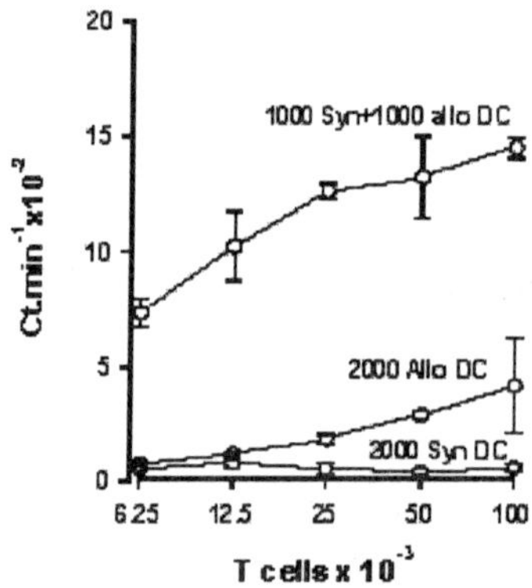

Figure 2. Requirement for DC of responder type in the human mixed leukocyte reaction. Peripheral blood mononuclear cells were cultured overnight on plastic and dendritic cells enriched on metrizamide gradients. The pellet cells were further depleted of dendritic cells by removal of HLA-DR bearing cells using antibody and complement. The remaining lymphocytes showed little evidence of background proliferation as assessed by the uptake of tritiated thymidine. The addition of 2000 DC syngeneic with the esponder lymphocytes or 2000 allogeneic DC caused little stimulation. However, when 1000 of each type of DC was added, a full primary mixed leukocyte reaction was observed with high levels of thymidine uptake. Cultures were 20 μl hanging drops in Terasaki plates which were exposed to tritiated thymidine (1 μg/ml, 2 Ci/mmol) for two hours on day 4 of culture and the thymidine uptake into the acid insoluble fraction measured by scintillation counting.

3. PRESENTATION OF PEPTIDES

Our earlier published work showed the requirements for DC exposed directly to antigens and those acquiring antigens indirectly for the primary stimulation of responses in syngeneic lymphocytes using contact sensitisers, ovalbumin conjugated to contact sensitiser and influenza virus. In each case, the two populations of DC were required. Since the contact sensitiser used was fluorescein isothiocyanate (FITC), it was possible to trace the transfer of this antigen between the directly pulsed cells and the non-pulsed dendritic cells. Supernatants of cells also contained primary stimulatory materials, which could be removed by antibodies to FITC, strongly supporting the idea that the transferred antigen is critical for primary T cell stimulation[1]. In other systems, supernatants of DC exposed to tumour antigens provide protection against *in vivo* tumour growth, supporting the evidence that materials shed from DC may be potent immunogens[10].

One of the antigens used in earlier experiments on antigen transfer between DC was influenza virus. More recently, we studied the requirement for two DC using a potent peptide epitope of influenza - the 147-160 (arginine minus) peptide already shown to stimulate primary proliferative and cytotoxic T cell responses [11]. Once again, mouse DC pulsed with antigen and DC not exposed to antigen were both required to see primary proliferative responses to this peptide (data not shown). Figure 3 shows that the DC pulsed with peptide shed material into the supernatants that stimulated primary proliferative response in T cells containing DC. Supernatants from DC not pulsed with antigen caused minimal amounts of syngeneic stimulation. These non-stimulatory DC supernatants with peptide added immediately before addition to the responder cells did not cause primary proliferative response. This data suggests that, for small peptides not requiring processing as well as for larger antigens, transfer of processed material from dendritic cells exposed directly to antigen to those not exposed directly to antigen is required for the stimulation of primary proliferative responses.

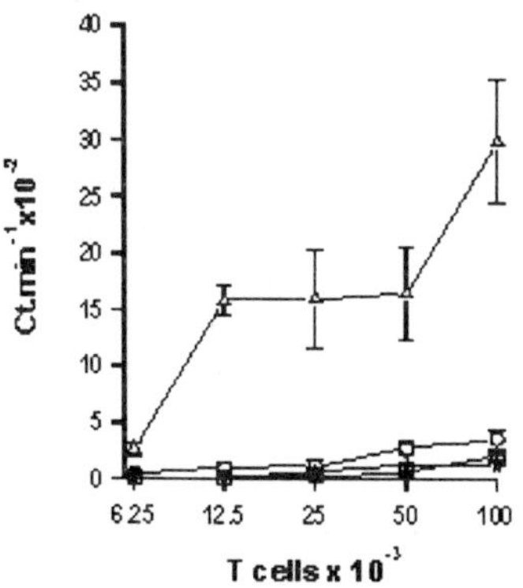

Figure 3. Stimulation of primary proliferative response to peptide using supernatants of antigen-pulsed dendritic cells. The supernatants of DC, exposed to the influenza peptide 147-160 (Arg^- peptide) for 2 hours and then incubated overnight at 10^6 DC/ml, when added in 1 μl aliquots to different numbers of lymph node lymphocytes stimulated primary proliferative responses as indicated by uptake of tritiated thymidine (∇). The supernatants of non-antigen pulsed DC (O) or of this supernatant with free peptide added (□) did not cause proliferation that was significantly different from that in T cells alone (☆). Thus, peptide alone or supernatants of normal dendritic cells did not stimulate primary responses but the supernatants of peptide-pulsed dendritic cells stimulated primary proliferative responses.

4. CONCLUSIONS

The functional hallmark of the dendritic cell is the capacity to stimulate primary allogeneic mixed leukocyte reactions. The basis for this test is the belief that the ability of DC directly to stimulate allogeneic lymphocytes is being tested. However, the major stimulus in this test may be from secondarily acquired antigens presented syngeneically to lymphocytes. This model of primary responses to foreign antigens transferred across an antigen gradient to responder DC may provide a good model for primary stimulation to antigens in syngeneic systems. Thus, foreign antigens acquired by 'antigenically naïve' DC from syngeneic DC previously exposed to the foreign antigens may be major route for primary T cell stimulation. A major question exercising many working on dendritic cells is the multiplicity of DC types now being described with suggestions of different lineage relationships, states of maturation and multiple interactions with different types of lymphocyte. It is not clear which of these multiple DC populations is actually able directly to stimulate primary T cell responses. Further analysis of this question may lead to a more restricted picture of what constitutes a dendritic cell able to stimulates primary responses. A second consequence is the development of a novel theory concerning the basic immunological question of the mechanisms for self/non-self discrimination. 'Self-processed' antigens from the direct environment of DC may be non-stimulatory. However, those antigens acquired ready-processed from other DC (non-self-processed) but not in the immediate environment are stimulatory. This indirect mechanism would prevent the development of immune responses to antigens common to the local environment.

REFERENCES

1. Knight, S. C., S. Iqball, M. S. Roberts, S. Macatonia, and P. A. Bedford. 1998. Transfer of antigen between dendritic cells in the stimulation of primary T cell proliferation. Eur.J.Immunol. 28:1636-1644-.
2. Bedford, P., K. Garner, and S. C. Knight. 1999. MHC class II molecules transferred between allogeneic dendritic cells stimulate primary mixed leukocyte reactions. Int.Immunol 11:1739-1744.
3. Crow, M. K. and H. G. Kunkel. 1982. Human dendritic cells: major stimulators of the autologous and allogeneic mixed leucocyte reactions Clin.Exp.Immunol 49:338-346.
4. Steinman, R. M. and M. D. Witmer. 1978. Lymphoid dendritic cells are potent stimulators of the primary mixed leukocyte reaction in mice. Proc.Natl.Acad.Sci.USA 75:5132-5136.

5. Weinberger, O., R. N. Germain, T. Springer, and S. J. Burakoff. 1982. Role of syngeneic Ia+ accessory cells in the generation of allospecific CTL responses J Immunol 129:694-697.
6. Mann, D. L. and L. Abelson. 1980. Monocyte function in mixed lymphocyte reactions Cell Immunol 56:357-364.
7. Benichou, G., R. C. Tam, L. R. Soares, and E. V. Fedoseyeva. 1997. Indirect T-cell allorecognition: perspectives for peptide-based therapy in transplantation Immunol Today 18:67-71.
8. Auchinloss, H. and H. Sultan. 1997. Antigen processing and presentation in transplantation. Curr.Opin.Immunol. 8:681.
9. Thery, C., A. Regnault, J. Garin, J. Wolfers, L. Zitvogel, P. Ricciardi-Castagnoli, G. Raposo, and S. Amigorena. 1999. Molecular characterization of dendritic cell-derived exosomes. Selective accumulation of the heat shock protein hsc73. J Cell Biol. 147:599-610.
10. Zitvogel, L., A. Regnault, A. Lozier, J. Wolfers, C. Flament, D. Tenza, P. Ricciardi-Castagnoli, G. Raposo, and S. Amigorena. 1998. Eradication of established murine tumors using a novel cell-free vaccine: dendritic cell-derived exosomes. Nat.Med. 4:594-600.
11. Macatonia, S. E., S. C. Knight, A. J. Edwards, S. Griffiths, and P. R. Fryer. 1987. Localization of antigen on lymph node dendritic cells after exposure to the contact sensitizer fluorescein isothiocyanate. *J.Exp.Med.* 166:1654-1667.

Neural regulation of dendritic cell function

GEORGES JM MAESTRONI
Center for Experimental Pathology, Istituto Cantonale di Patologia, 6601 Locarno, Switzerland

1. INTRODUCTION

DC are a trace population of bone marrow-derived antigen-presenting cells, irregular in shape and widely distributed in both lymphoid and non-lymphoid tissues (1, 2). Those having migrated to non-lymphoid tissues such as the epidermal layer of the skin, the respiratory and gastrointestinal systems and interstitial regions of solid organs are considered immature. On the contrary, fully mature DC are located in lymphoid organs. After antigen internalization and inflammation, DC leave the tissues interfacing with the external environment and enter the lymphatic vessels to reach the lymphoid organs and undergo maturation (1-3). While still immature the primary function of DC is to capture and process antigens, then to present the antigenic peptides and activate specific T cells (1, 2). In fact, DC have adhesion molecules to ensure T cell contact, high surface levels of Major Histocompatibility Complex II molecules for peptide presentation and costimulatory molecules such as CD80-B7/1 and CD86-B7/2. T cells may in turn induce DC maturation via CD40 binding (1, 2). The ability of DC to migrate from areas of antigen encounter to sites of T cell priming is fundamental to their capacity of stimulating an immune response; however, how DC know where to go is still rather obscure. The major route of DC entry into lymph nodes are the afferent lymphatic vessels (3, 4). Chemokines expressed by endothelial cells in lymphatics and lymph node venules and chemokine receptors in DC seem to contribute to DC migration as chemoattractants and by triggering integrin-dependent adhesive

Progress in Basic and Clinical Immunology, Edited by Mackiewicz *et al.*
Kluwer Academic/Plenum Publishers, New York, 2001

interactions (4-6). However, the primary force that drives DC displacement is the lymphatic circulation. Lymph flow is regulated by spontaneous contraction of lymphatic vessel smooth muscle that in turn is stimulated by sympathetic nerves and ARs (7). The AR mediate the functional effects of epinephrine and norepinephrine by coupling to several of the major signaling pathways modulated by G proteins. The AR family includes nine different gene products: three β (β_1, β_2, β_3), three α_2 (α_{2A}, α_{2B}, α_{2C}) and three α1 (α_{1a}, α_{1b}, α_{1d}) receptor subtypes. The α1-ARs are present in several tissues including brain, heart, blood vessels, liver, kidney, prostate and spleen where they mediate a variety of physiological effects such as cardiac inotropy and chronotropy, vasocontraction, glycogenolysis and the contractions of the urinary tract (8). On the other hand, the interaction between sympathetic nerves and cells of the immune system has been demonstrated in terms of distribution of tyrosine hydroxylase positive fibers in lymphoid organs, expression of ARs on cells of the immune system and immunomodulatory effects of the main sympathetic neurotransmitter NE (9-11). We reported that catecholamines can also exert important hematopoietic effects via α1-ARs expressed in bone marrow progenitor cells (12-16). Relevant to the present study, NE has been shown to stimulate lymphoid cell mobilization via α1-ARs (17).

2. RESULTS

2.1 Langerhans Cells Migration

We studied whether NE participates in determining the emigration pathway of skin DC such as epidermal Langerhans cells. We used the fluorescent molecule FITC as an antigen to induce migration of

Langerhans cells to regional lymph nodes. Mice were painted with FITC on the back after shaving and the effect of adrenergic agents was evaluated in terms of number of cells positive for both FITC and CD86 (B7-2) found 24 hours later in the draining lymph nodes. The results obtained show that topical application of the α1-adrenergic antagonist prazosin but not the β-adrenergic antagonist propranolol inhibited migration of Langerhans cells to the draining lymph nodes (Fig 1). In addition, the i.p. injection of yohimbine, an α2- adrenergic antagonist which increases the noradrenergic tone, resulted in a significant increase of migrated Langerhans cells. Altogether these results suggest that NE is involved in skin DC migration via α1-ARs.

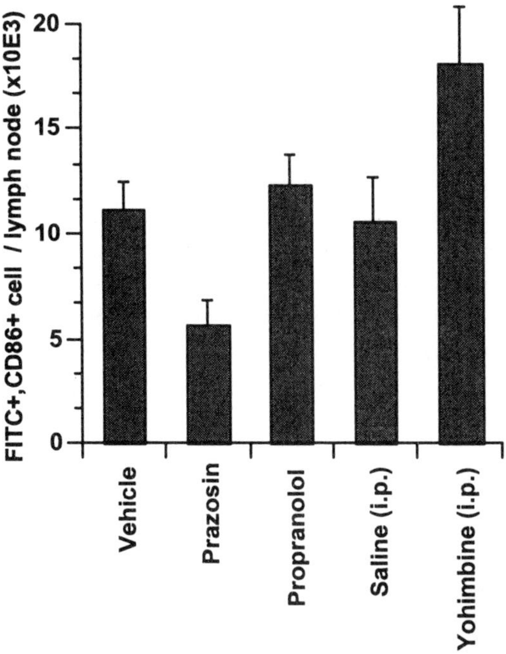

Figure 1. Effect of adrenergic antagonists on Langerhans cells migration. The mean values plus the standard deviation of migrated epidermal Langerhans cells after FITC painting of the skin and treatment with adrenergic antagonists are shown. Data are from 5 experiments (15 mice per group). a: $p< 0.01$ (ANOVA).

2.2 Emigration of Skin DC in Organ Cultures

A strong stimulation of skin DC was noted when NE was added in the culture medium. On average a three-fold increase of migrated DC was found in presence of NE and a four-fold increase was found using the chemokine 6Ckine as positive control (Table I). As expected the α1-AR antagonist prazosin inhibited the NE effect (Table I). These results confirmed that NE can mobilize skin DC via α1-ARs.

Table I. Effect of NE in the emigration of DC from skin explants

	No of ears	Emigrated DC ($x10^3$)
MEDIUM	12	39 ± 21.8
6Ckine (120 ng/ml)	12	167.8 ± 47.7 [a]
NE (10^{-6} M)	14	131.3 ± 14.8 [a]
NE (10^{-6} M) + PRA (10^{-8} M)	14	56.1 ± 18
PRA (10^{-8} M)	12	36.2 ± 16.3

The values represent the mean number of cells emigrated from one ear skin dorsal halve ± the standard deviation during 24 h incubation. 6Ckine was used as positive control. PRA: prazosin a: p< 0.001 vs Medium,. NE + PRA, PRA (ANOVA)

2.3 CHS Response to FITC

To investigate whether the adrenergic inhibition of skin DC migration in vivo results in an altered development of DC-dependent immune response, we measured the CHS response to FITC after sensitization in presence of either prazosin or propranolol . Figure 2 shows that prazosin but not propranolol treatment during sensitization inhibited the CHS response expressed as net ear swelling. This indicated that the prazosin-induced inhibition of DC migration resulted in a reduced sensitization to FITC.

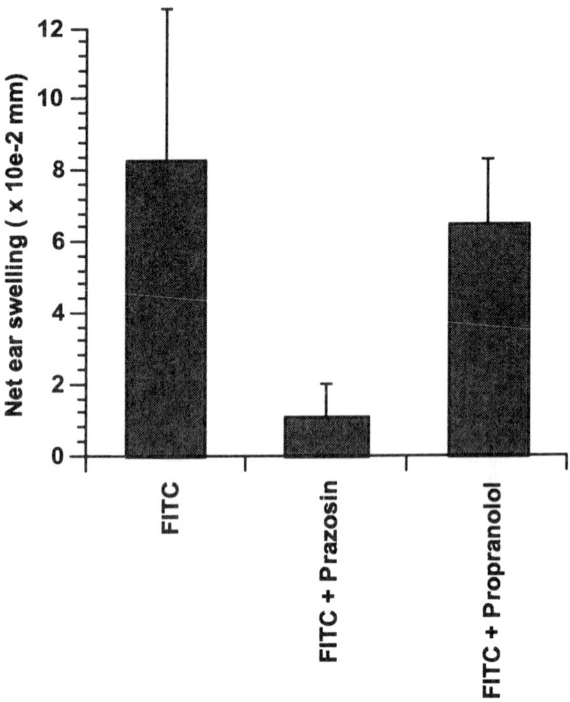

Figure 2. Effect of adrenergic antagonists on the CHS response to FITC. Mice (n = 7 / group) were sensitized with FITC in presence or absence of adrenergic antagonists and 6 days later were challenged on the right ear. The left ear was painted with vehicle as a control. The mean values plus the standard deviation of the net ear swelling is reported. The CHS response was significantly lower in mice sensitized with FITC in presence of prazosin (a: p< 0.02, ANOVA)

2.4 In Vitro DC Migration

To study in greater detail the possibility that NE is involved in DC migration, we set up experiments in a chemotaxis microchamber using NE or the synthetic β-adrenergic agonist isoproterenol as chemoattractants. Fig. 3 shows that NE but not isoproterenol is indeed a powerful chemoattractant for bone marrow-derived DC. The DC generated from bone marrow cultures were heterogeneous for their expression of MHC class II and B7-2, i.e. for their degree of maturation. With this cell population containing immature DC, NE 10^{-6} M (319.3 ng/ml) exerted a chemotactic activity which was intermediate in comparison to those exerted by RANTES (100 ng/ml) and the secondary lymphoid tissue chemokine 6Ckine (120 ng/ml) which has been recently suggested to play a role in migration and homing of mature DC (18). Consistently, 6Ckine was highly chemotactic with DC brought to maturation by CD40 stimulation while NE apparently did not attract mature DC (Fig. 3). In line with the results obtained in vivo and with the lack of effect of isoproterenol, prazosin neutralized the chemotactic effect of NE.

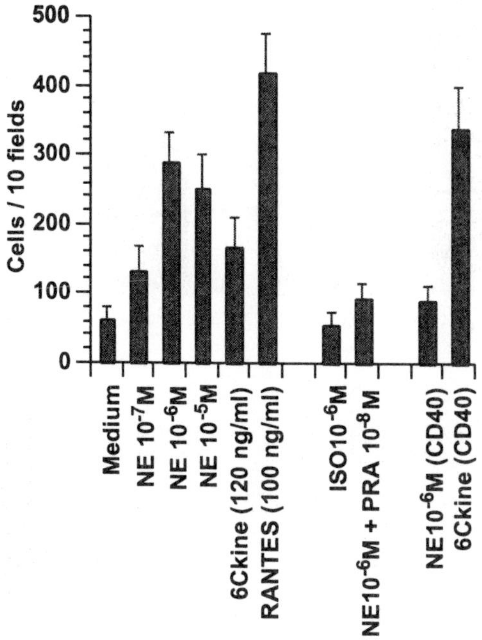

Figure 3. NE-mediated chemotaxis. Data are from 7 experiments. Medium, NE, isoproterenol (ISO) RANTES and 6Ckine were added in the lower wells of the chemotactic chamber. Prazosin (PRA) was added together with DC in the upper wells. DC harvested by bone marrow cultures or after CD40 stimulation (CD40) were seeded in the upper wells.

Checkerboard analysis revealed that not only is NE a chemoattractant for DC, but it may also induce chemokinesis (data not shown). When seeded in the upper chamber together with the cells, NE prevented spontaneous (control) migration but not the chemotactic activity of RANTES (data not shown). However, although less than toward a NE gradient (NE in lower wells only), DC also migrated in a constant NE concentration (10^{-6} M NE both in the upper and lower wells). These results indicate that NE is both a chemoattractant and a chemokinetic factor for immature, but not for mature DC.

2.5 Expression of α1-Ars In DC

The prazosin sensitivity of DC migration and the lack of effect of β-adrenergic agents both in vivo and in vitro imply the participation of α1-ARs. This type of AR has been indeed reported to mediate the effect of catecholamines on lymphatic vessels (19). However, our studies suggest that DC may likewise express α1-ARs. To elucidate this point, we investigated the presence of mRNA coding for the three α1-ARs subtypes (a, b, d) in bone marrow-derived DC before and after CD40 stimulation. RT-PCR analysis revealed the expression of the α1b-AR mRNA in bone marrow-derived DC. Apparently, the other two α1-ARs subtypes are not expressed (Fig.4). The α1b-AR mRNA expression was, however, almost undetectable in DC stimulated by anti-CD40 antibodies (Fig. 4). This is most likely the reason why NE does not attract mature, CD40-stimulated DC (Fig.3). Presumably, the α1b-AR is expressed in an immature fraction of bone marrow-derived DC. This would agree also with the in vivo effect of prazosin on epidermal Langerhans cells (Fig.1) that are considered immature DC (20).

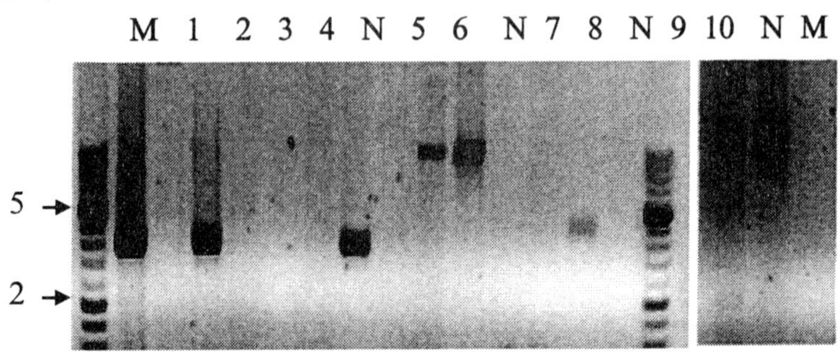

Figure 4. RT-PCR of α1-AR genes in immature and mature DC. Immature DC are intended DC just harvested from bone marrow cultures, mature DC are DC after CD40 stimulation. Murine brain is used as positive control. M: molecular weight markers; N: negative control (no RNA); 1-4: hypoxanthine-phosphoribosyl-transferase of immature DC (1) and brain (3),

expected size: 390 bp; 2, 4: mock controls (no reverse transcriptase) 5, 6: α1a-AR in immature DC and brain respectively, expected size: 375 bp; 7,8: α1b-AR in immature DC and brain, expected size 687 bp; 9,10: α1d-AR in immature DC and brain, expected size: 428 bp; 10,11: α1b-AR in mature DC and brain. The specificity of the PCR products was controlled by Southern blotting and hybridization with digoxigenin-labeled specific probes (data not shown).

3. DISCUSSION

Altogether, these findings suggest that α1b-ARs expressed in DC drive at least part of their emigration pathway to regional lymph nodes. In vivo, the effect of prazosin and yohimbine suggests that endogenous NE plays indeed a role in DC migration. Prazosin and propranolol were administered topically to possibly target Langerhans cells or other epidermal structures while yohimbine was injected i.p. because its well known sympathomimetic activity depends on blockade of both peripheral and central presynaptic α2-ARs. In addition, NE greatly stimulated skin DC emigration in organ cultures and the NE effect was neutralized by prazosin. This indicates that the effect of prazosin and yohimbine in vivo (Fig.1) was not dependent on an altered FITC labeling of DC. Finally, preincubation of DC with the irreversible α1b-AR antagonist chloroethylclonidine resulted in impaired migration when DC were adoptively transferred. It should be noted that after the chloroethylclonidine exposure, DC were viable and retained the ability to migrate in vitro against RANTES but not against NE (data not shown). Therefore, the impaired migration of these DC in vivo was probably due to the irreversible inactivation of the α1b-AR and this confirmed a role for NE in DC migration in vivo. Most interesting, the inhibition of DC migration induced by prazosin was followed by an impaired DC-dependent immune response as shown in the CHS experiments (Fig. 2). Probably, the impaired DC migration resulted in a reduced antigen presentation and T cell activation.

In vitro, NE exerted a powerful chemoattractant/chemokinetic effect on bone marrow-derived, immature DC via their α1b-AR. The fact that CD40-stimulated, mature DC show a very low expression of the α1b-AR may explain why NE did not act on these cells and suggests that, unlike 6Ckine (5), NE is not involved in the homing of mature DC in lymph nodes. 6Ckine is, in fact, strongly expressed in the high endothelial venules of lymph nodes and has been shown to mediate both chemotaxis and adhesion of mature but not immature DC (5).

Possibly, the rich sympathetic innervation of lymphatic smooth muscle (7) creates a NE gradient able to recruit immature DC from non-lymphoid tissues. Nerve fibers are in fact present in the tunica externa and media of afferent lymphatic vessels. Thus, the sympathetic innervation of lymphatic vessels would have the dual role of stimulating smooth muscle contraction, which in turn promotes lymph flow, and of recruiting DC. Nevertheless, an alternative physiological interpretation of the results obtained may also be proposed. Since NE appears to be also chemokinetic (Fig. 4) and DC seem to lose their sensitivity to NE during maturation, it might be that under condition of enhanced sympathetic activity (stress, anxiety, cold exposure), increased DC chemokinesis enhances the ability of DC to sample local antigens. This would result in an increased number of maturing DC that can be attracted by relevant chemokines such as 6Ckine and reach the draining lymph nodes. In any case, NE might interact with the chemoattractant activity of chemokines that are expressed at sites of inflammation to activate antigen uptake (21). This, however, does not seem to apply for RANTES (Fig. 3). A better understanding of the role of NE in DC migration requires more detailed studies on the interaction between the α1b-AR, antigenic activation and locally produced inflammatory cytokines and chemokines (4).

In conclusion we show that immature DC express α1b-ARs which participate in cell mobilization and migration to regional lymph nodes. This finding should be considered in studies concerning skin diseases, allergy and autoimmune disorders. As far as it concerns skin diseases, psoriasis and atopic dermatitis may worsen with anxiety [Sirinek, 1991 #528], a behavioral condition that can be mimicked pharmacologically by yohimbine which is known to augment catecholamine release. The fact, that yohimbine accelerates skin DC migration might be relevant in our understanding of these elusive yet widespread skin diseases. In addition, our finding might open new pharmacological possibilities for modulating the immune response.

ACKNOWLEDGEMENTS

The skilful technical assistance of Ms Elisabeth Hertens and Ms Paola Galli is gratefully acknowledged.

REFERENCES

1.Shortman, K. and Caux, C. Dendritic cell development: multiple pathways to nature's adjuvants. Stem Cells, 15 : 409-419, 1997.

2.Sallgaller, M. L. and Lodge, P. A. Use of cellular and cytokine adjuvants in the immunotherapy of cancer. J. Surg. Oncol., 68 : 122-138, 1998.

3.Weinlich, G., Heine, M., Stössel, H., Zanella, M., Stoizner, P., Ortnet, U., Smolle, J., Koch, F., Sepp, N. T., Schuler, G. and Romani, N. Entry into lymphatics and maturation in situ of migrating murine cutaneous dendritic cells. J. Invest. Dermatol., 110 : 441-448, 1998.

4.Bancherau, J. and Steinman, R. M. Dendritic cells and the control of immunity. Nature, 392 : 245-252, 1998.

5.Kellermann, S.-A., Hudak, S., Oldham, E. R., Liu, Y.-J. and McEvoy, L. M. The CC chemokine receptor-7 ligands 6Ckine and macrophage inflammatory protein-3β are potent chemoattractants for in vitro and in vivo-derived dendritic cells. J. Immunol., 162 : 3859-3864, 1999.

6.Warnock, R. A., Campbell, J. J., Dorf, M. E., Matsuzawa, A., McEvoy, L. M. and Butcher, E. C. The role of chemokines in the microenvironmental control of T versus B cell arrest in Peyer's patch high endothelial venules. J. Exp. Med., 191 : 77-88, 2000.

7.McHale, N. G. Lymphatic innervation. Blood Vessels, 27 : 127-136, 1990.

8.Graham, R. M., Perez, D. M., Hwa, J., Piascik, M. T., and . Alpha 1-adrenergic receptor subtypes. Molecular structure, function, and signaling. Circ. Res., 78 : 737-749, 1996.

9.Madden, K. S., Sanders, V. M. and Felten, D. L. Catecholamine influences and sympathetic neural modulation of immune responsiveness. Annu. Rev. Pharmacol. Toxicl., 35 : 417-448, 1995.

10.Feldman, R. D., Hunninghake, G. W. and MacArdle, W. L. Beta-adrenergic-receptor-mediated suppression of interleukin-2 receptors in human lymphocytes. J. Immunol., 139 : 3355-3359, 1987.

11.Felten, S. Y. and Felten, D. L. Innervation of lymphoid tissue. *In* : R. Ader, D. L. Felten and N. Cohen (eds.), Psychoneuroimmunology II., San Diego: Academic Press, 1991.

12.Maestroni, G. J. M., Conti, A. and Pedrinis, E. Effect of adrenergic agents on hematopoiesis after syngeneic bone marrow transplantation in mice. Blood, 5 : 1178-182, 1992.

13.Maestroni, G. J. M. and Conti, A. Noradrenergic modulation of lymhohematopoiesis. Int. J. Immunopharmacol., 16 : 117-122, 1994.

14.Maestroni, G. J. M. and Conti, A. Modulation of hematopoiesis via alpha-1 adrenergic receptors on bone marrow cells. Exp. Hematol., 22 : 314-321, 1994.

15.Maestroni, G. J. M., Togni, M. and Covacci, V. Norepinephrine protects mice from acute lethal doses of carboplatin. Exp. Hematol., 25 : 491-494, 1997.

16.Maestroni, G. J. M. Catecholaminergic regulation of hematopoiesis in mice. Blood, 92 : 2971-2973., 1998.

17.Rogausch, H., Del Rey, A., Oertel, J. and Besedovsky, H. Norepinephrine stimulates lymphoid cell mobilization from the perfused rat spleen via β–adrenergic receptors. Am. J. Physiol., 276 : R724-R730, 1999.

18.Saeki, H., Moore, A. M., Brown, M. J. and Hwang, S. T. Cutting Edge: Secondary lymphoid tissue chemokine (SLC) and CC chemokine receptor 7 (CCR7) participate in the emigration pathway of mature dendritic cells from skin to regional lymph nodes. J. Immunl., 162 : 2472-2475, 1999.

19.Dobbins, D. E. Catecholamine-mediated lymphatic constriction: involvement of both alpha1- and alpha2-adrenoreceptors. Am. J. Physiol., 263 : H473-478, 1992.

20.Schuler, G. and Steinman, R. Murine epidermal Langerhans cells mature into potent immunostimulatory dendritic cells in vitro. J. Exp. Med., 161 : 526-546, 1985.

21.Baggiolini, M. Chemokines and leukocyte traffic. Nature, 392 : 565-568, 1998.

A central role for heat shock proteins in host deficiency

PRAMOD K. SRIVASTAVA
University of Connecticut School of Medicine

1. INTRODUCTION

We have suggested previously that heat shock proteins play a central role in host defense. Specifically, we posit that the release of HSPs from cells is the primary event for initiation of the innate and adaptive immunological cascades.

2. RELEASE OF HEAT SHOCK PROTEINS FROM MAMMALIAN CELLS: CONSEQUENCES FOR INNATE IMMUNITY

We have recently shown (Basu et al., 2000) that necrotic but not apoptotic cell death leads to the release of biologically potent HSPs from cells. The released HSPs stimulate macrophages and dendritic cells to secrete cytokines and induce expression of antigen presenting and co-stimulatory molecules on the dendritic cells. These events may also be recapitulated in vivo (Binder et al., 2000). The quantities of HSPs shown to be necessary to stimulate APCs *in vitro* are well within the range expected to be released locally as a result of cell lysis *in vivo*. Typically, 1 g of tissue yields approximately 30 μg gp96, 200 μg hsp70 and 400 μg hsp90. These recoveries are somewhere in the range of 25%. Therefore, 1 g of tissue contains ~2.5 mg HSPs. If one assumes that tissue lysis *in vivo* occurs not in solution but in a semi-liquid physical state, then the lysis of as little as 1 mg of cells (approximately 10^5-10^6 cells, depending on the cell type) ultimately leads to the release of ~2 μg HSP in a volume of ~1-2 μl or less. This represents a concentration of 1-2 mg/ml – a higher concentration than that used in our *in vitro* studies. Considerations of quantity are therefore compatible with an *in vivo* role of HSPs in the activation of APCs. We have shown that the HSPs also interact with these APCs through the highly conserved NFκB pathway. As HSPs are intracellular, abundant and soluble, their presence in the extracellular milieu and the consequent activation of APCs constitutes an excellent mechanism for response to cell death.

The lipopolysaccharides (LPS) of gram-negative bacteria have been shown to possess properties similar to those reported by us for HSPs. The HSPs are clearly more ancient and more ubiquitous than LPS, as even the earliest forms of life contain HSPs, while LPS is unique to gram negative bacteria. We suggest that the HSP-mediated and LPS-mediated activation of APCs represent utilization of similar mechanisms for similar objectives, although from different starting points. The mechanism of response to external danger may indeed be modeled on the more primitive mechanism of response to cellular disintegration that is signaled, we suggest, by release of internal molecules such as HSPs. Janeway has suggested that pattern recognition receptors (PRRs) present on APCs serve to act as sentinels of the immune system against primordial non-self and its descendants (Medzhitov and Janeway, 1997). HSPs are highly conserved between self and non-self organisms. The possibility that the ligands for the HSPs responsible for the HSP-APC interaction may also serve as PRRs acting as sentinels of internal danger is attractive and helps reconcile the differences between the self/non-self and danger models of immune response.

3. RELEASE OF HEAT SHOCK PROTEINS FROM MAMMALIAN CELLS: CONSEQUENCES FOR ADAPTIVE IMMUNITY

HSPs isolated from mammalian cells have been shown to be associated with peptides including antigenic peptides. This principle has been demonstrated in tumor and viral systems (see Table 1) and has been reviewed extensively elsewhere (Srivastava et al., 1998). HSP-peptide complexes, whether isolated from cells or reconstituted *in vitro* (Blachere et al., 1997), can be used to immunize effectively against cells that express the HSP-chaperoned peptides as T-cell epitopes. The uniqueness of HSPs as peptide chaperone-immunogens lies in the fact that extremely small quantities of peptides (nanograms or picograms) are sufficient for eliciting potent CD8+ T-cell responses, but only if the peptides are chaperoned by the HSPs. Peptides alone or chaperoned by non-HSP proteins such as albumin do not elicit such responses. These observations make HSPs the first adjuvants of mammalian origin. They have been injected into tens of thousands of mice, frogs and rats, and as described in the next section, in over one hundred patients, and have been found to be safe and well-tolerated.

The first insight into the mechanism by which immunization with HSP-peptide complexes elicits antigen-specific CD8+ T-cells came from depletion studies which showed that priming of immune response by HSP-peptide complexes was exquisitely sensitive to abrogation of phagocytic cell function (Udono et al., 1994). Subsequently, it was shown that macrophages, but not B cells, fibroblasts or other non-professional antigen presenting cells (APC) take up gp96-peptide complexes and re-present the gp96-chaperoned peptides on the MHC I molecules of the macrophages; re-presentation does not occur by transfer of peptides from the gp96 molecules to MHC I on the cell surface (Suto and Srivastava, 1995, Castellino et al., 2000). The observation that extremely small quantities of HSP-peptide complexes were effective in eliciting specific immunity led to the suggestion that professional APCs possess HSP-receptors which take up HSP-peptide complexes with specificity (Srivastava et al., 1994). The identity of the receptor for the gp96 HSP has recently been revealed (Binder et al, 2000). Further details of the mechanism, including the identity of the macrophage compartment that takes up the HSP-peptide complexes and the mechanism by which the peptides arrive at the endoplasmic reticulum (ER) are unclear, although our studies reveal the requirement of proteasomes and transporter associated protein (TAP) for processing and presentation of gp96-chaperoned peptides (Basu et al, 2001). The mechanism of immunogenicity of other HSP preparations, the hsp90 and hsp70-peptide complexes, also remain to be clarified.

Table 1. Defined cytotoxic T lymphocyte (CTL) epitopes that were eluted from HSPs derived from infected/transfected cells, or immunological studies which demonstrated HSP-peptide binding.

Epitope/Antigen	MHC I	Reference
VSV	K^b	Nieland et al., 1996; Suto & Srivastava, 95
Ovalbumin	K^b	Breloer et al., 1998
	K^b	Blachere et al., 1997
PRL1a	L^d	Ishii et al., 1999
SV40	D^b, K^b	Blachere et al., 1997
	D^b,K^b	Blachere et al., 1993

β Galactosidase	L^d	Arnold et al., 1997; Arnold et al., 1995
Minor H	K^d, K^b	Arnold et al., 1997
	K^d, K^b	Arnold et al., 1995
Influenza	K^b	Blachere et al., 1997
		Heikema et al., 1997
LCMV	K^b	Ciupitu et al., 1998
Human Melanoma		
gp100	A3	Castelli et al., 2000
gp100	Cw8	Castelli et al., 2000
MART-1	A2	Castelli et al., 2000

4. CONCLUDING REMARKS

This area of work began in 1982 (Srivastava 1982) with the strange observation that HSPs – the most ubiquitous and highly conserved group of molecules in living systems – were able to elicit potent and antigen-specific immune responses. At face value, the HSPs would be the worst imaginable candidates for tumor antigens because of their ubiquity and conservation. Work from our and other laboratories has dispelled some of the skepticism elicited by the early observations, as the broader outlines of the mechanisms behind the phenomenology have become less opaque. Surly, several important questions remain to be addressed. Regardless, it is now clear that the ability of HSPs to chaperone peptides and to stimulate APCs has conferred on these ubiquitous, abundant molecules, extraordinary immunological properties.

REFERENCES

1. Arnold, D., Faath, S., Rammensee, H., and Schild, H., 1995, Cross-priming of minor histocompatibility antigen-specific cytotoxic T cells upon immunization with the heat shock protein gp96. J Exp Med 182, 3:885-9.
2. Arnold, D., Faath, S., Rammensee, H., and Schild, H., 1997, Influences of transporter associated with antigen processing (TAP) on the repertoire of peptides associated with the endoplasmic reticulum- resident stress protein gp96. J Exp Med 186, 3:461-6.
3. Basu, S., Binder, R., Suto, R., Anderson, K., and Srivastava, P.K., 2000, Mammalian heat shock proteins signal cell death through activation of the NFkB pathway in antigen presenting cells. FASEB J Abstracts 14(6):A945.
4. Basu, S., Binder, R.J., Srivastava, P.K., 2001, CD91 is a common receptor for heat shock proteins gp96, hsp90, hsp70 and calreticulin, Immunity, 14, 1-20.
5. Blachere, N., Udono, H., Janetzki, S., Li, Z., Heike, M., and Srivastava, P.K., 1993, Heat shock protein vaccines against cancer. J Immunotherapy 14, 4:352.
6. Blachere, N.E., Li, Z., Chandawarkar, R., Suto, R., Jaikaria, N., Basu, S., Udono, H. and Srivastava, P.K., 1997, Heat shock protein-peptide complexes, reconstituted in vitro, elicit

peptide-specific cytotoxic T lymphocyte response and tumor immunity. J Exp Med 186, 8:1315-22.
7. Breloer, M., Marti, T., Fleischer, B., and von Bonin, A., 1998, Isolation of processed, H-2Kb-binding ovalbumin-derived peptides associated with the stress proteins HSP70 and gp96. Eur. J. Immunol. 28:1016-21.
8. Charaka, 500 B.C, published 1957, Charaka Samhita, Motilal Banarasi Das Publishers, Allahabad.
9. Ciupitu, A.M., Petersson, M., O.D., C., Williams, K., Jindal, S., Kiessling, R., and Welsh, R., 1998, Immunization with a lymphocytic choriomeningitis virus peptide mixed with heat shock protein 70 results in protective antiviral immunity and specific cytotoxic T lymphocytes. J. Exp. Med. 187, 5:685-91.
10. Castellino, F., Boucher, P., Eichelberg, K., Mayhew, M., Rothman, J., Houghton, A., and Germain, R., 2000, Receptor-mediated uptake of antigen/heat shock protein complexes results in major histocompatibility complex class I antigen presentation via two distinct processing pathways. J. Exp. Med 191(11): in press.
11. Gallucci, S., Lolkema, M., and Matzinger, P., 1999, Natural adjuvants: endogenous activators of dendritic cells. Nat. Med. 5(11): 1249-55.
12. Hanson, D. and Murphy, P. (1984). Demonstration of interleukin-1 activity in apparently homogenous specimens of the pI 5 form of the rabbit endogenous pyrogen. Infect. Immun. 45: 483-90.
13. Heikema, A., Agsteribbe, E., Wilschut, J., and Huckriede, A., 1997, Generation of heat shock protein-based vaccines by intracellular loading of gp96 with antigenic peptides. Immunol. Lett. 57, 1-3:69-74.
14. Ishii, T., Udono, H., Yamano, T. Ohta, H., Uenaka, A., Ono, T., Hizuta, A., Tanaka, N., Srivastava, P.K. and Nakayama, E., 1999, Isolation of MHC class I-restricted tumor antigen peptide and its precursors associated with heat-shock proteins hsp70, hsp90, and gp96. J. Immunol. 162(3):1303-9.
15. Janetzki S, Polla D, Rosenhauer V, Lochs H, Srivastava PK., 2000, Immunization of cancer patients with autologous cancer-derived heat shock protein gp96 : A pilot study. Intl. Journal of Cancer , 88, 232-238.
16. Lindquist, S. and Craig, E., 1988, The heat-shock proteins. Annu. Rev. Genet. 22: 631-77.
17. Luheshi, G. and Rothwell, N., 1996, Cytokines and fever. Int. Arch. Allergy Immunol. 109:301.
18. Dinarello, C., Cannon, J., and Wolff, S., 1988, New concepts in the pathogenesis of fever. Rev. Infect. Dis. 10(1):168-89.
19. Masso-Welch P., Black J., Erikson, J., and Repasky, E., 1999, Polarized expression of immunoglobulin, spectrin, and protein kinase C beta II occurs in B cells from normal BALB/c autoimmune lpr, and anti-ssDNA transgenic, tolerant mice. J. Leukoc. Biol. 66(4):617-24.
20. Medzhitov, R. and Janeway, C., Jr., 1997, Innate immunity: the virtues of a nonclonal system of recognition. Cell. 91:295-8.
21. Nieland, T., Tan, M., Monne-van Muijen, M., Koning, F., Kruisbeek, A. and van Bleek, G., 1996, Isolation of an immunodominant viral peptide that is endogenously bound to the stress protein GP96/GRP94. Proc Natl Acad Sci U S A 93, 12:6135-9.
22. Old, L.J. 1985, Tumor necrosis factor (TNF) Science. 230:630-2.
23. Ritossa, F. (1962). A new puffing pattern induced by temperature shock and DNP in Drosophila. Experientia 18:571-73.
24. Saper, C. and Breder, C., 1994, The neurologic basis of fever. N. Engl. J. Med. 330: 1889-6.

25. Sauter B., Albert M., Francisco L., Larsson, M., Somersan ,S., and Bhardwaj, N., 2000, Consequences of cell death: exposure to necrotic tumor cells, but not primary tissue cells or apoptotic cells, induces the maturation of immunostimulatory dendritic cells. J. Exp. Med. 191(3):423-34.
26. Srivastava, P.K., Studies on cell surfaces during normal and abnormal growth: purification of a tumor-associated antigen and a tumor-rejection-antigen from a rat hepatoma, 1982, Doctoral Thesis at the Osmania University, Hyberabad.
27. Srivastava, P.K., Ménoret, A., Basu, S., Binder, R., McQuade, K., 1998, Heat shock proteins come of age: Primitive functions acquire new roles in an adaptive world. Immunity (8): 657-665.
28. Srivastava, P.K. and Heike, M., 1991, Tumor-specific immunogenicity of stress-induced proteins: Convergence of two evolutionary pathways of antigen presentation? Semin. Immunol. 3, 57-64.
29. Srivastava, P.K. and Maki, R., 1991, Stress-induced proteins in immune response to cancer Curr. Top. Microbiol. Immunol. 167, 109-123.
30. Srivastava, P.K., Udono, H., Blachere, N., and Li, Z., 1994, Heat shock proteins transfer peptides during antigen processing and CTL priming. Immunogenetics. 39:93-98.
31. Suto, R. and Srivastava, P.K., 1995, A mechanism for the specific immunogenicity of heat shock protein-chaperoned peptides. Science 269:1585-8.

CYTOKINES

Allele specific regulation of cytokine genes: Monoallelic expression of the IL-1A gene

CORNELIS L. VERWEIJ, JEAN-PIERRE BAYLEY, ALEIDA BAKKER AND ERIC L. KAIJZEL
Department of Rheumatology, Leiden University Medical Center, P.O.box 9600, 2300 RC Leiden, The Netherlands (e-mail:<verweij@abcoude.com>)

1. INTRODUCTION

The host immune response strongly controls the susceptibility and outcome of inflammatory and infectious diseases in humans. Cytokines play an important role in this response as crucial intercellular signaling molecules that are responsible for multidirectional communication among immune and inflammatory cells engaged in host defense. They exert their effects by binding to high-affinity receptors expressed on target cells thereby inducing biochemical signals within these cells which profoundly change their behaviour. It has become clear that cytokines not only play important roles in tissue homeostasis but also in the pathogenesis of many immune related disorders. A large body of evidence indicated that the cytokine profile, examplified by the balance between inflammatory and anti-inflammatory activities, is a determining factor in the progress of the immune response and the maintenance of tissue homeostasis and might provide an explanation for interindividual differences in the host immune response. A critical question to be answered is which molecular mechanism underlies the imbalance of pro- and anti-inflammatory activity in immune related disease. Clinically useful information should come from understanding the molecular regulatory steps underlying the imbalance in the cytokine profile that would allow the identification of people who display an imbalance in their cytokine profile enabling clinicians to predict outcomes and to tailor treatment.

2. GENETIC BASIS FOR INTERINDIVIDUAL VARIATION IN CYTOKINE PRODUCTION

Evidence exists that disease susceptibility and outcome are determined by host genetic factors. It is estimated that approximately 1 common polymorphism in every 300 nucleotides exists. If only a minority of these turn out to be of functional relevance across the approximately 30,000 genes in the human genome the functional variants would constitute a enormous source as genetic factors involved in disease susceptibility and variability. Besides single genes defects with devastating consequence of great importance for the clinicians is the potentially considerable number of gene variants with subtle effects on the regulation or function of specific immunological mediators. Subtle functional mutations in eg. the promoter region of inflammatory genes might increase or decrease the likelihood of developing severe inflammatory complications. Together, a combination of these variants may yield a trait that do not obey simple rules of mendelian segregation seen for monogenic disorders. The involvement of many different genes means that the contribution of a single gene variant may be relatively small and may depend on other loci as well as environmental factors. Knowledge on which genetic variants do influence disease via a subtle effect on gene regulation or protein function would be of considerable practical relevance to tailor treatment. Moreover, insight in such functional genetic variants is of great value for novel therapeutic intervention. These considerations have lead to great enthusiasm and a massive undertaking in both academia and pharmaceutical industries for systemic genetic analysis of common immune diseases.

The finding of interindividual variation in the amount of cytokines produced by peripheral blood mononuclear cells isolated from normal individuals[1-4] may provide a clue as to why patients have an imbalance in their cytokine profile. To estimate whether genetic influences were involved in the distinct cytokine production profiles we analysed cytokine production in whole blood cultures of monozygotic twins and siblings after stimulation with endotoxin. We observed increased correlations for IL-10 and TNF production in monozygotic twins when compared with siblings[1]. These data are in accordance with those of other investigators who reported on associations between genetic markers and cytokine production levels. Also the production of IL-1B and IL-1RA vary between individuals and seems to be genetically determined[4].

3. CLINICAL RELEVANCE OF GENETICALLY DETERMINED CYTOKINE PRODUCTION PROFILES

The above observations suggest that the host genetic background contributes considerable to the profile of cytokines produced upon a challenge with an offending agent and hence mediate divergent clinical outcomes. When cytokine production capacity of relatives within families was classified as low and high based on dichotomy around the median it was calculated that families with low TNF production had a 10-fold increased risk for fatal meningococcal disease[1]. Families with high IL-10 production had a 20-fold increased risk for fatal disease. Families with both characteristics had the highest risk. From these data it is concluded that a genetically determined pro-inflammatory cytokine profile is important in the initial recovery phase of an infectious disease. This is in agreement with animal studies where an anti-inflammatory cytokine profile during the initial phase of infection dampens the non-specific host response and allows growth of micro-organisms. Analogously, IL-10 attenuates the clearance of various pathogens[5,6]. Moreover, TNF receptor knock-out mice are highly susceptible to infection[8]. Whereas recombinant TNF can protect animals against lethal Gram negative bacterial sepsis[7]. For inflammatory auto-immune diseases the opposite is seen. Absence of IL-10 leads to a chronic arthritis[9]. Thus the same profile may be beneficial in one condition and detrimental in another depending on the clinical burden. Persons with an anti-inflammatory cytokine profile may be less able to mount a robust immune response to eliminate the infectious agent and will develop fulminant disease. On the other hand a shift towards the pro-inflammatory side may underlie the pathology in polygenic diseases characterised by chronic inflammation and tissue destruction.

4. CYTOKINE POLYMORPHISMS AND DISEASE

In the last decade the cytokine genes themselves, with TNF and IL-1beta as prototype pro-inflammatory cytokines have received considerable attention as carriers of functional relevant genetic variation. The search for heterogeneity within cytokine genes has uncovered extensive polymorphism.

In the gene encoding TNF a total of nine bi-allelic single nucleotide polymorphisms (SNPs) have been identified; one in the first intron at position +489, one at position +70 in the 5'untranslated region and seven in the 5'regulatory region. The TNF gene is located on chromosome 6 in the

MHC locus. This region of the genome is highly polymorphic and many disease with an auto-immune component are associated with MHC alleles. The TNF –308 G to A transition polymorphism is the first genetic variant identified within the TNF promoter. The rare A allele is strongly associated with the HLA-A1-B8-DR3-DQ2 haplotype, which is associated with auto-immune diseases and the high TNF producer phenotype. Allele distribution studies in stratified patient groups revealed significant associations with disease outcome in infectious diseases. The most significant association has been obtained in malaria. Gambian children who are homozygous for the TNF-308A allele have increased susceptibility to cerebral malaria. It was estimated that TNF-308A homozygotes have a relative risk of 4.0 to develop cerebral malaria and 7.7 for death and sequela[10]. The –376A allele is associated with susceptibility to cerebral malaria in both Gambian and Kenyan children, and this association is entirely independent of that observed for the TNF-308A allele. For the –238 A polymorphism significant associations of the GA genotype have been described in patients with juvenile psoriasis and psoriatic arthritis[11]. The +489 SNP is associated with common variable immune deficiency independent of HLA[12]. In rheumatoid arthritis we observed a significant association of TNF genotypes and disease severity. In a cohort of RA patients wherein joint damage was monitored at disease entry, and after 3, 6 and 12 years, a significant reduced rate of joint damage was seen in +489 GA and –238 GA heterozygous patients[13,14].

As differences in disease susceptibility and/or outcome may result from a disturbed immune response the association of cytokine alleles with disease has strengthened the speculation on functionality of cytokine gene polymorphisms. Although these data have been interpreted to indicate that the TNF polymorphisms control transcription, the functional significance of the polymorphisms remain controversial when evaluating the results from several studies using promoter gene constructs linked to reporter genes in combination with T-, B- and monocytic cell lines[15-18].

The IL-1 gene family is clustered together on chromosome 2q12-21, and includes the IL-1A, IL-1B and IL-1RN genes. IL-1 receptor antagonist is a natural IL-1beta antagonist. Evidence exists that the ratio of IL-1beta/IL-1 receptor antagonist influences the outcome of inflammatory diseases. IL-1A contains at least two bi-allelic SNPs; one in the promoter region at –889 and one in exon 5 at +4845. These two SNPs are complete linkage. Four SNPs have been described in the IL-1B gene at position –511, -30, +3867 and +3953. Genetic heterogeneity in the IL-1RN gene is caused by variable number of tandem repeats (VNTR) of 86 bp in intron 2 and SNPs at positions +2017 in exon 2, +2072 in intron 2, +3600 in intron 3 and +5111 in exon 4. IL-1 A polymorphisms at postion –889 and +4845 associations with chronic polyarthritis and chronic iridocyditis in juvenile chronic arthritis have been reported. For IL-1B and IL-1RN polymorphisms associations with a wide range of chronic and autoimmune conditions (eg. Infectious bowel disease, periodontitis, Sjogren's syndrome, IDDM, psoriasis and RA). In analogy to the TNF polymorphisms for the IL-1 gene cluster polymorphisms the functional relevance is uncertain, although an association between IL-1B and IL-1RN polymorphism and a lower IL-1beta/IL-1 receptor antagonist ratio is described.

5. ALLELE SPECIFIC TRANSCRIPT QUANTIFICATION (ASTQ)

As it could be argued that promoter studies in cell lines are not representative for the physiological situation a method to compare differences in allelic TNF transcript production in primary cells was developed. This method, called allele specific transcript quantification (ASTQ), is based on genetic variation that exists in the transcribed region of the gene that allows molecular discrimination between the two allelic transcripts in a heterozygous individual.

In general, each of the two genes in a diploid organism contributes equally to the total production of a specific transcript. However, exceptions can arise when mutations alter allele specific mRNA production. The presence of transcriptionally different TNF alleles would lead to unequal contribution of each allele to the total TNF mRNA pool. The intragenic polymorphisms at position +70 (C-insertion)[19] and +489 (TaiI RFLP)[20] provide the opportunity to distinguish between the allelic (pre-)mRNAs[21,22]. For this analysis healthy controls and patients with RA who are heterozygous for either the +70 or +489 polymorphism were selected. PBMC were isolated and stimulated with LPS to activate monocytes and with anti-CD3 and anti-CD28 to stimulate T cells. Total RNA was harvested and RT-PCR on TNF (pre-)mRNA was performed. For the +70 alleles quantification of the respective TNFmRNA RT-PCR products, based

on the one nucleotide in length, revealed no significant difference in transcript production between the two alleles[21]. This result was confirmed in an analysis wherein the +489 polymorphism was used to distinguish between the allelic transcripts[22]. Since the +489 polymorphism is located within intron I, ASTQ analysis was performed on TNF precursor-mRNA. To distinguish between the TNF allelic precursor RT-PCR products the PCR product was digested with TaiI. The relative amount of allele-specific restriction fragments is indicative for the difference in allelic TNF pre-mRNA production. To exclude interference of heteroduplex products, which are formed in the final annealing step of the PCR reaction and would lead to

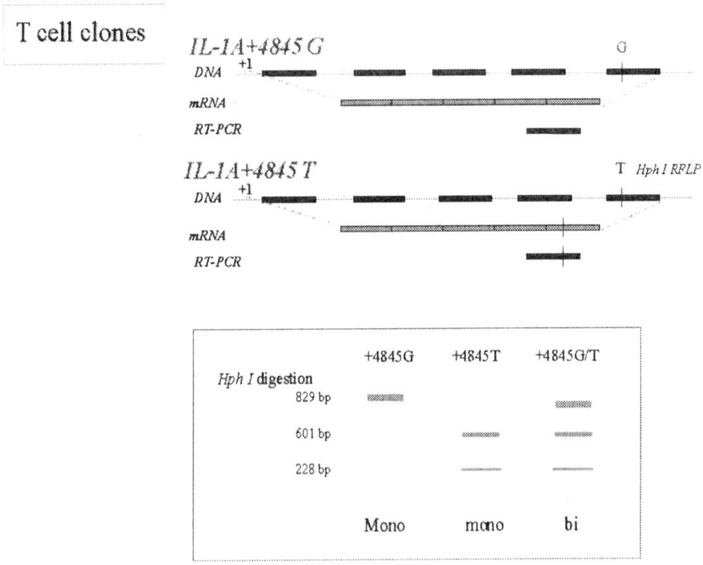

Figure 1. Schematic representation of the procedure for allele specific transcript quantification (ASTQ) analysis using the IL-1A +4845 G to T (RFLP) polymorphism in exonV. The T at position +4845 creates a HphI restriction site which is not recognized in the G allele. RT-PCR was performed with a primer set spanning IL-1A intron IV on mRNA isolated from a T cell clone of a IL-1A +4845 heterozygous individual stimulated for 24 hr with anti-CD3, anti-CD28 and PMA. The PCR product is subsequently digested with HphI and fractionated on a 1.5% agarose gel. Shown are the characteristic digestion patterns that appear for monoallelic expression of the +4845G allele (829 bp), the +4845T allele (601 bp and 228 bp) and biallelic +4845GT expression (829 bp, 601 bp and 228 bp).

an overrepresentation of the non-cleavable product, ^{32}P-dCTP was included in the final DNA-synthesis cycle of the PCR reaction. By this means, which was named final cycle labeling (FCL) PCR, only de-novo formed product was labeled, and thus homoduplex, PCR products that are representative of the relative amount of original pre-mRNA RT templates. Analysis of the radiolabeled RT-PCR products excludes the disturbing effects of heteroduplexes revealed no significant difference between the allelic TNF-pre RT-PCR products. Similar results were obtained when ASTQ analysis was applied on synovial biopsie tissue derived RNA from patients with RA where TNF is induced by physiological stimulation. Since some of the individuals and patients tested were also heterozygous for SNPs at promoter position –308, -863, -857 or –1031, these data argue against functional relevance of these SNPs, thereby confirming results from promoter reportergene studies wherein no differences in the activity of allelic promoters was observed. Moreover, the data indicate that the existence of transcriptionally distinct TNF alleles is not a likely explanation for the occurence of interindividual variation in TNF production.

Therefore, it is more likely that disease associations that exist with TNF polymorphisms are not direct, but result from linkage disequilibrium with functional variants of the MHC region in proximity of the TNF gene, in particular the class III region that contains a remarkable high density of genes with an immunologic function.

6. MONOALLELIC EXPRESSION OF THE IL-1A GENE

Most interestingly, recently an example of an extreme situation of allelic regulation of cytokine genes in the mouse was described. Classical examples of extreme allelic gene regulation include genes subject to allelic exclusion such as immunoglobulin and T cell receptor genes, X-linked genes and olfactory receptor genes. In the mouse model it was demonstrated that

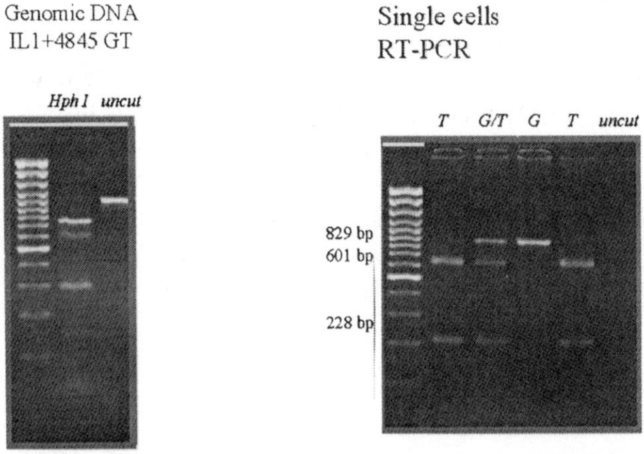

Figure 2. ASTQ analysis of IL-1A transcript production in T cell clones derived of a +4845 GT heterozygous individual. In the left panel the digestion pattern of the undigested genomic PCR product and the digested genomic PCR product of the +4845 heterozygous individual person containing fragments for the respective allelic PCR fragments is shown.

The right panel reveals the results with RT-PCR products that were obtained from 4 different T cell clones of the heterozygous individual. These results reveal monoallelic expression in 3 of the clones (one T and two G) and one clone with biallelic expression.

Individual cells were to express only one or the other of the parental IL-2 and IL-4 alleles[23,24]. In analogy to the situation in mice mono-allelic expression of the IL-1A genes in T cells in healthy individuals was observed. For this purpose T cell clones of an individual who was heterozygous for the IL-1A +4845 GT polymorphism was selected. The T allele of this RFLP is cleavable with HphI, whereas the G allele is not (figure 1). ASTQ analysis performed on RT-PCR products of anti-CD3/anti-CD28/PMA stimulated T cells (24hr) revealed mono-allelic expression in some of the T cell clones tested (figure 2). The same result was consistently found in three independent experiments. Based on these findings a novel mechanism of cytokine gene regulation, that treats each allele independently, is proposed. Evidence exists that allele silencing or activation remains constant in a clonal lineage. This phenomenon may provide a novel mechanism that generates a diverse repertoire of cytokines produced by immune cells from a limited amount of precursors from which the appropriate phenotype may be selected.

The frequency of mono-allelic expression suggests that the activation/silencing of each allele is independently regulated by a stochastic process. In this respect this phenomenon is different from genomic imprinting of genes in a parent-dependent manner, which represents a specialized form of gene regulation which may be vitally important for mammalian development. The mechanisms which underlie allelic imprinting and the molecular nature of the imprint itself remain elusive but most likely include epigenetic modifications of DNA, such as methylation and chromatin structural changes. In addition cytokine genes might influence these processes. Imbalances in the homeostasis of allelic expression may lead to polarized cytokine profiles with pathology as a consequence.

7. CONCLUDING REMARKS

Evidence is increasing that genetic differences control disease susceptibility and outcome. Examples of single gene defects that result in gross phenotypic abnormalities exist but are relatively rare. Of more general importance for common immune related diseases are subtle differences in the regulation and function of specific immunological mediators. A large body of data indicates that genetically determined variation in cytokine production capacity between individuals exists and is clinically relevant. In order to explain the genetic basis for interindividual variation in cytokine production capacity cytokine gene variants were identified that served a role as genetic markers for disease susceptibility and/or severity. As such these markers may serve an important role in disease prognosis and to tailor treatment. Further studies are required to determine whether the relevant cytokine variants contribute directly to the pathophysiology of the disease through disturbance of the cytokine homeostasis or is at best a genetic marker of another (unknown) polymorphism in the cytokine gene or another immunological relevant gene in close proximity. ASTQ analysis does not provide evidence for the existence of trancriptionally distinct TNF alleles as an explanation for the occurence of interindividual variation in TNF production.

Additionally our analyses suggest that IL-1 genes are mono-allelically expressed in some T cells and bi-allelically expressed in others, raising interesting questions regarding gene regulation. Thus cytokine genes may be regulated in a stochastic manner that results in 0, 1 or 2 alleles of a given cytokine gene expressed in each cell. This type of regulation could account for the wide variety of different combinations of cytokine expressed in individual cells and therefore plays an important role of the generation of cells with a range of different effector functions. Imbalances in the homeostasis of allelic expression, eg. as a consequence of genetic differences between cytokine genes (in combination with environmental factors), may lead to polarized cytokine profiles/effector functions with pathology as a consequence.

REFERENCES

1. Westendorp, R.G.J., Langermans, J.A.M., Huizinga, T.W.J., Elouali, A.H., Verweij, C.L., Boomsma, D.I., Vandenbrouke, J.P., 1997, Genetic influence on cytokine production and fatal meningococcal disease. Lancet 349: 170-173.
2. Jacob, C.O., Fronek, Z., Lewis, G.D., Koo, M., Hansen, J.A., McDevitt, H.O., 1990, Heritable major histocompatibility complex class II-associated differences in production of TNFα: relevance to genetic predisposition to systemic lupus erythematosus. Proc Natl Acad Sci USA 87: 1233-1237.
3. Pociot, F., Briant, L., Jongeneel, C.V., Molvig, J., Worsaae, H., Abbal. M., Thomson, M., Nerup, J., Cambon-Thomsen, A., 1993, Association of TNF and class II MHC alleles with the secretion of TNF-alpha and TNF-beta by human mononuclear cells: a possible link to insulin-dependent diabetes mellitus. Eur J Immunol 23: 224-232
4. Bendtzen, K., Morling, N., Fonsgaard, A., Svenson, M., Jakobsen, B., Odum, A., Soejgaard, A. 1988, Association between HLA-DR2 and production of tumor necrosis factor α and interleukin 1 by mononuclear cells activated by lipopolysaccharide. Scand J Immunol 28: 599-606.

5. Fernandes, D.M., Baldwin, C.L., 1995, Interleukin 10 downregulates protective immunity to *Brucella abortus*. Infect Immun 63:1130-1133
6. Gazznelli, R.T., Wysocka, M., Hieny, S. et al., 1996, In the absence of endogenous IL-10, mice acutely infected with *Toxoplasma gondii* succumb to a lethal immune response dependent on CD4+ T cells and accompanied by overproduction of IL-12, IFNy, and TNFa. J Immunol 157: 798-805
7. Alexander, H.R., Sheppard, B.C., Jensen, J.C., et al., 1991, Treatment with recombinat human tumor necrosis factor alpha protects rats against lethality, hypotension, and hypothermia of gram-negative sepsis. J Clin Invest 88: 34-39
8. Rothe, J., Lesslauer, W., Lotscher, H., et al., 1993, Mice lacking the tumour necrosis factor receptor I are resistant to TNF-mediated toxicity but highly susceptible to infection by *Listeria monocytogenes*. Nature 364: 798-802
9. Kuhn, R., Lohler, J., Rennick, D., Rajewsky, K., Muller, W., 1993, Interleukin-10-deficient mice develop chronic enterocolitis. Cell 75:263-269
10. McGuire, W., Hill, A.V.S., Allsopp, C.E.M., Greenwood, B.M., Kwiatkowski, D., 1994, Variation in the TNFα promotor region associated with susceptibility to cerebral malaria. Nature 371: 508-512
11. Hohler, T., et al., 1997, A TNF-alpha promoter polymorphism is associated with juvenile onset psoriasis and psoriatic arthritis. J Invest Dermatol 109:562-565
12. Mullighan, C.G., Fanning, G.C., Chapel, H.M., Welsh, K.I., 1997, TNF and lymphotoxin-alpha polymorphisms associated with common variable immunodeficiency: role in the pathogenesis of granulomatous disease. J Immunol 159:6236-6241
13. van Krugten, M.V., Huizinga, T.W.J., Kaijzel, E.L., Drossears-Bakker, K.W., van de Linde, P., Zanelli, E., Hazes, J.M.W., Zwinderman, A.H., Breedveld, F.C., Verweij, C.L. ,1999, Association of the TNF +489 polymorphism with susceptibility and radiographic damage in rheumatoid arthritis patients. Genes Immunity 1: 1-6
14. Kaijzel, E.L., van Krugten, M.V., Brinkman, B.M.N., Huizinga, T.W.J., Breedveld, F.C., and Verweij, C.L. 1998, Functional analysis of a human tumor necrosis factor alpha promoter polymorphism related to joint damage in rheumatoid arthritis. Molec. Med. 4: 724-733
15. Brinkman, B.M.N., Zuijdgeest, D., Kaijzel, E.L., Breedveld, F.C., Verweij, C.L., 1996, Relevance of the tumor necrosis factor alpha (TNF alpha) - 308 promoter polymorphism in TNF alpha gene regulation. J Inflamm 46: 32-41.
16. Stuber, F., Udalova, I.A., Book, M., Drutskaya, L.N., Kuprash, D.V., Turetskaya, R.L., Schade, F.U., Nedospasov, S.A.,1996, -308 tumor necrosis factor (TNF) polymorphism is not associated with survival in severe sepsis and is unrelated to lipopolysaccharide inducibility of the human TNF promoter. J Inflamm 46: 42-50.
17. Wilson, A.G., Symons, J.A., McDowell, T.L., McDevitt, H.O., Duff, G.W., 1997, Effects of a polymorphism in the human tumor necrosis factor alpha promoter on transcriptional activation. Proc Natl Acad Sci USA 94: 3195-3199.
18. Kroeger, K.M., Carville, K.S., Abraham, L.J., 1997, The –308 tumor necrosis factor promoter polymorphism effects transcription. Mol Immunol 134:391-399
19. Brinkman, B.M.N., Kaijzel, E.L., Huizinga, T.W.J., Giphart, M.J., Breedveld, F.C., Verweij CL., 1995, Detection of a C-insertion polymorphism within the human tumor necrosis factor alpha (TNFA) gene. Hum Genet 96: 493.
20. D'Alfonso, S., Momigliano, R.P., 1996, An intragenic polymorphism in the human tumor necrosis factor alpha (TNFA) chain-encoding gene. Immunogenetics 44: 321-322
21. Brinkman, B.M.N., Huizinga, T.W.J., Breedveld, F.C., and Verweij, C.L. 1996, Allele-specific quantification of TNFA transcripts in rheumatoid arthritis. Hum. Genet. 97: 813-818
22. Kaijzel, E.L., Bayley, J.P., van Krugten, M.V., Smith, L., van de Linde P., Bakker, A.L., Huizinga, T.W.J., and Verweij, C.L. 2001, Allele specific quantification of tumor

necrosis factor (TNF) transcription and the role of promoter polymorphisms in rheumatoid arthritis and healthy individuals. Genes Immun. in press

23. Hollander, G., Zuklys, S., Morel, C., Mizoguchi, E., Mobisson, K., Simpson, S., Terhorst, C., Wishart, W., Golan, D.E., Bhan, A.K., and Burakoff S.J., 1998, Monoallelic expression of the interleukin-2 locus. Science 279: 2118-2121
24. Bix, M., and Locksley, R., 1998, Science 281: 1352-1354

Effect of polysaccharide sulfates on the production of interleukin-8 in an *ex vivo* model

PAWEŁ P. JAGODZINSKI, WIESŁAW H. TRZECIAK
Department of Biochemistry and Molecular Biology University School of Medical Sciences 6, Swięcickiego St., 60-781 Poznań, Poland

1. INTRODUCTION

Bacterial infections as well as immunological diseases result in activation of various endogenous mediators including cytokines (1). One of these cytokines is interleukin–8 (IL-8) which attracts neutrophils, basophils and T-cells, induces adherence to vascular endothelium and extravasation into tissue spaces (1). It has been evidenced that the levels of IL-8 in body fluids are elevated in the patients with inflammatory diseases: cardiac failure, rheumatoid arthritis, and infections of the renal, pulmonary, and urinary tracts (2,3). IL-8 belongs to C-X-C chemokine family and is produced by a variety of cell types, including endothelial cells, hepatocytes, keratinocytes and monocyte-derived macrophages in response to lipopolysaccharides and inflammatory cytokines: tumor necrosis factor alpha (TNF-α) and IL-1 (1,4). Numerous medicines have been used to stimulate the immune system. The root of Panax ginseng had been known in East Asia, as an elixir, used as an antiseptic, stomachic, tonic and sedative drug for thousands of years (5). It has recently been reported that acidic polysaccharides extracted from the root of Panax ginseng, stimulate IL-8 synthesis in monocyte-derived macrophages and may augment the activation and chemotaxis of neutrophils in the incidence of sepsis (5).

Progress in Basic and Clinical Immunology, Edited by Mackiewicz *et al.*
Kluwer Academic/Plenum Publishers, New York, 2001

In the present study, we examined the effects of high molecular weight dextran sulfate (HMDS), low molecular weight dextran sulfate (LMDS) and 40 kD dextran (DS40) on the production of IL-8 in an ex vivo model.

2. MATERIALS AND METHODS

HMDS (500 kDa) was obtained from Pharmacia Biotech (Uppsala, Sweden). LMDS (8 kDa), DS40 (40 kDa) and lipopolysaccharide (LPS) were purchased from Sigma Chemical Co. (St. Louis, USA). Blood from healthy donors was drawn into heparinized 10 ml vacutainers. The whole blood was diluted 1:10 in RPMI 1640 GibcoBRL (Grand Island, USA) medium supplemented with 2mM glutamine and 50 μg/ml gentamicin sulfate. Blood samples were incubated in the absence or presence of 10 μg/ml of LPS without or with the addition of HMDS, LMDS or DS40 in the concentrations of: 0.1, 0.3, 1, 3, 10, 30 and 100 μg/ml. After 24 h of incubation the culture supernatants were harvested and IL-8 production was determined by enzyme-linked immunosorbent assay (ELISA) using reagents purchased from PharMigen, (San Diego, USA).

3. RESULTS AND DISCUSSION

Our results demonstrate that HMDS stimulates IL-8 production in a dose-dependent fashion. The HMDS in the concentration of 100 μg/ml resulted in stimulation of IL-8 production to a similar level as LPS in the concentration of 10 μg/ml (Fig. 1). In contrast, LMDS and DS40 did not effect IL-8 production in an *ex vivo* model (Fig.1). It was also demonstrated that the simultaneous addition of HMDS and LPS inhibited the production of IL-8. The mixture of HMDS in the concentration of 30 μg/ml and LPS in the concentration of 10μg/ml decreased IL-8 production to the control level (Fig 2). However, the mixture of LPS and LMDS or LPS and DS40 did not affect on the production of IL-8.

It has been reported that polysaccharides, such as krestin and lentinan, exhibit immunomodulating activity and are used to medicate the cancer in Japan (6,7).

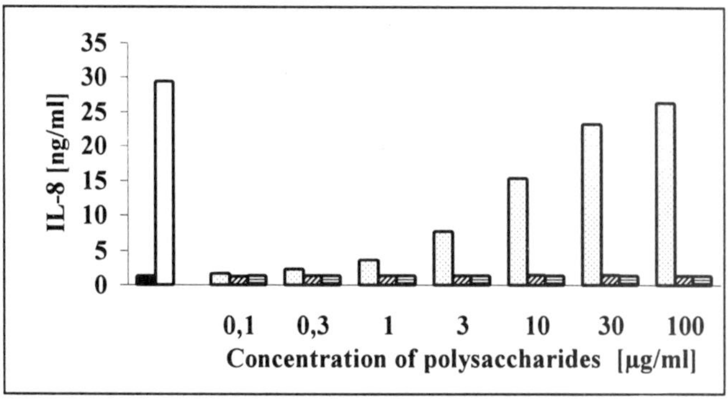

Figure1. Effects of polysaccharides on IL-8 production in ex vivo model. Whole blood was diluted 1:10 in RPMI 1640 and incubated in the absence- or the presence of HMDS- , LMDS- or DS40- The white bar represents blood samples incubated in the presence of LPS in concentration of 10 µg/ml. The values are means from five independent experiments with SD < 15%.

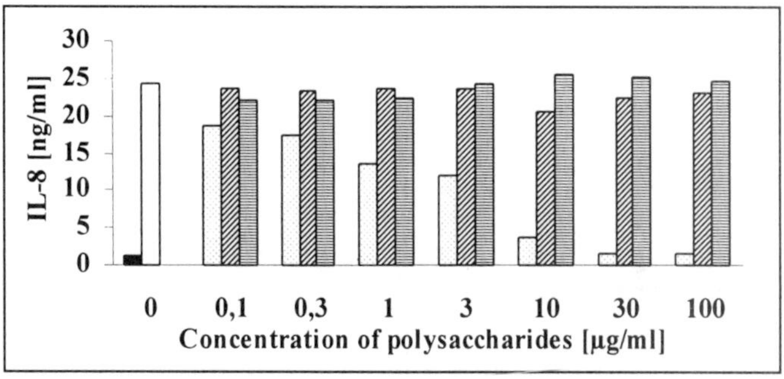

Figure 2. Inhibition effects of HMDS on LPS-stimulated IL-8 production in ex vivo model. Whole blood was diluted 1:10 in RPMI 1640 medium and mixed with LPS (10µg/ml) and incubated in the absence- or presence of HMDS- , LMDS- or DS40-. The black bar presents blood samples incubated in the medium without any stimulants. The values are means from five independent experiments with SD < 15%.

Since the *ex vivo* model is most similar to *in vivo* conditions (1), we decided to mix whole blood with RPMI 1640 medium and challenged inducible IL-8 properties of HMDS, LMDS as well as DS40. We found that HMDS stimulates IL-8 formation in similar fashion to LPS, a known stimulator of IL-8 biosynthesis (Fig 1). Our observation was consistent with the effect of low molecular weight heparin (5 kDa) on the whole blood that resulted in formation of IL-8 (8). It has also been shown that the acidic polysaccharides extracted from *Panax ginseng* stimulate IL-8 production in human monocyte-derived macrophages *in vitro* (5). Our finding as well as the results of other investigators (5,8) suggest that polysaccharides containing different acidic side-chain groups might enhance biosynthesis of IL-8 under *ex vivo* as well as *in vitro* conditions. We also observed that despite the stimulatory effects of HMDS and LPS on the formation of IL-8 both compounds antagonise each other in the biosynthesis of IL-8 in an *ex vivo* model. We presume that LPS and HMDS, might bind each other in an unknown way resulting in the formation of molecules that fail to stimulate production of IL-8 in an *ex vivo model.* However, more detailed studies should be conducted to provide the exact explanation of the stimulatory effect of acidic polysaccharides as well as the antagonism between LPS and HMDS molecules in IL-8 formation.

ACKNOWLEDGMENTS

Supported by grant No. 501-1-08-05 from K. Marcinkowski University School of Medical Sciences, Poznań.

REFERENCES

1. DeForge, L.E., and Remick D.G., 1991, Kinetics of TNF, IL-6, and IL-8 gene expression in LPS-stimulated human whole blood. Biochem Biophys Res Commun 174: 18-24.
2. Harada, A., Sekido, N., Akahoshi, T., Wada, T., Mukaida, N., and Matsushima, K., 1994, Essential involvement of interleukin-8 (IL-8) in acute inflammation. J Leukoc Biol 56: 559-564.
3. Sekido, N., Mukaida, N., Harada, A., Nakanishi, I., Watanabe, Y., and Matsushima, K., 1993, Prevention of lung reperfusion injury in rabbits by a monoclonal antibody against interleukin-8. Nature 365: 654-657.
4. Rollins, B.J., Chemokines. 1997, Blood 90: 909-928.
5. Sonoda, Y., Kasahara, T., Mukaida, N., Shimizu, N., Tomoda, M., and Takeda, T., 1998, Stimulation of interleukin-8 production by acidic polysaccharides from the root of Panax ginseng. Immunopharmacology 38: 287-294.
6. Chihara, G., Hamuro, J., Maeda, Y., Arai, Y., and Fukuoka, F., 1970, Fractionation and purification of the polysaccharides with marked antitumor activity, especially lentinan, from Lentinus edodes (Berk.) Sing. (an edible mushroom). Cancer Res 30: 2776-2781.
7. Tsukagoshi, S., Hashimoto, Y., Fujii, G., Kobayashi, H., Nomoto, K., and Orita, K., 1984, Krestin (PSK). Cancer Treat Rev 11: 131-155.
8. Call, D. R., and Remick, D. R., 1998, Low molecular weight heparin is associated with greater cytokine in a stimulated whole blood model. Shock 10: 192-197.

Coordination of interleukin-6 biology by membrane bound and soluble receptors

STEFAN ROSE-JOHN
Department of Biochemistry, Christian-Albrechts-Universität zu Kiel, Oslhausenstr. 40, D-24098 Kiel, Germany

1. INTRODUCTION

On target cells IL-6 first binds to the IL-6 receptor (IL-6R). The complex of IL-6 and IL-6R associates with the signaltransducing membrane protein gp130, thereby inducing its dimerization and initiation of signaling[1]. gp130 is expressed by all cells in the body whereas IL-6R is mainly expressed by hepatocytes, monocytes/macrophages and lymphocytes. A naturally occurring soluble form of the IL-6R (sIL-6R), which has been found in various body fluids, is generated by two independent mechanisms, limited proteolysis of the membrane protein and translation from an alternatively spliced mRNA[2]. Interestingly, the sIL-6R together with IL-6 stimulates cells which only express gp130[3,4], a process which has been named transsignaling[2,5]. Recently, it has been shown that the sIL-6R strongly sensitizes target cells[6]. Early hematopoietic progenitor cells[5,7], many neural cells[8,9], smooth muscle cells[10] and endothelial cells[11], among others, are only responsive to IL-6 in the presence of sIL-6R[12].

Progress in Basic and Clinical Immunology, Edited by Mackiewicz *et al.*
Kluwer Academic/Plenum Publishers, New York, 2001

1.1 Initial Comments

Cytokine receptors exist in membrane bound and soluble form. Interestingly, both forms bind their ligands with comparable affinity. While most soluble receptors are antagonists in that they compete for the ligands with their membrane counterparts, some soluble receptors are agonists. In this case, the complex of ligand and soluble receptor binds on target cells to a second receptor subunit and initiates signal transduction. Soluble receptors of the IL-6 family of cytokines are agonists[13-15]. *In vivo,* the IL-6/sIL-6R complex stimulates several types of target cells which are not stimulated by IL-6 alone, since they do not express the membrane bound IL-6R. Such cells include endothelial cells[11], hematopoietic progenitor cells[16], osteoclasts[17] and neuronal cells[18].

2. THE CONCEPT OF DESIGNER CYTOKINES

Using the information on membrane bound and soluble cytokine receptors, we have constructed chimeric proteins in which receptor recognition modules have been altered or exchanged and in which cytokines have been fused to their soluble cytokine receptors. Furthermore, chimeric receptor proteins have been constructed which contain cytokine binding modules of gp130, LIFR or OSMRß. This approach has allowed the definition of cytokine binding modules on receptor proteins[19,20].

Furthermore, we have constructed a fusion protein consisting of the domains of IL-6 and sIL-6R which are necessary for biological function. The two proteins are fused by a flexible polypeptide linker (Fig. 1). The recombinant protein was folded correctly and showed biological activity. The fusion protein which we call Hyper-IL-6 is 100-1000 times more active than the separate proteins IL-6 and sIL-6R. Many cells including hematopoietic progenitor cells, neuronal cells, endothelial cells, smooth muscle cells which do not respond to IL-6 show a remarkable response to IL-6/sIL-6 R[21,22].

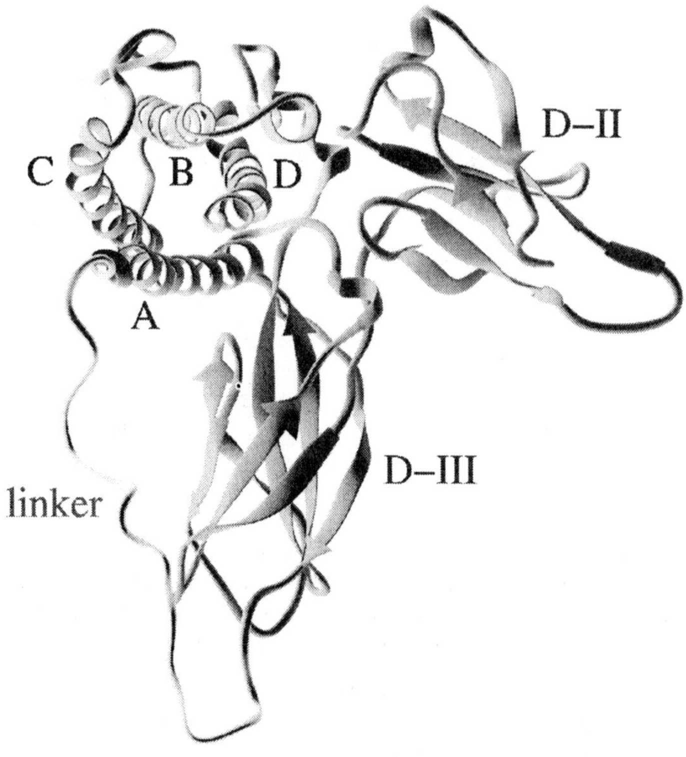

Figure 1. Hyper-IL-6: a highly active designer cytokine consisting of IL-6 and soluble IL-6R. Molecular model of the fusion protein of IL-6 and sIL-6R (Hyper-IL-6) consisting of IL-6 and sIL-6R fused by a flexible peptide linker. A, B, C, D denote the four helices of IL-6; D-II and D-III are the two cytokine-binding receptor domaines of the sIL-6R which were used for the construction of the fusion protein.

3. THE ROLE OF SOLUBLE GP130

The role of a soluble form of gp130 (sgp130) was also analyzed. It turned out that sgp130 exclusively inhibits IL-6 responses mediated by the sIL-6R without interfering with responses via the membrane bound IL-6R[23]. Therefore we postulate that sgp130 is the natural inhibitor of IL-6/sIL-6R complexes (Fig. 2).

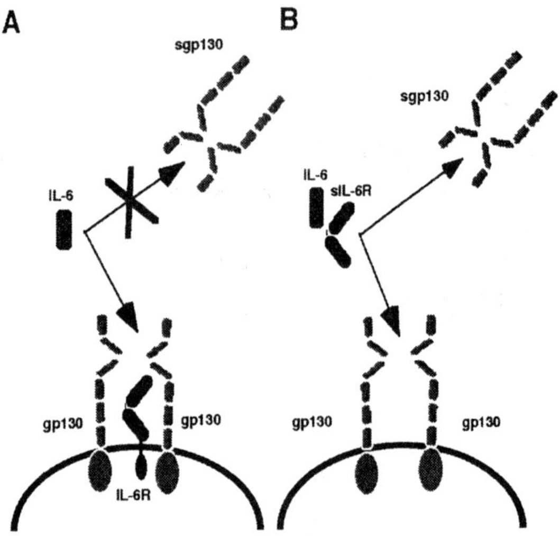

Figure 2. Schematic view of the inhibitory mechanism of sgp130. (A) sgp130 has no access to IL-6 complexed by IL-6R and two molecules of membrane bound gp130. (B) The IL-6/sIL-6R complex can bind to both, membrane bound and sgp130. Consequently, a molar excess of sgp130 leads to competitive inhibition of the IL-6/sIL-6R response.

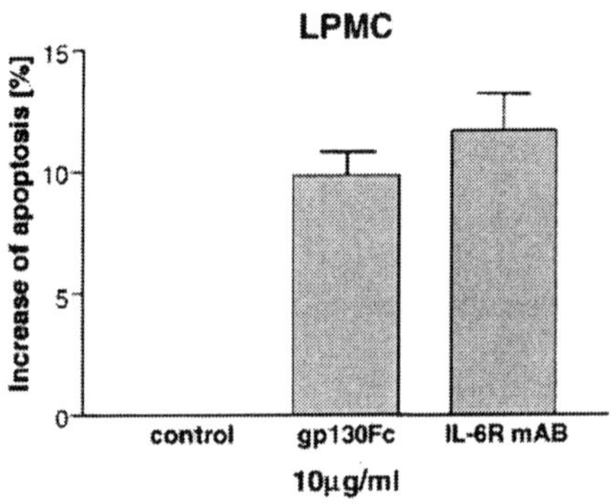

Figure 3. Apoptosis of lamina propria mononuclear cells (LPMC) of Crohn patients upon treatment with sgp130. LPMCs were isolated and cultured for 48 h in the presence or absence of 10 µg/ml of a neutralizing mAB specific for human IL-6R or 10 µg/ml sgp130Fc. Subsequently, cells were stained for annexin V and propidiumiodide and analyzed by FACS. The increase in apoptotic (annexin V positive and propidiumiodide negative) cells is shown. The data presented are means of triplicate measurements with standard errors shown as vertical bars.

A functional role of sIL-6R has recently been demonstrated in chronic inflammatory bowl disease (Morbus Crohn). We could show that T-cells of Morbus Crohn patients are extremely resistant to Apoptosis and show activation of the JAK-STAT signal transduction pathway. These T-cells produce large amounts of IL-6 but lack membrane bound IL-6R. Surprisingly, treatment of these cells with a neutralizing monoclonal antibody to IL-6R induced apoptosis. Moreover treatment of the cells with sgp130 showed the same effect (Fig. 3). These results clearly show that IL-6 is involved in apoptosis resistance of T-cells of Morbus Crohn patients. Moreover, the data demonstrate that sIL-6R and not the membrane bound IL-6R is responsible for T-cell stimulation. Most likely, the sIL-6R is produced by lamina propria macrophages or neutrophiles[23,24]

4. CONCLUSION

We conclude that sgp130 is the natural inhibitor of IL-6 responses dependent on sIL-6R. Furthermore, recombinant sgp130 is expected to be a valuable therapeutic tool to specifically block disease states in which sIL-6R transsignaling responses exist, e.g. in Morbus Crohn Disease.

NOTES

There are inclusions in this text from a number of different articles which which are cited in the reference section.

ACKNOWLEDGMENTS

The work from our laboratory was supported by grants from the Deutsche Forschungsgemeinschaft Bonn, Germany.

REFERENCES

1. Taga, T. & Kishimoto, T. gp130 and the Interleukin-6 Family of Cytokines. *Annu. Rev. Immunol.* **15**, 797-819 (1997).
2. Rose-John, S. & Heinrich, P.C. Soluble receptors for cytokines and growth factors: generation and biological function. *Biochem. J.* **300**, 281-90 (1994).
3. Taga, T., Hibi, M., Hirata, Y., Yamasaki, K., Yasukawa, K., Matsuda, T., Hirano, T. & Kishimoto, T. Interleukin-6 triggers the association of its receptor with a possible signal transducer, gp130. *Cell* **58**, 573-81 (1989).
4. Mackiewicz, A., Schooltink, H., Heinrich, P.C. & Rose-John, S. Complex of soluble human IL-6-receptor/IL-6 up-regulates expression of acute-phase proteins. *J. Immunol.* **149**, 2021-7 (1992).
5. Peters, M., Müller, A. & Rose-John, S. Interleukin-6 and soluble Interleukin-6 Receptor: Direct Stimulation of gp130 and Hematopoiesis. *Blood* **92**, 3495-3504 (1998).

6. Peters, M., Jacobs, S., Ehlers, M., Vollmer, P., Müllberg, J., Wolf, E., Brem, G., Meyer zum Büschenfelde, K.H. & Rose-John, S. The function of the soluble interleukin 6 (IL-6) receptor in vivo: sensitization of human soluble IL-6 receptor transgenic mice towards IL-6 and prolongation of the plasma half-life of IL-6. *J. Exp. Med.* **183**, 1399-406 (1996).
7. Peters, M., Schirmacher, P., Goldschmitt, J., Odenthal, M., Peschel, C., Dienes, H.P., Fattori, E., Ciliberto, G., Meyer zum Büschenfelde, K.H. & Rose-John, S. Extramedullary expansion of hematopoietic progenitor cells in IL-6/sIL-6R double transgenic mice. *J. Exp. Med.* **185**, 755-766 (1997).
8. März, P., Cheng, J.-C., Gadient, R.A., Patterson, P., Stoyan, T., Otten, U. & Rose-John, S. Sympathetic Neurons can produce and respond to Interleukin-6. *Proc. Natl. Acad. Sci. USA* **95**, 3251-3256 (1998).
9. März, P., Otten, U. & Rose-John, S. Neuronal Activities of IL-6 Type Cytokines often Depend on Soluble Cytokine Receptors. *Eur. J. Neurosci.* **11**, 2995-3004 (1999).
10. Klouche, M., Bhakdi, S., Hemmes, M. & Rose-John, S. Novel Path of activation of primary human smooth muscle cells: upregulation of gp130 creates an autocrine activation loop by IL-6 and its soluble receptor. *J. Immunol.* **163**, 4583-4589 (1999).
11. Romano, M., Sironi, M., Toniatti, C., Polentarutti, N., Fruscella, P., Ghezzi, P., Faggioni, R., Luini, W., van Hinsbergh, V., Sozzani, S., Bussolino, F., Poli, V., Ciliberto, G. & Mantovani, A. Role of IL-6 and its soluble receptor in induction of chemokines and leukocyte recruitment. *Immunity* **6**, 315-325 (1997).
12. Kallen, K.J., Galle, P., R. & Rose-John, S. IL-6 dependent biology and therapy: where do we stand and what are the options? *Exp. Opin. Invest. Drugs* **8**, 1-23 (1999).
13. Althoff, K., Reddy, P., Peschon, J., Voltz, N., Rose-John, S. & Müllberg, J. Contribution of the Amino Acid Sequence at the Cleavage Site to the Cleavage Pattern of Transmembrane Proteins. *Eur. J. Biochem.* **267**, 2624-2631 (2000).
14. Althoff, K., Müllberg, J., Aasland, D., Voltz, N., Kallen, K.-J., Grötzinger, J. & Rose-John, S. Recognition sequences and structural elements contribute to shedding susceptibility of membrane proteins. *Biochem. J.* **353**, 663–672 (2001).
15. Müllberg, J., Althoff, K., Jostock, T. & Rose-John, S. The Importance of Shedding of Membrane Proteins for Cytokine Biology. *Eur. Cyt. Netw.* **11**, 27-38 (2000).
16. Audet, J., Miller, C.L., Rose-John, S., Piret, J.M. & Eaves, C.J. Distinct role of gp130 activation in promoting self-renewal divisions by mitogenically stimulated murine hematopoietic cells. *Proc. Natl. Acad. Sci. USA*, in press (2001).
17. Tamura, T., Udagawa, N., Takahashi, N., Miyaura, C., Tanaka, S., Yamada, Y., Koishihara, Y., Ohsugi, Y., Kumaki, K., Taga, T., Kishimoto, T. & Suda, T. Soluble interleukin-6 receptor triggers osteoclast formation by interleukin 6. *Proc. Natl. Acad. Sci. USA* **90**, 11924-8 (1993).
18. Brunello, A.G., Weissenberger, J., Kappeler, A., Franke, S., Peters, M., Rose-John, S. & Weis, J. Astrocytic Alterations in Interleukin-6/soluble Interleukin-6 Receptor a Double-Transgenic Mice. *Am. J. Pathol.* **157**, 1485-1493 (2000).
19. Kallen, K.-J., Grötzinger, J., Lelièvre, E., Vollmer, P., Aasland, D., Renné, C., Müllberg, J., Meyer zum Büschenfelde, K.-H., Gascan, H. & Rose-John, S. Receptor recognition sites of cytokines are organized as exchangeable moduls: transfer of the LIFR binding site from CNTF to IL-6. *J. Biol. Chem.* **274**, 11859-11867 (1999).
20. Kallen, K.-J., Grötzinger, J. & Rose-John, S. New Perspectives in the Design of Cytokines and Growth Factors. *Trends Biotechnol.* **18**, 455-461 (2000).
21. Fischer, M., Goldschmitt, J., Peschel, C., Kallen, K.J., Brakenhoff, J.P.J., Wollmer, A., Grötzinger, J. & Rose-John, S. A Designer Cytokine with High Activity on Human Hematopoietic Progenitor Cells. *Nature Biotech.* **15**, 142-145 (1997).

22. Renné, C., Kallen, K.-J., Müllberg, J., Jostock, T., Grötzinger, J. & Rose-John, S. A new type of Cytokine Receptor Antagonist directly targeting gp130. *J. Biol. Chem.* **273**, 27213-27219 (1998).
23. Jostock, T., Müllberg, J., Özbek, S., Atreya, R., Blinn, G., Voltz, N., Fischer, M., Neurath, M.F. & Rose-John, S. Soluble gp130 is the natural inhibitor of soluble IL-6R transsignaling responses. *Eur. J. Biochem.* **268**, 160-167 (2001).
24. Atreya, R., Mudter, J., Finotto, S., Müllberg, J., Jostock, T., Wirtz, S., Schütz, M., Bartsch, B., Holtmann, M., Becker, C., Strand, D., Czaja, J., Schlaak, J.F., Lehr, H.A., Autschbach, F., Schürmann, G., Nishimoto, N., Yoshizaki, K., Ito, H., Kishimoto, T., Galle, P.R., Rose-John, S. & Neurath, M.F. Blockade of IL-6 transsignaling abrogates established experimental colitis in mice by suppression of the antiapoptotic resistance of lamina propria T cells. *Nature Med.* **6**, 583-588 (2000).

Termination and modulation of IL-6-type cytokine signaling

PETER C. HEINRICH, JOHANNES BODE, MANUELA DECKER, LUTZ GRAEVE, ASTRID MARTENS, GERHARD MÜLLER-NEWEN, STEFAN PFLANZ, FRED SCHAPER, JOCHEN SCHMITZ
Department of Biochemistry, Technical University RWTH Aachen, Pauwelsstraße 30, Aachen, Germany

1. INTRODUCTION

The family of Interleukin-6(IL-6)-type cytokines comprises IL-6, IL-11, leukemia inhibitory factor (LIF), oncostatin M (OSM), ciliary neurotrophic factor (CNTF), cardiotrophin-1 (CT-1) and the recently described novel neurotrophin-1/B-cell stimulatory factor 3/cardiotrophin-1-like cytokine. These cytokines play an important role in hematopoiesis, inflammation, the acute phase response, and bone and heart development as well as neurogenesis. The redundant effects can be attributed to the shared use of the common signal transducing receptor chain glycoprotein (gp) 130. Gp130 is homodimerized by IL-6 and IL-11 upon binding to their ligand-specific α-receptors. The other cytokines of this family trigger the heterodimerization of gp130 with LIF receptor (LIF-R) or the OSM-specific receptor (OSM-R).

Early in 1994 the major steps in IL-6-type cytokine signaling have been elucidated[1-2].

A schematic representation of our present view on the gp130/Jak/ STAT signaling[3] is shown in figure 1.

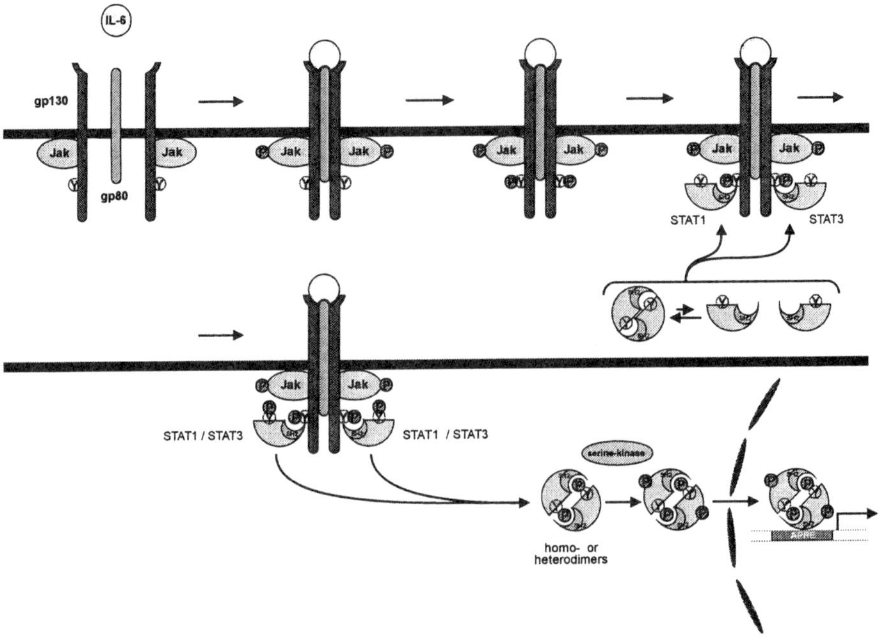

Figure 1. IL-6 signalling via the gp130/Jak/STAT pathway.

The signal transducer gp130 associates with tyrosine kinases of the Janus family (Jak1, Jak2 and Tyk2). Upon ligand binding and receptor dimerization, Jaks are activated and in turn phosphorylate gp130 on several cytoplasmic tyrosine residues which then provide docking sites for SH2-domain-containing molecules such as transcription factors of the STAT family (STAT3 and STAT1). Upon phosphorylation the STATs translocate as dimers into the nucleus where they bind to promoter regions of specific response genes. Additionally, the tyrosine phosphatase SHP-2 becomes recruited to gp130 via tyrosine residue 759[3].

In this presentation two important questions in respect to the Jak/STAT signal transduction pathway will be addressed: (1) How is IL-6-type cytokine signaling terminated? and (2) How is IL-6-type cytokine signaling modulated?

Several interesting mechanisms for termination of the Jak/STAT signal transduction pathway have been proposed.

2. TYROSINE PHOSPHATASES IN THE NUCLEUS

Thus far, there has only been one single report on the dephosphorylation of activated STATs in the nucleus[4].

3. STAT DEGRADATION VIA THE NUCLEAR PROTEASOME

The degradation of STAT1 by the nuclear proteasome has been reported by Kim and Maniatis[5]. Experiments in our laboratory failed to demonstrate the degradation of STAT3 in the nucleus.

4. TYROSINE PHOSPHATASES DEPHOSPHORYLATE RECEPTOR-ASSOCIATED PROTEINS

The ubiquitously expressed tyrosine phosphatase SHP-2 has been shown to interact with grb2, GAB1, GAB2, SIRP, IRS1, and Jak kinases. SHP-2 is activated by tyrosine phosphorylation by a variety of receptors such as PDGF-R, EGF-R, c-kit, insulin-R, IL-2-R, IL-3-R, IL-5-R, Epo-R, IFNAR, GM-CSF-R, M-CSF-R, leptin-R, gp130.

Several laboratories found SHP-2 to be activated upon interleukin-6 (IL-6) action. This activation occurs via the recruitment of SHP-2 to phosphorylated tyrosine 759 (Y759) of the signal transducer gp130[6]. When Y759 of gp130 is exchanged by phenylalanine STAT activation is prolonged[7]. In a series of experiments using heterodimeric receptor chimeras we have shown that Y759 of a single gp130 receptor chain can attenuate signal transduction. Furthermore, SHP-2- and STAT-recruitment sites do not have to be located on the same gp130 receptor chain but within the same receptor complex[8].

5. SYNTHESIS OF JAK/STAT FEEDBACK INHIBITORS

Tyrosine 759 of gp130 not only binds and activates the tyrosine phosphatase SHP-2 but also the feedback inhibitor molecule SOCS-3. SOCS-3 belongs to a family of so called suppressors of cytokine signaling also known as JAB or SSI[9-11]. Presently, seven SOCS proteins are known. They are composed of a C-terminal SOCS box, an SH2-domain, an extended SH2-subdomain and a kinase inhibitory region. The sequence of 30 amino acids before the SH2-domain is important for function.

We have found that SOCS-3 specifically binds to the phosphotyrosine peptide around Y759 of gp130 (Fig. 2). No binding of SOCS-3 occurs when Y759 is unphosphorylated[12-13].

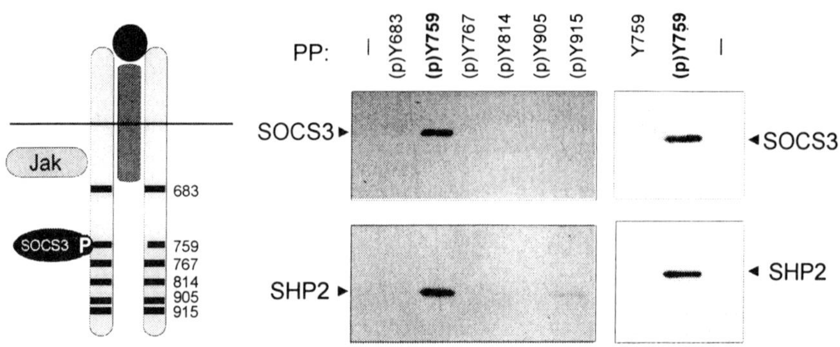

Figure 2. SOCS3 and SHP2 bind to the phosphotyrosine motif 759 of gp130. Cellular extracts of COS7 cells transfected with an expression vector for SOCS3 were incubated with biotinylated phosphotyrosine peptides corresponding to the individual cytoplasmic tyrosine motifs of gp130. After precipitation with NeutrAvidin®-coupled agarose the proteins were subjected to Western blot analysis.

Since SHP-2 also binds to the pY759 peptide of gp130 the question arose whether SOCS-3 binding is mediated through SHP-2. Since SHP-2 depletion from the cell lysate containing SHP-2 and SOCS-3 did not affect SOCS-3 binding, we concluded that SOCS-3 interacts directly with pY759 of gp130[12]. Whether and how SOCS-3 and SHP-2 are competing for binding to pY759 on the cytoplasmic tail of gp130 is presently under investigation.

6. SPECIFIC INHIBITION OF STAT PROTEINS BY PROTEIN INHIBITORS OF ACTIVATED STATS

PIAS (protein inhibitors of activated STATs) have first been identified by the group of Ke Shuai[14]. These proteins interact specifically with tyrosine-phosphorylated STATs and inhibit DNA binding. The N-terminal 50 amino acids of PIAS confer the protein to bind only STAT dimers. Within the PIAS molecule - between amino acids 392 and 541 - there is a STAT interaction domain.

When HepG2 cells were transfected with an acute phase protein promoter-luciferase reporter gene construct, a robust induction of luciferase activity is observed upon IL-6 stimulation. Cotransfection of the hepatoma cells with increasing amounts of cDNA coding for PIAS3 resulted in a strong inhibition of IL-6-induced luciferase activity (Fig. 3, left panel).

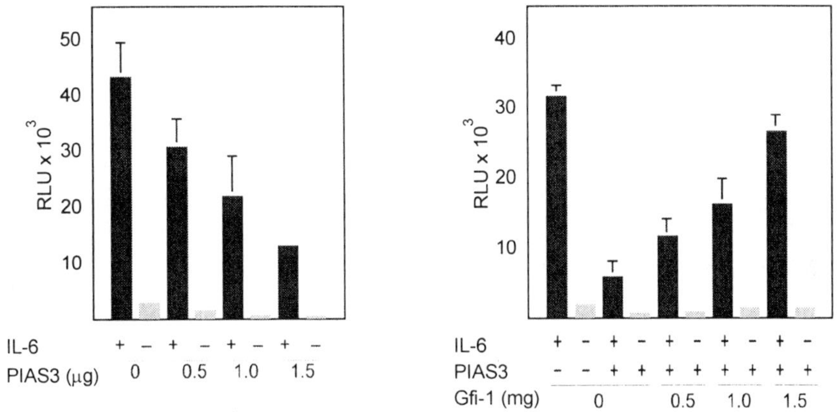

Figure 3. Gfi-1 relieves STAT3-mediated transcriptional transactivation from PIAS3 block. HepG2 cells were transfected with the α_1-antichymotrypsin-gene promoter luciferase reporter, a STAT3 expression vector and the indicated amounts of PIAS expression vector (left panel) or a constant amount of PIAS3 expression vector and the indicated amounts of Gfi-1 expression vector (right panel). Cells were treated with IL-6 and luciferase activity was determined.

The group of Tarik Möröy has identified the Zn-finger protein Gfi-1 (growth factor independence), which is able to releave the PIAS3-mediated block of STAT3-induced luciferase gene activation[15]. As shown in Figure 3, right panel, the expression of increasing amounts of Gfi-1 results in increased reporter gene induction.

7. EXPRESSION OF IL-6-, IL-11-, CNTF-α-RECEPTORS

Whereas the signal transducer gp130 as well as the LIF-receptor are widely expressed on many different cell types, IL-6-, IL-11- and CNTF-α-receptor expression is strictly regulated, i.e. the regulation of IL-6-, IL-11-, CNTF-α-receptor expression might represent an effective way to regulate signaling through these cytokines.

8. INTERNALIZATION OF CYTOKINE/RECEPTOR COMPLEXES

In order to escape from being overstimulated most plasma membrane receptors are internalized after ligand binding and initiation of signaling. We have shown a constitutive internalization for the IL-6-type cytokine signal transducer gp130 as well as for the LIF-R[16-17]. A di-leucine motif (L786, L787) in the middle of the cytoplasmic tail of gp130 was found to be responsible for the internalization of gp130. The constitutive internalization of neutralizing as well as of agonistic monoclonal antibodies against gp130 has been shown by confocal laser scanning microscopy in COS-7 cells expressing wild-type gp130. No internalization was observed with cells transfected with gp130 in which the di-leucine motif had been exchanged by alanine residues. Similar results were obtained after biotinylation of surface gp130 and subsequent internalization.

9. TWO SORTING MOTIFS WITHIN THE CYTOPLASMIC REGION OF THE IL-6 RECEPTOR α-CHAIN

Whereas the cytoplasmic tail of gp130 contains binding sites for Jak kinases, recruitment sites for SHP-2, SOCS3, STAT1 and STAT3 as well as an internalization motif, no function could be attributed to the cytoplasmic region of the IL-6 α-receptor (gp80). We have shown recently that the cytoplasmic part of gp80 is responsible for the basolateral expression of the IL-6 α-receptor gp80[18]. Madin Darby canine kidney (MDCK) cells stably transfected with wild-type gp80 showed a basolateral expression whereas gp80 which lacks its cytoplasmic domain is expressed apical. Successive truncation of the cytoplasmic tail of gp80 led to the identification of two sorting sequences: one containing tyrosine 408 and the other leucine 427 and isoleucine 428.

10. RECEPTOR SHEDDING

An efficient way for cells to escape from being overstimulated by cytokines or growth factors is receptor shedding, i.e. by limited proteolysis. Except for a few receptors the shedding proteases as well as the exact cleavage sites between the extracellular and transmembrane regions have not yet been characterized.

ACKNOWLEDGMENTS

The experimental work referred to in this article was supported by grants from the Deutsche Forschungsgemeinschaft (SFB 542) and the Fonds der Chemischen Industrie (Frankfurt a.M.).

REFERENCES

1. Lütticken, C., Wegenka, U. M., Yuan, J., Buschmann, J., Schindler C., Ziemiecki, A., Harpur, A.G., Wilks, A. F., Yasukawa, K., Taga, T., Kishimoto, T., Barbieri, G., Pellegrini, S., Sendtner, M., Heinrich, P. C., and Horn, F., 1994, Association of transcription factor APRF and protein kinase Jak 1 with the Interleukin-6 signal transducer gp 130. *Science* **263**: 89-92.
2. Stahl, N., Boulton, T. G., Farruggella, T., Ip, N. Y., Davis, S., Witthuhn, B. A., Quelle, F. W., Silvennoinen, O., Barbieri, G., Pellegrini, S., Ihle, N. J., and Yancopoulos G. D., 1994. Association and activation of Jak-Tyk kinases by CNTF-LIF-OSM-IL-6 β receptor components. *Science* **263**: 92-95.
3. Heinrich P. C., Behrmann I., Müller-Newen G., Schaper F., and Graeve L., 1998. Interleukin-6-type cytokine signalling through the gp130/Jak/STAT pathway. *Biochem. J.* **334**: 297-314.
4. Haspel R. L., Salditt-Georgieff M., and Darnell Jr., J. E., 1996.The rapid inactivation of nuclear tyrosine phosphorylated Stat1 depends upon a protein tyrosine phosphatase. *EMBO J.* **15**: 6262-6268.
5. Kim T. K. and Maniatis T., 1996. Regulation of interferon-gamma-activated STAT1 by the ubiquitin-proteasome pathway. *Science* **273**: 1717-1719.
6. Stahl N., Farruggella T. J., Boulton T. G., Zhong Z., Darnell Jr. J. E., and Yancopoulos G. D., 1995. Choice of STATs and other substrates specified by modular tyrosine-based motifs in cytokine receptors. *Science* **267**: 1349-1353.
7. Schaper F., Gendo C., Eck M., Schmitz J., Grimm C., Anhuf D., Kerr I. M., and Heinrich P. C., 1998. Activation of the protein tyrosine phosphatase SHP2 via the interleukin-6 signal transducing receptor protein gp130 requires tyrosine kinase Jak1 and limits acute-phase protein expression. *Biochem. J.* **335** : 557-565.
8. Anhuf D., Weissenbach M., Schmitz J., Sobota R., Hermanns H. M., Radtke S., Linnemann S., Behrmann I., Heinrich P. C., and Schaper F., 2000. Signal transduction of IL-6, leukemia-inhibitory factor, and oncostatin M: structural receptor requirements for signal attenuation. *J. Immunol.* **165**: 2535-2543.
9. Endo T. A., Masuhara M., Yokouchi M., Suzuki R., Sakamoto H., Mitsui K., Matsumoto A., Tanimura S., Ohtsubo M., Misawa H., Miyazaki T., Leonor N., Taniguchi T., Fujita T., Kanakura Y., Komiya S., and Yoshimura A., 1997. A new protein containing an SH2 domain that inhibits JAK kinases. *Nature* **387**: 921-924
10. Starr R., Willson T. A., Viney E. M., Murray L .J., Rayner J. R., Jenkins B. J., Gonda T. J., Alexander W. S., Metcalf D., Nicola N. A., and Hilton D. J., 1997. A family of cytokine-inducible inhibitors of signalling. *Nature* **387**: 917-921.
11. Naka T., Narazaki M., Hirata M., Matsumoto T., Minamoto S., Aono A., Nishimoto N., Kajita T., Taga T., Yoshizaki K., Akira S., and Kishimoto T., 1997. Structure and function of a new STAT-induced STAT inhibitor. *Nature* **387**: 924-929.
12. Schmitz J., Weissenbach M., Haan S., Heinrich P. C., and Schaper F., 2000. SOCS3

exerts its inhibitory function on interleukin-6 signal transduction through the SHP2 recruitment site of gp130. *J. Biol. Chem.* **275**: 12848-12846.

13. Terstegen L., Gatsios P., Bode J. G., Schaper F., Heinrich P. C., and Graeve L., 2000. The inhibition of interleukin-6-dependent STAT activation by mitogen-activated protein kinases depends on tyrosine-759 in the cytoplasmic tail of gp130. *J. Biol. Chem.* **275**: 18810-18817.
14. Chung C. D., Liao J. Y., Liu B., Rao X. P., Jay P., Berta P., and Shuai K., 1997. Specific inhibition of Stat3 signal transduction by PIAS3. *Science* **278**: 1803-1805.
15. Rödel B., Tavassoli K., Karsunky H., Schmidt T., Bachmann M., Schaper F., Heinrich P., Shuai K., Elsässer H. P., and Möröy T., 2000. The zinc finger protein gfi-1 can enhance STAT3 signaling by interacting with the STAT3 inhibitor PIAS3. *EMBO J.* **19**: 5845-5855.
16. Dittrich E., Haft C. R., Muys L., Heinrich P. C., and Graeve L., 1996. A di-leucine motif and an upstream serine in the interleukin-6 (IL-6) signal transducer gp130 mediate ligand-induced endocytosis and down-regulation of the IL-6 receptor. *J. Biol. Chem.* **271**: 5487-5494
17. Thiel S., Behrmann I., Dittrich E., Muys L., Tavernier J., Wijdenes J., Heinrich P. C., and Graeve L. 1998. Internalization of the interleukin 6 signal transducer gp130 does not require activation of the Jak/STAT pathway. *Biochem. J.* **330**: 47-54.
18. Martens A. S., Bode J. G., Heinrich P. C., and Graeve L., 2000. The cytoplasmic domain of the interleukin-6 receptor gp80 mediates its basolateral sorting in polarized madin-darby canine kidney cells. *J. Cell. Sci.* **113**: 3593-3602.

Cytokine-induced STAT signalling through the cytoplasmic compartment

PRAVIN B. SEHGAL
Departments of Cell Biology & Anatomy, and Medicine, New York Medical College, Valhalla, New York, USA

1. INTRODUCTION

The standard model for cytokine-induced signalling through the cytoplasmic compartment by the family of proteins designated "STATs" ("signal transducers and activators of transcription") posits that STAT proteins exist in the cytoplasmic compartment as monomers which are activated by tyrosine (Tyr) phosphorylation by receptor-associated Janus family kinases (JAKs), the Tyr-phosphorylated STATs dimerize and then the STAT dimers translocate to the nucleus[1]. In previous work from this laboratory we have evaluated whether STAT proteins existed in the cytoplasmic compartment as free monomers and whether these then dimerized upon Tyr-phosphorylation following cytokine induction[2,3]. We used gel-filtration chromatography through Superose-6 columns for sizing STAT protein complexes, and observed that STAT1, STAT3, STAT5a, and STAT5b existed in complexes of size 200-400 kDa and 1-2 MDa in the cytosolic compartment of hepatocytes (rat liver or human Hep3B hepatoma cell lines)[2,3]. Upon stimulation with interleukin-6 (IL-6) there was no appreciable shift in size of the Tyr-phosphorylated STAT3 that would indicate the occurrence of a simple monomer to dimer transition[2,3]. These observations, among others, led us to propose that STAT proteins existed in the cytoslic compartment not as free monomers but as high molecular weight complexes of size 200-400 kDa ("statosome I") and 1-2 Mda ("statosome

Progress in Basic and Clinical Immunology, Edited by Mackiewicz *et al.*
Kluwer Academic/Plenum Publishers, New York, 2001

II") in association with other proteins which regulated STAT function and trafficking through the cytoplasmic compartment[2,3] (Fig. 1).

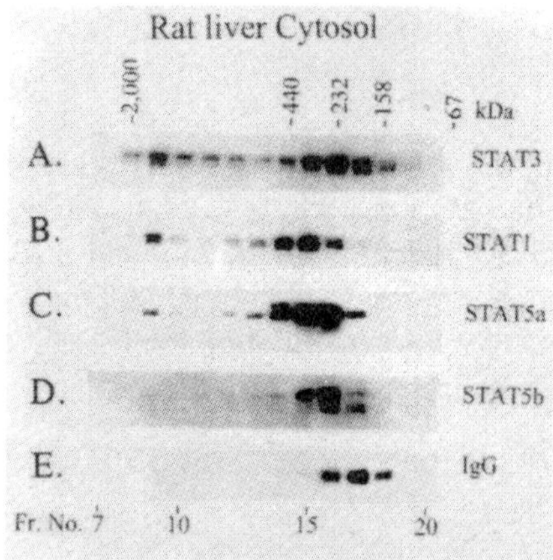

Figure 1. Suprose-6 FPLC analyses of STAT proteins in rat liver cytosol. Aliquots of 200 μl of rat liver cytosol (the 100K xg supernatant) was fractionated through Superose-6 FPLC and the elution of various STAT proteins evaluated by SDS-PAGE and Western blotting of 100 μl aliquots of each eluate fraction. Panels A-D show the elution of STAT3, STAT1, STAT5a and STAT5b. Panel E shows the elution of murine anti-STAT3 mAb (IgG)(approx. 160-180 kDa) off the same column in a separate run. From ref. 2.

In this article we briefly discuss data which address several issues: (1) the reliability of Superose-6 FPLC for estimating the size of STAT proteins; (2) the analysis of cytosolic STAT protein complexes by two-dimensional polyacrylamide gel electrophoresis (2-D PAGE); (3) the extent of cytoplasm to nucleus translocation of STAT3 in response to IL-6; and, (4) the possible association of STAT3 with sedimentable cytoplasmic structures, including organelles.

2. RESULTS AND DISCUSSION

2.1 Reliability of estimating the size of STAT proteins by gel filtration FPLC

The Western blot data in Fig. 1 show that various STAT proteins in the cytosolic postmicrosomal fraction of rat liver hepatocytes elute off a Superose-6 FPLC column with a bimodal distribution: the bulk of the STAT proteins elute in complexes of apparent size 200-400 kDa while a smaller amount of STAT proteins is present in complexes of size 1-2 MDa[2]. In interpreting protein-sizing data such as in Fig. 1, it has been suggested that the use of globular proteins (bovine serum albumin, aldolase, catalase, ferritin) as markers for estimating the size of STAT proteins in solution is inappropriate on the grounds that STAT proteins may have an extended shape[4]. Thus even though the bulk of STAT proteins elute in the 200-400 kDa region off Superose-6 columns, it has been argued that this material is a free monomer[4], and that an approach to validate the gel-filtration sizing of STAT proteins would be to express a recombinant non-Tyr-phosphorylated monomer STAT protein, express a recombinant Tyr-phosphorylated STAT dimer and then verify the gel-filtration properties of the respective recombinant monomer and dimer.

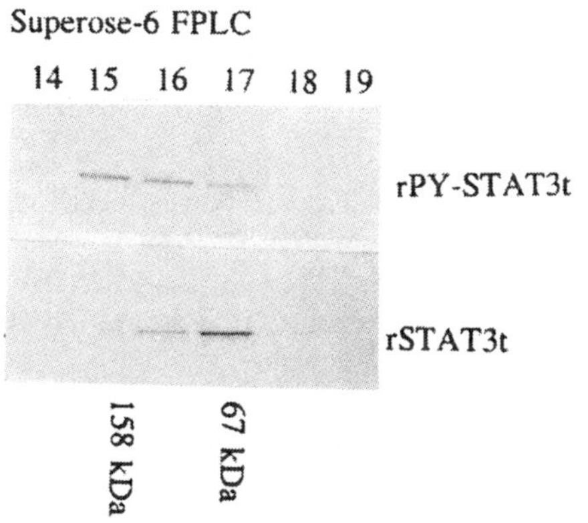

Figure 2. Superose-6 FPLC of recombinant monomeric STAT3t ("rSTAT3t") and recombinant dimeric Tyr-phosphorylated STAT3t ("rPY-STAT3t) produced in E. coli as described by Becker *et al.* (ref. 5). Figure illustrates Coomassie blue-stained SDS-PAGE of the purified recombinant proteins as compared to the elution of aldolase (158 kDa) and bovine serum albumin (67 kDa).

The data in Fig. 2 verify that that the elution profiles of recombinant E.coli-derived STAT3t monomer and the recombinant Tyr-phosphorylated-STAT3t dimer expressed matches those expected of the monomer and the dimer (approximately 70 kDa for the monomer and 140 kDa for the dimer) even though the globular proteins catalase (232 kDa), aldolase (158 kDa) and bovine serum albumin (67 kDa) were used for calibration. Additionally, we have verified that the Tyr-phosphorylated STAT3t dimer possesses DNA-binding activity (data not shown). These data obtained in our laboratory confirm similar conclusions reached earlier by Becker et al.[5], and further support our interpretation of the data in Fig. 1 as indicating the absence of free monomeric STAT proteins in the cytosolic compartment, and support our proposal of the statosome model. Similar conclusions about the role of "accessory proteins" in forming high-molecular weight complexes of STAT1 in the cytosol of HeLa cells, including the reliability of STAT sizing data derived from gel filtration chromatography, were also reached by Lackmann et al[6].

2.2 Two-dimensional PAGE of STAT3-containing cytosolic complexes

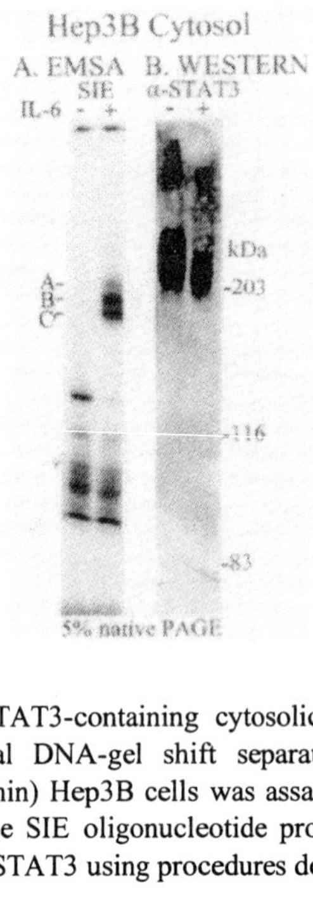

Figure 3. Western blotting of STAT3-containing cytosolic complexes separated through native PAGE (5%) using typical DNA-gel shift separation conditions. Cytosol from uninduced and IL-6-induced (30 min) Hep3B cells was assayed in a DNA-binding assay in panel A (10 μl aliquots) using the SIE oligonucleotide probe and using Western blotting (approximately 50 μl aliquots) for STAT3 using procedures described in ref. 2.

We have used the technique of two-dimensional PAGE to further investigate cytosolic STAT3-containing complexes. We carried out native 5% PAGE in the first dimension under conditions used in standard DNA-binding gel-shift assays[2]. Western blotting of such native gels revealed the presence of STAT3 in two complexes which migrated slower than the DNA-bound SIF-A, B and C complexes (which include the IL-6-inducible STAT3 homodimer, STAT1/3 heterodimer and STAT1 homodimer respectively) Fig.3). In native gels, the apparent mobility of these complexes corresponded to sizes > 200 kDa (although the migration of proteins in native gels need not correspond to their size, a comparison of Fig. 1 with Fig. 3 suggests that the STAT3 complex in the 200-400 kDa region in Fig. 3 apparently corresponds to statsosome I while the slower migrating complex >>500 kDa may correspond to statosome II). Fig. 4 shows that these native complexes when analysed in the second dimension by 7.5% PAGE under reducing and denaturing conditions release Western-blottable STAT3 of molecular mass 91 kDa. Similar data were obtained for STAT1 in cytosolic complexes in native PAGE in the first dimension and upon SDS-PAGE in the second dimension (data not shown).

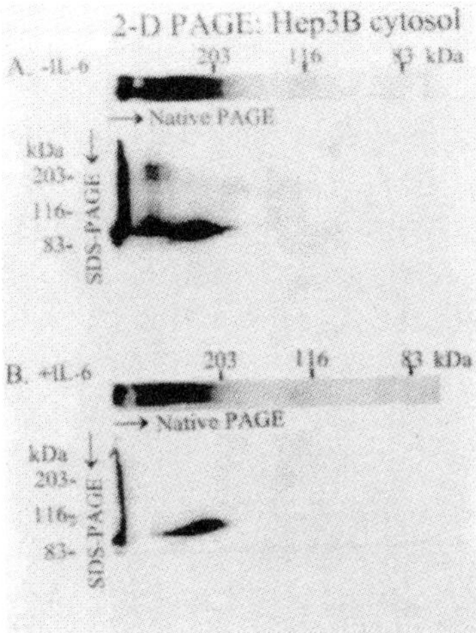

Figure 4. Two-dimensional PAGE and Western blotting analyses of statosome I and II complexes present in the cytosol of Hep3B cells. Aliquots (approximately 50µl) of cytosol from uninduced and IL-6 induced Hep3B cells were separated by native PAGE as in Fig. 3 in the first dimension and then through SDS-PAGE (7.5%) in the second dimension, and STAT3 complexes probed by Western blotting.

However, STAT1 and STAT3 were largely included in different cytosolic complexes in that anti-STAT3 antibody "supershifted" only STAT3 but not STAT1 when assayed by native PAGE and Western blotting (Fig. 6 in ref. 2), and when assayed by gel-filtration FPLC (Fig. 8 in ref. 2). While the proteins in these complexes remain to be identified, we have previously reported that anti-STAT3 antibody "coshifts" several proteins including the glucose regulated protein 58 (GRP58) together with STAT3 and that antibody to GRP58 inhibits the DNA-binding activity of the SIF-A complex. Collum et al[7] have also recently reported the identification of a protein designated "StIP1" which associates with nonphosphorylated STAT3 in the cytosol.

2.3 Extent of cytoplasm to nucleus translocation of STAT3 in response to IL-6

It has become customary in discussions of cytokine-induced STAT protein translocation to think of a large-scale bulk movement of STATs from the cytoplasm to the nucleus. As presented in the published literature this is typically illustrated using immunofluorescence data for cytokine-induced cytoplasm to nucleus translocation which appear to show the emptying of respective STATs from the cytoplasm and their accumulation in the nucleus[1]. Nevertheless, when biochemical assays have been used for assaying for STAT proteins, such as ^{35}S-methionine labelling or Western blotting, at best only 15-30% of the bulk of the respective STAT1 or STAT3 proteins have been observed to be translocated to the nucleus (e.g. STAT1 translocation in interferon-gamma-induced HeLa cells[8] or STAT3 translocation in IL-6-induced hepatoma Hep3B cells[2]). Furthermore, when assayed biochemically or by immunofluorescence only approximately half of the cytoplasmic pool of Tyr-phosphorylated STAT3 in IL-6-induced Hep3B cells appears to be translocated to the nucleus[2,9].

Thus, upon cytokine stimulation only a minority fraction of the cytoplasmic STAT proteins are translocated to the nuclear compartment, and it has been argued that in particular cell systems, perhaps as much as 90% of the cytosolic STAT1 is unavailable for signal transduction[6]. As assayed by gel-filtration analyses, Tyr-phosphorylated STAT3 in IL-6-treated Hep3B cytoplasm was found predominantly in complexes which correspond to statosome I (200-400 kDa) and statosome II (1-2 MDa) complexes[2]. Similarly Tyr-phosphorylated STAT1 in interferon-γ-induced HeLa cell cytosol was found in complexes of size 200-300 kDa[6], and Tyr-phosphorylated STAT3 and STAT5 were found in complexes of size 200-400 kDa and >1 MDa in the cytosol of cells induced with colony stimulating factor 1[10].

The disparity between the biochemical results and the immunofluorescence data concerning the extent of STAT protein translocation in response to cytokines may reside in variable immunological accesibility of the respective STAT proteins in the different cellular compartments. Rayanade et al[9,11] have reported the phenomenon of "STAT-masking" in which the immunological accesibility of STAT proteins assayed using confocal immunofluorescence analyses was markedly reduced in the cytoplasm and nucleus of IL-6-treated Hep3B cells expressing a wt-like mutant of p53 (Val-135), even though Western blotting assays for STAT3 revealed no loss of STAT3 from any compartment.

2.4 Association of STAT proteins with sedimentable cytoplasmic structures, including organelles

Further support for the existence of the large 1-2 MDa statosome II complexes (see Fig. 1) derives from the discovery of 100,000 x*g* sedimentable complexes of STAT1 and STAT3 in the cytosol of IL-6-treated Hep3B cells from within which structures DNA-binding activity can be released in cell-free DNA-shift assays. The possibility that STAT proteins, in particular Tyr-phosphorylated STAT3, may be associated with cytoplasmic organelles such as plasma membrane, mitochondria and/or endoplasmic reticulum or other intracytoplasmic organelles is suggested by the observation that the "mitochondrial pellet" ("MP" in Fig. 2 in ref. 2) contained 5-10% of the total cellular STAT3 and up to 20% of the cellular Tyr-phosphorylated STAT3 in IL-6-treated Hep3B cells, as assayed by Western blotting for these proteins.

The possibility that STAT proteins might be involved in plasma membrane to organelle signalling or organelle to nucleus signalling is a tantalizing and exciting issue to evaluate.

3. CONCLUSIONS

Recent experimental data from this and several other laboratories[2,3,6,10] have cast doubt on aspects of the standard model[1] of STAT signalling. We and others[2,3,6,10] have found that the bulk of the STAT proteins existed in the cytosolic compartment as high-molecular weight complexes (termed "statosomes" by us[2,3]) in association with various accessory proteins. The statosome model of STAT signalling proposes that the signalling function of STAT proteins through the cytoplasmic compartment is regulated by these cytosolic accessory proteins. Association of STAT proteins with cytoplasmic organelles and with mediating organellar function is a novel possibility that deserves evaluation.

ACKNOWLEDGEMENTS

Research in this laboratory was supported by Research Grant CA-82647 from the National Institutes of Health. We thank Dr. Christoph W. Muller for providing the recombinant STAT3 constructs.

REFERENCES

1. Darnell, J.E., Jr., 1997, STATs and gene regulation. *Science* 277:1630-1635.
2. Ndubuisi, M.I., Guo, G.G., Fried, V.A., Etlinger, J.D. and Sehgal, P.B., 1999, Cellular physiology of STAT3: where's the cytoplasmic monomer? *J. Biol. Chem.* 274: 25499-25509.
3. Sehgal, P.B., 2000, STAT-signalling through the cytoplasmic compartment: consideration of a new paradigm. *Cell. Signalling* 12: 525-535.
4. Qureshi, S.A., Salditt-Georgieff, M., and Darnell, J.E., Jr., 1995, Tyrosine-phosphorylated Stat1 and Stat2 plus a 48-kDa protein all contact DNA in forming interferon-stimulated-gene factor 3. *Proc. Natl. Acad. Sci. USA* 92: 3829-3833.
5. Becker, S., Corthals, G.L., Aebersold, R., Groner, B., and Muller, C.W., 1998, Expression of a tyrosine phosphorylated, DNA binding STAT3β dimer in bacteria. *FEBS Lett.* 441: 141-147.
6. Lackmann, M., Harpur, A.G., Oates, A.C., Mann, R.J., Gabriel, A., Meutermans, W., Alewood, P.F., Kerr, I.M., Stark, G.R., and Wilks, A.F., 1998, Biomolecular interaction analysis of IFNγ-induced signaling events in whole-cell lysates: prevalence of latent STAT1 in high-molecular weight complexes. *Growth Factors* 16:39-51.
7. Collum, R.G., Brutsaert, S., Lee, G., and Schindler, C., 2000, A Stat3-interacting protein (StIP1) regulates cytokine signal transduction. *Proc. Natl. Acad. Sci. USA* 97: 10120-10125.
8. Haspel, R.L., Salditt-Georgieff, M., and Darnell, J.E., Jr., 1996, The rapid inactivation of nuclear tyrosine phosphorylated STAT1 depends upon a protein tyrosine phosphatase. *EMBO J.* 22:6262-6268.
9. Rayanade, R.J., Ndubuisi, M.I., Etlinger, J.D., and Sehgal, P.B., 1998, Regulation of IL-6 signaling by p53: STAT3- and STAT5-masking in p53-Val-135-containing human hepatoma Hep3B cell lines. *J. Immunol.* 161:325-334.
10. Yeung, Y.G., Wang, Y., Einstein, D.B., Lee, P.S.W., and Stanley, E.R., 1998, Colony-stimulating factor-1 stimulates the formation of multimeric cytosolic complexes of signaling proteins and cytoskeletal components in macrophages. *J. Biol. Chem.* 273:17128-17137.
11. Rayanade, R.J., Patel, K., Ndubuisi, M.I., Sharma, S., Omura, S., Etlinger, J.D., Pine, R., and Sehgal, P.B., 1997, Proteasome- and p53-dependent masking of signal transducer and activator of transcription (STAT) factors. *J. Biol. Chem.* 272:4659-4662.

Cytokine-mediated growth inhibition of human melanoma cells

MARCIN KORTYLEWSKI[*,#], PETER C. HEINRICH[*], ANDRZEJ MACKIEWICZ[#], and IRIS BEHRMANN[*]
[*]Department of Biochemistry, RWTH Aachen, Germany; [#]Department of Cancer Immunology at GreatPoland Cancer Center, University School of Medical Sciences, Poznan, Poland

1. INTRODUCTION

Interleukin-(IL)-6 and oncostatin M (OSM), closely related cytokines sharing gp130 as a common receptor signal transducing subunit[1], are known for their antiproliferative action on melanocytes[2] and melanoma cells from early phases of tumor growth[3,4]. In contrast, cells from advanced stage melanomas in most cases acquire a so called „multicytokine resistance" phenotype becoming unresponsive to several cytokines including IL-6 and/or OSM. Therefore, it seems plausible that local paracrine growth inhibition plays an important role for the prevention of the first *in situ* stages of melanoma development. We and others suggest that in the case of melanoma cells Jak/STAT signaling can be critical for the negative regulation of their growth[5,6].

2. MOLECULAR MECHANISM OF gp130-MEDIATED GROWTH INHIBITION

As a cellular model to study the antiproliferative action of IL-6 and OSM we have chosen human A375 melanoma cells. Both cytokines significantly inhibit growth of A375 cells, although the effect of OSM is more

Progress in Basic and Clinical Immunology, Edited by Mackiewicz *et al.*
Kluwer Academic/Plenum Publishers, New York, 2001

pronounced. A very early effect that can be observed upon stimulation of cells with IL-6-type cytokines is the activation of latent cytoplasmic STAT factors, which subsequently translocate to the nucleus. We observed that in A375 cells the level of activation of STAT3 and STAT1 factors correlated with the growth inhibitory effects of IL-6 and OSM. To investigate the role of the STATs for the growth inhibitory action of IL-6 type cytokines in greater detail, we took advantage of chimeric receptors consisting of the extracellular region of the erythropoietin (EPO) receptor fused to the transmembrane and intracellular parts of gp130[7]. It enabled us to study signals elicited by the cytoplasmic part of gp130 or muteins thereof independently of endogeneous wild type gp130 in A375 cells. A truncated chimeric receptor retaining only the membrane-proximal region of gp130 did neither activate STATs nor mediate growth arrest of stable transfectants. These functions were restored by the addition of short STAT recruitment modules comprising critical tyrosine residues from gp130 (Y767, Y814).

Moreover, we used dominant negative forms of STAT1 and STAT3 to discern between their roles in mediating the growth inhibition[8]. Overexpression of dominant negative forms of STAT3 but not of STAT1 abrogated the inhibitory effect of IL-6 as well as of OSM in A375 cells. Therefore, STAT3 seems to play a crucial role in transmitting the antiproliferative effects of IL-6-type cytokines.

In further studies, we have identified the cyclin-dependent kinase inhibitor p27/Kip1 gene as a novel target of positive regulation by IL-6 and OSM. p27/Kip1, a cyclin-dependent kinase inhibitor, is known to prevent cell cycle progression by inhibiting the activity of cyclin E-associated kinase (cdk2)[9]. We observed STAT3-dependent upregulation of p27 mRNA by IL-6 and OSM, which correlated with an accumulation of p27 protein. Our finding implicates a possible importance of p27/Kip1 for melanoma development which corresponds to reports demonstrating an inverse relation between p27-levels and tumor thickness[10] as well as the silencing of p27 gene by its promoter methylation in a significant proportion of melanomas[11].

3. ROLE OF MAPK IN CONTROL OF p27/KIP1 EXPRESSION

The mitogen-activated protein kinases (MAPK) Erk1 and Erk2 play a crucial role in the regulation of cell growth and differentiation. A number of studies has suggested the involvement of the MAPK cascade in promoting melanoma development. *Ras* mutations activating the MAPK cascade were observed in about 20% of primary melanomas, and at even higher rates in the case of metastatic and recurrent melanomas[12,13].

We have shown that the gp130-mediated activation of tyrosine phosphatase SHP-2, often acting as an adaptor to the Ras/MAPK pathway, did not affect the growth behavior of transfected human A375 melanoma cells[6]. Erk1 and Erk2 kinases turned out to be constitutively active. Using PD98059, a specific inhibitor of MEK1 kinase, we investigated the role of persistently activated MAP kinases for cell growth. The inhibition of MAPK activity induced a dose-dependent growth arrest in the G0/G1 phase. Correspondingly, we observed potent upregulation of the cyclin-dependent kinase inhibitor p27/Kip1 resulting at least in part from its increased stability. Similar effects were also observed in the case of another human melanoma cell line, WM239. Our findings suggest that constitutively active Erk1/2 kinases contribute to the growth of melanoma cells by decreasing the stability of the p27/Kip1 inhibitor. The efficient growth inhibitory action of PD98059, a specific inhibitor of Erk1/2 activation, underlines the potential of novel therapeutic approaches targeting members of the Ras/Raf/MAPK pathway in the treatment of human melanoma. Moreover, our study emphasizes the role of p27/Kip1as a plausible key player in the control of melanoma cell proliferation (Fig. 1).

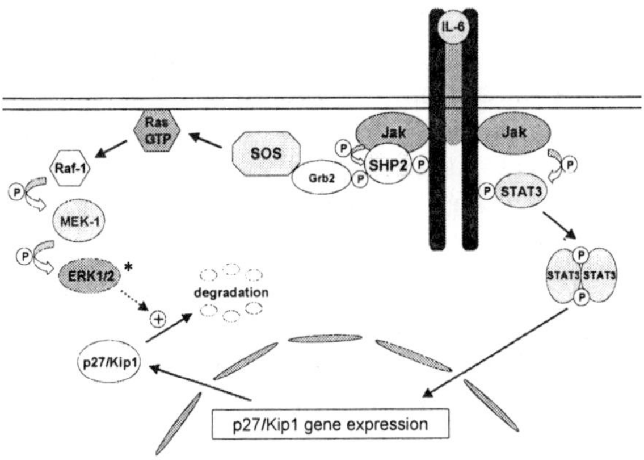

Figure 1. p27/Kip1 as a plausible target of regulation by opposing signals via Jak/STAT and MAPK pathways (*constitutively active in A375 and WM239 melanoma cells).

ACKNOWLEDGMENTS

This work has been supported by grants from the START program of the RWTH Aachen, the State Committee for Scientific Research (Warsaw), the

Deutsche Forschungemeinschaft (Bonn), and the Fonds der Chemischen Industrie (Frankfurt). We like to thank Heike Hermanns for her help with the preparation of the manuscript.

REFERENCES

1. Heinrich, P.C., Behrmann, I., G, M.-N., Schaper, F., Graeve, L.,1998, Interleukin-6-type cytokine signalling through the gp130/Jak/STAT pathway. *Biochem J*, 334:297-314.
2. Swope, V.B., Abdel-Malek, Z., Kassem, L.M., Nordlund, J.J.,1991, Interleukins1α and 6 and tumor necrosis factor-α are paracrine inhibitors of human melanocyte proliferation and melanogenesis. *J Invest Dermatol*, 96:180-5.
3. Lu, C., Vickers M. F., Kerbel R. S., 1992, Interleukin 6: a fibroblast-derived growth inhibitor of human melanoma cells from early but not advanced stages of tumor progression. *Proc. Natl. Acad. Sci. USA*, 89:9215-9219.
4. Lu, C., Rak J. W., Kobayashi H., Kerbel R. S., 1993, Increased resistance to oncostatin M-induced growth inhibition of human melanoma cell lines derived from advanced-stage lesions. *Cancer Res.* 53:2708-2711.
5. Oh, J.-W., Katz A., Haroch S., Eisenbach L., Revel M., Chebath J., 1997, Unmasking by soluble IL-6 receptor of IL-6 effect on metastatic melanoma: growth inhibition and differentiation of B16-F10.9 tumor cells. *Oncogene*, 15:569-577.
6. Kortylewski, M., Heinrich, P. C., Mackiewicz, A., Schniertshauer, U., Klingmuller, U., Nakajima, K., Hirano, T., Horn, F., Behrmann, I., 1999, Interleukin-6 and oncostatin M-induced growth inhibition of human A375 melanoma cells is STAT-dependent and involves upregulation of the cyclin-dependent kinase inhibitor p27/Kip1. *Oncogene*, 18:3742-53.
7. Gerhartz, C., Heesel, B., Sasse, J., Hemmann, U., Landgraf, C., Schneider-Mergener, J., Horn, F., Heinrich, P.C., Graeve, L., 1996, Differential activation of acute phase response factor/STAT3 and STAT1 via the cytoplasmic domain of the interleukin 6 signal transducer gp130. *J Biol Chem*, 271:12991-8.
8. Nakajima, K., Yamanaka, Y., Nakae, K., Kojima, H., Ichiba, M., Kiuchi, N., Kitaoka, T., Fukada, T., Hibi, M., Hirano, T., 1996, A central role for Stat3 in IL-6-induced regulation of growth and differentiation in M1 leukemia cells. *Embo J*, 15:3651-8.
9. Sherr C.J., Roberts.J.M., 1999, CDK inhibitors: positive and negative regulators of G1-phase progression. *Genes Dev,* 13:1501-1512.
10. Florenes, V.A., Maelandsmo, G.M., Kerbel, R.S., Slingerland, J.M., Nesland, J.M., Holm, R., 1998, Protein expression of the cell-cycle inhibitor p27Kip1 in malignant melanoma: inverse correlation with disease-free survival. *Am J Pathol*, 153:305-12..
11. Worm J., Bartkova J., Kirkin A.F., Straten P., Zeuthen J., Bartek J., Guldberg P., 2000, Aberrant $p27^{Kip1}$ promoter methylation in malignant melanoma. *Oncogene*, 19:5111-5115.
12. Ball, N. J., Yohn, J. J., Morelli, J. G., Norris, D. A., Golitz, L. E., Hoeffler, J. P.,1994, Ras mutations in human melanoma: a marker of malignant progression. *J Invest Dermatol,* 102:285-90.
13. Jafari, M., Papp, T., Kirchner, S., Diener, U., Henschler, D., Burg, G., Schiffmann, D., 1995, Analysis of ras mutations in human melanocytic lesions: activation of the ras gene seems to be associated with the nodular type of human malignant melanoma. *J Cancer Res Clin Oncol*, 121:23-30.

Interleukin-6, tumor necrosis factor α and interferon γ in patients with anorexia nervosa

RENATA KOMOROWSKA-PIETRZYKOWSKA*, ANDRZEJ RAJEWSKI*, MAGDALENA SOBIESKA# and KRZYSZTOF WIKTOROWICZ#

**Department of Child and Adolescent Psychiatry, 27/33 Szpitalna Street, #Chair of Biology and Environmental Protection, ½ Długa Street, University of Medical Sciences, Poznań, Poland*

1. INTRODUCTION

Several factors influence the immune system in Anorexia Nervosa, among them the inadequate supply of the alimentary compounds and disturbances in the neuroendocrine system. The previously reported changes in some cytokines' concentrations were regarded not only as an effect of the disease but were postulated to be one of the reasons of AN.

2. MATERIAL AND METHODS

20 patients with AN according to DSM-IV criteria (15 restricting type; 5 bulimic type):

Body Mass Index (BMI) before treatment 10.6 - 17.9

Duration of illness 2 - 60 months

Depression severity 7 - 16 points (Hamilton Depression Scale- HDS)

Patients were treated with psychotherapy, only those with severe depressive symptoms were shortly given mianserin (15 mg) for not longer than four weeks.

Progress in Basic and Clinical Immunology, Edited by Mackiewicz *et al.*
Kluwer Academic/Plenum Publishers, New York, 2001

Serum concentrations of IL-6, TNF α and IFN γ, before and after the treatment were assessed using ELISA method with respective kits from R&D, USA.

3. RESULTS

Patients were divided into subgroups as follows:
C - whole investigated group
1A – patients with BMI<15, 1B –patients with BMI ∃ 15
2A – patients with disease duration shorter than 12 months
2B – patients with disease duration equal or longer than 12 months
3A – patients with HDS <13
3B – patients with HDS ∃ 13
4A – patients with restricting type of Anorexia
4B – patients with bulimic type of Anorexia
TNF α was not detected in any investigated sample.

The concentration of IL-6 was elevated in all sera samples against normal values. Significantly higher values were observed in patients with more pronounced depressive symptoms and they decreased after treatment, but not in patients suffering from AN longer than one year.

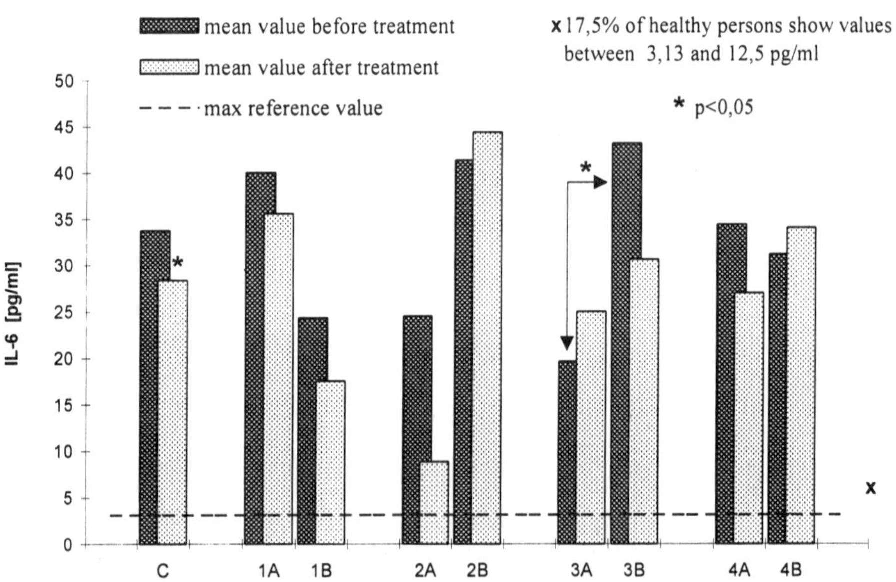

Figure 1: Mean IL-6 concentrations before and after treatment

Mean concentration of IFN γ was also elevated against normal values. Significantly higher values were observed in patients with BMI<15. The concentration of IFN γ increased after treatment.

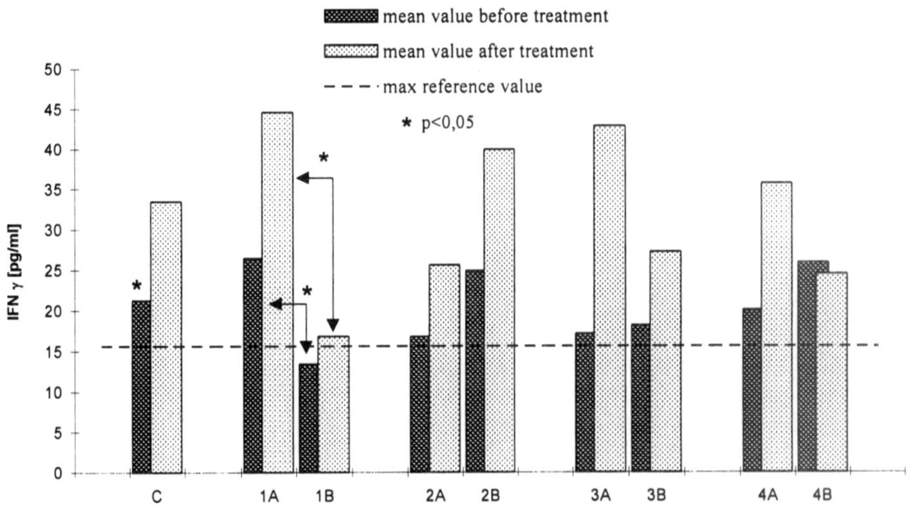

Figure 2: Mean IFN γ concentrations before and after treatment

4. CONCLUSIONS

(i)Increased concentration of IFN γ and IL-6 was shown in Anorexia Nervosa. (ii) IL-6 level was significantly higher in patients with more pronounced depressive symptoms, than in patients with HDS score below 13. (iii) Serum concentration of IFN γ was significantly elevated in patients showing more symptoms of emaciation, than in patients with BMI above 15. Weight restoration did not eliminate alterations in the cytokine concentrations.

The increase of serum concentrations of IL-6 and IFN γ is an indication of a disregulation in the cytokine network in patients suffering from anorexia, as any inflammatory stimulus may be excluded on the basis of normal blood morphology, ESR and not elevated TNF α. Both IL-6 (previously called interferon- ∃2) and IFN γ seem to be stimulated by the same, non-inflammatory stimulus, probably an alteration in the neurotransmitters. Increased concentration of IFN γ may contribute to low incidence of viral infection in AN patients. On the other hand, persisting elevated levels of this cytokine may lead to autoimmune disturbances. In the presented data the level of IFN γ did not normalize after restoration of body weight, what could indicate that the stimulating factor is still present. Similarly, an elevated concentration of IL-6 persisted despite the improvement of body mass and it was independent of any treatment. It was already described that this may lead to inhibition of lipogenesis (what could promote cachexia) and to enhancement of osteoporotic processes. An increase of IL-6 may be caused by improper alimentary behavior, but may also indicate the disturbed neurohormonal balance. Similar alterations were previously described for depressive patients.

REFERENCES

1. Maes M., Scharpe S., Melzer H.Y. et al.: Increased neopterin and interferon γ secretion and lower availability of L-tryptophan in major depression: further evidence for an immune response. Psychiatry Res. 1994, 54(2), 143-160
2. Holden R.J., Pacula I.S.: The role of Tumor Necrosis Factor α in the pathogenesis of Anorexia Nervosa and Bulimia Nervosa, Cancer Cachexia and Obesity. Med. Hypotheses 1996, 47, 423-438
3. Kaschka W.P.: Psychoneuroimmunology and neuroendocrinology – an integrative view. Current Update in Psychoimmunology. G. Wieselman (ed.) Springer-Verlag, Wien, New York 1997.
4. Monteleone P. Maes M., Fabrazzo M., Tortorella A., Lin B., Bosmans E., Kenis G., Maj M.: Immunoendocrine findings in patients with eating disorders. Neuropsychobiology 1999, 40, 115-120.
5. Schattner A., Tepper R., Steibock M., Hahn T., Schonfeld A: Tumour necrosis factor, interferon gamma and cell-mediated cytotoxity in anorexia nervosa. Clin. Exp. Immunol. 1990, 32(4), 183-184.
6. Chandra R.K.: Nutrition and Immunology. New York, Liss, 1988.
7. Służewska A., Rybakowski J.K., Bosmans E., Maes M., Sobieska M.: Some interleukins, their receptors and alpha-1-acid glycoprotein as indicators of immune activation in depression. Behav. Pharmacol. 1995, 6, 66-88.

Interleukin-1 system in testis - quantitative analysis

Expression of immunomodulatory genes in male gonad

NATALIA ROZWADOWSKA, DOROTA FISZER, MACIEJ KURPISZ
Institute of Human Genetic, Polish Academy of Sciences, Poznan, Poland

1. INTRODUCTION

There is a growing body of evidence suggesting that interleukin-1 and other cytokines may influence mammalian testis function. IL-1α activity seems to be tissue specific, and it appears in literature as a testicular interleukin-1 (tIL-1)[1]. Its activity was detected both in testicular interstitium and seminiferous epithelium. Being secreted in para- or autocrine manner, IL-1 inhibits steroidogenesis in Leydig cells, what suggests the modulatory role of this cytokine in LH-dependent testosterone synthesis. Sertoli cells are also capable to produce IL-1. The level of interleukin-1 expression in these cells is distinctly connected with the intensity of DNA synthesis in gametogenic cells. Thus IL-1 could be a nutritional factor, important for activity of seminiferous epithelium. Its expression both in Sertoli and Leydig cells depends on the local concentrations of hCG, FSH and LH and the other cytokines (e.g. TNFα) or growth factors in testis. Hence, IL-1 appears as another element of regulatory network essential for maintenance of testis physiology.[2]

Progress in Basic and Clinical Immunology, Edited by Mackiewicz *et al.*
Kluwer Academic/Plenum Publishers, New York, 2001

1.1 Initial Comments

Most of the data, concerning testicular IL-1 expression, come from animal models. We decided to investigate this problem in humans, due to the different organisation of seminiferous epithelium, which do not allow the extrapolation of results from rodents. We tried to estimate the levels of mRNA specific for IL-1α, IL-1β, IL-1R1 (IL-1 receptor 1) and IL-1RA (IL-1 receptor antagonist) genes in different functional fractions of human testicular cells. We used quantitative PCR with isotopic detection to determine the activity of IL-1 genes system.

2. MATERIALS AND METHODS

Testicular cells were isolated from human testis, obtained from individuals who had undergone orchidectomy for treatment of prostatic cancer, by using combined enzymatic (collagenase) and mechanical treatment. Then the cells were purified and fractionated on discontinuous Percoll gradient.[3]

Total RNA was extracted from fractionated cells applying GTC (guanidium isothiocyanate) method.

Standard RNA (cRNA) was prepared by *in vitro* transcription of two suitable plasmids. Plasmid pAW109 was used to obtain cRNA for genes coding for IL-1α and IL-1β and pBSK for genes coding for IL-1R1 and IL-1RA.

To obtain cDNA, the SuperScript reverse transcriptase with oligo dT_{15} primer was applied. Reaction contained 3μg of studied RNA and known number of copies of cRNA

The amplification of serial dilutions of cDNA, was performed. PCR mixture contained isotopic deoxynuleotide (^{32}P dCTP). PCR reaction product was electropohoresed on 10% polyacrylamide gels. After drying, the gels were read on Phosphoimaging detection system.[4]

3. RESULTS

The higher level of transcription for IL-1α and IL-1RA was observed in seminiferous epithelium as comparing to the interstitial compartment (Fig. 1, Table 1). On the other hand expression of genes for IL-1β and IL-1RI was stronger in the interstitium. than in intratubular fraction.

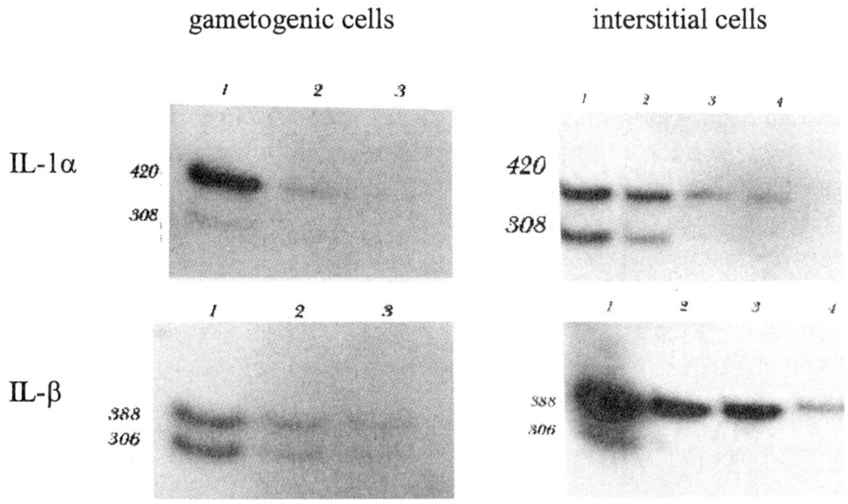

Figure 1. Visualisation of quantitative PCR products on 10% polyacrylamide gel. Tracks 1-4 show serial dilutions of cDNA (420bp, 388bp) with internal standards (cRNA – 308bp, 306bp).

Table 1. Number of copies of specific mRNA in 1 ng of total isolated RNA from different cell fractions.

GENES	INTRATUBULAR CELLS	INTERSTITIAL CELLS	PBL'S
INTERLEUKIN-1 ALFA	357,4	48,5	-
INTERLEUKIN-1 BETA	12,8	133,8	-
INTERLEUKIN-1 RECEPTOR I	10,3	92,2	31,6
INTERLEUKIN-1 RECEPTOR ANTAGONIST	211,2	138,4	569

4. CONCLUSIONS

Obtained results strongly indicated that human testicular cells originated both from seminiferous epithelium and interstitial tissue are capable to synthesise IL-1. Data indicated that the strongest transcription for IL-1α and IL-1RA genes takes place in the intratubular compartment of the testis. Probably pattern of this expression creates a specific paracrine system, which may control spermatogenesis without (in spite of high concentration of IL-1α) inflammatory reactions.

mRNA levels for genes of IL-1 system in extratubular compartment do not differ among each other. However high expression of genes coding for IL-1β and IL-1R1 in interstitium might possibly indicate the role of translated molecules as signalling factors of immune system.

REFERENCES

1. Khan S.A., Soder O. et al., 1987, The rat testis produces large amounts of an interleukin-1-like factor. Int. J. Androl. 10:459-503
2. Kurpisz M., Janitz M., 1995, Antigens and immunomodulatory factors in spermatogenesis. In: Immunology of Human Reproduction, Eds. Kurpisz M., Fernandez N. Bios Scientific Publishers, Ch.3: 33-52
3. Janitz M., Fiszer D., Łukaszyk A., Skorupski W., Kurpisz M., 1995, Analysis of mRNA expression for interleukin-1 genes on human testicular cells. *Immunol. Letters* 48: 139-143
4. Wang A.M., Doyle M.V., Mark D.F., 1989, Quantitation of mRNA by the polymerase chain reaction. *Proc. Natl. Acad. Sci.*; 86: 9717-21

IMMUNODEFICIENCIES

Mapping genes underlying complex disorders: progress on IgA deficiency and common variable immunodeficiency

I. VORECHOVSKY, A. D. B. WEBSTER, L. HAMMARSTROM
University College London, Royal Free Campus, London, UK and Karolinska Institute at NOVUM, Huddinge, Sweden

1. IGAD/CVID AS THE MOST COMMON PRIMARY IMMUNODEFICIENCIES SHARING GENETIC SUSCEPTIBILITY

IgA deficiency (IgAD, MIM 137100) is the most frequent primary immunodeficiency in humans (for review see Burrows and Cooper, 1997; Hammarstrom et al., 2000). It is characterized by the absence of IgA in serum and mucosal secretions due to an as yet unidentified defect of terminal lymphocyte differentiation. Affected individuals may suffer from susceptibility to infections and autoimmune complications. While IgAD is defined by a laboratory measurement and is usually asymptomatic, common variable immunodeficiency (CVID, MIM 240500) is characterized clinically by overt susceptibility to infections and by frequent inflammatory and autoimmune symptomatology. In addition to the lack of IgA, CVID patients have decreased levels of additional isotypes in serum.

Our previous systematic study (Vorechovsky et al., 1995) indicated a higher than expected prevalence of CVID among close relatives of IgAD patients, consistent with previously suggested shared pathogenesis of the two distinguishable primary immunodefiiencies (Olerup et al., 1992; Volanakis et al., 1992). A substantial proportion of families containing both IgAD and CVID was found in multiple-case families obtained by screening family

Progress in Basic and Clinical Immunology, Edited by Mackiewicz *et al.*
Kluwer Academic/Plenum Publishers, New York, 2001

members of IgAD patients for serum Ig levels (Vorechovsky et al., 1995). In multiple-case families with a dominant transmission of CVID/IgAD, CVID was usually present in the parental generation followed by the occurrence of IgAD in descendants (Vorechovsky et al., 1995). This observation is consistent with the hypothesis that CVID may develop later in life as a rare and more severe manifestation of a common, complex genetic defect. This hypothesis has been supported by a description of a gradual decline of IgG levels in serum that progressed at similar ages in affected siblings (Johnson et al., 1997) and the existence of IgG subclass deficiencies in a subset of IgAD patients (Oxelius et al., 1981). It is now well documented that CVID may develop from IgAD over time (Espanol et al., 1996; Ishizaka et al., 1989).

2. IGAD/CVID AS COMPLEX GENETIC TRAITS

IgAD and CVID do not segregate in families in a recognizable Mendelian pattern. While most multiple-case families show a dominant transmission of the defect (Vorechovsky et al., 1995), the inheritance pattern in some families resemble a recessive transmission (Koistinen, 1976; Wilton et al., 1985), suggesting - but not necessarily proving – locus heterogeneity. Indeed, extensive clinical heterogeneity of CVID and distinct inheritance patterns lead to a suggestion that CVID probably represents a group of genetic defects and that no single mechanism is likely to account for the disease pathogenesis. Attempts have been made to classify CVID into several classes (type A, B and C) (Spickett et al., 1997), but distinct pathogenetic mechanisms underlying phenotypic differences remain to be shown. The lack of the long-term follow-up of IgAD/CVID patients might help explain some of the observed heterogeneity, with the observed progression of milder forms of CVID to a more severe disease over time, or IgAD to IgG subclass deficiencies and overt CVID.

Unclear segregation pattern in families and putative multifactorial nature of IgAD/CVID has hampered the genetic dissection of these disorders. Although a number of cellular abnormalities were reported in CVID, functional studies of CVID over more than two decades have failed to identify the primary defect. Since the disease phenotype is persistent (Koskinen et al., 1994; Vorechovsky et al., 1995), the phenocopy rate is low and the relative risk to siblings (λ_s) estimated at 50 (Vorechovsky et al., 1995) indicates a strong degree of familial clustering, chromosome susceptibility loci underlying this complex trait should be detectable by genetic linkage analysis, followed by positional candidate gene strategies to identify the culprit molecules. Such an approach would obviate the need for an insight into disease pathogenesis.

2.1 The role of HLA

Numerous case-control studies have previously shown associations of HLA alleles with both IgAD and CVID (Ambrus et al., 1977; De La Concha et al., 1999; Hammarstrom et al., 1983; Machulla et al., 2000; Olerup et al., 1990; Schaffer et al., 1989; Wilton et al., 1985), suggesting the existence of a predisposing locus or loci in this region. Further support for the presence of a susceptibility mutation(s) in the MHC (designated *IGAD1*) awaited the evidence for genetic linkage as a significantly increased allele sharing in affected individuals and positive family-based allelic associations, as demonstrated by transmission disequilibrium tests (TDT) (Vorechovsky et al., 1999a; Vorechovsky et al., 2000). TDTs reduce the confounding effect of the population stratification or admixture on putative allelic associations in case-control studies. With a higher number of multiple-case families, the evidence for the presence of susceptibility gene(s) for IgAD/CVID in the MHC is now strong (Vorechovsky et al., 2000) and has been supported by both linkage and association studies.

However, although independent studies agree that the MHC contains a susceptibility gene(s) for IgAD/CVID, there is no consensus as to the exact location within the MHC. Fine mapping of *IGAD1* would facilitate a search for a genuine predisposing mutation(s), but this has been hindered by a high gene density in the region, excessive polymorphism, lower than average recombination fractions and several hot spots for meiotic crossover events in the MHC. The location of *IGAD1* in the class III region has been supported by the observed absence of IgAD among 43 Sardinian DR3 homozygotes who share class II but not class III alleles with the IgAD-associated Northern European haplotype (Cucca et al., 1998). A recent analysis of ancestral haplotypes in a large kindred with 3 CVID patients, 3 cases with IgAD and 2 cases with lower IgA levels (Schroeder et al., 1998) suggested that the region between the class III microsatellites designated *821/823* (Hsieh et al., 1997) and the HLA-B locus contained the susceptibility gene. However, our haplotype analysis based on the short tandem repeat haplotypes across the MHC does not favour this location and placed the disease gene to a more proximal region, extending between the telomeric part of the class II region and the centromeric part of the class III region (Vorechovsky et al., 2000). This long-lasting controversy (French et al., 1991; French and Dawkins, 1990; Olerup et al., 1991) has been difficult to resolve due to high linkage disequilibrium in the region, particularly on the extended HLA A1, -B8, -DR3 haplotypes. These haplotypes were shown to provide most of the

MHC-conferred susceptibility, although several other haplotypes show a disease association (Vorechovsky et al., 2000; Machulla et al., 2000).

Although a mere strength of allelic association in the MHC is unlikely to narrow down the region and point to the culprit gene, recent studies show the power of linkage disequilibrium fine-mapping even in mixed populations (Collins, 2000; Eaves et al., 2000) and in regions with marked differences of linkage disequilibrium measures, as exemplified by studies on type 1 diabetes (Herr et al., 2000). With a mosaic of completely sequenced MHC haplotypes available to the public (Consortium, 1999), it will now become possible to resolve this issue using linkage disequilibrium studies and a dense set of suitable polymorphic markers across the MHC in multiple-case families. Statistical methods for fine mapping using linkage disequilibrium analyses of ancestral haplotypes in general pedigrees have now become available (MacLean et al., 2000) and it is hoped that this approach will narrow down the disease gene to a smaller area amenable to further testing.

Indirect evidence suggests that the MHC is a major locus in determining the disease susceptibility and the role of putative non-MHC genes is only minor. First, the differences in the prevalence of IgAD among ethnic groups as determined by screening of blood donors for Ig levels appear to correspond to the prevalence of the susceptibility HLA A1, -B8, -DR3 haplotype (Table 1). A gradient in the prevalence of this haplotype can also be observed in European populations, with Welsh and Irish haplotype frequencies at the top and the Eastern Mediterranean frequencies at the bottom of the range; however, it remains to be shown that this gradient could be mirrored in the prevalence of IgAD.

Table 1. Population prevalence of IgAD and HLA-A1, B8, DR3 haplotypes in different ethnic groups

Ethnic group	Population prevalence of IgAD	Allele frequencies of DR3	Allele frequencies of B8	Haplotype frequencies of HLA-A1, B8, DR3
European Caucasians	1/300-700	Avg. 11%	Avg. 9%	2-12% (see Fig. 1)
Latin	1/1000 (Brazil)	8%	4%	1.7%
Han population in China	1/2600	6%	1.5%	0.3%
African Americans	1/6000	13%	4%	1.5%
Japanese	1/18500	0.3%	0%	0%

Source: Bone Marrow Donors Worldwide (www.bmdw.org and www.swmed.edu; Burrows and Cooper, 1997).

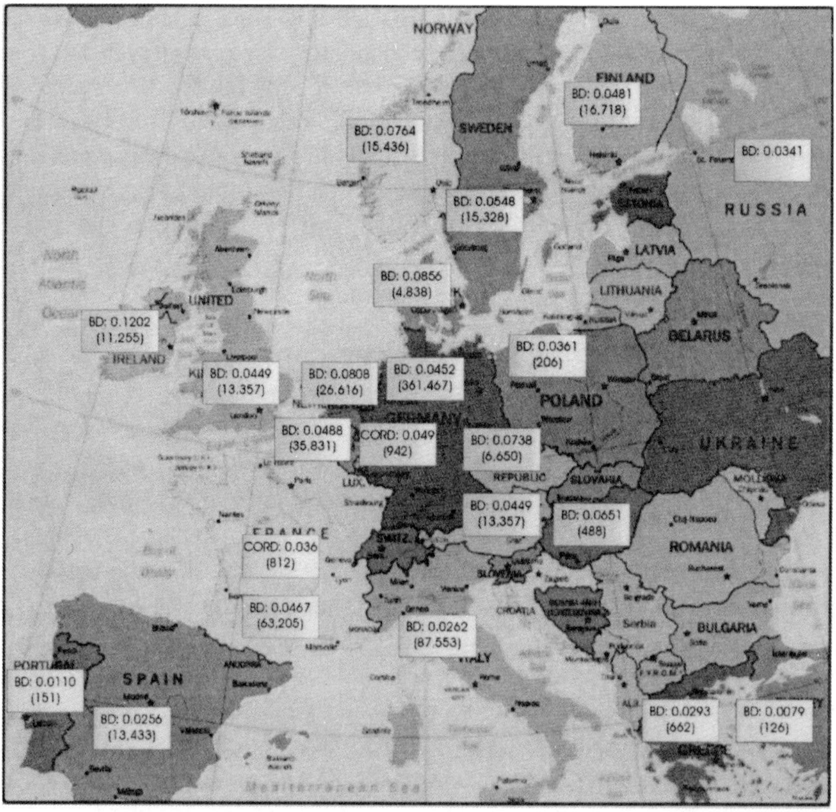

Figure 1. Frequencies of HLA-A1, B8, DR3 haplotypes in European populations. Legend: BD, frequencies estimated in blood donors; CORD, frequencies estimated from cord blood samples. Source: Bone Marrow Donors Worldwide (www.bmdw.org and www.swmed.edu). The numbers of analyzed donors are in brackets.

Second, based on allele-sharing data in multiple-case families and with a tacit assumption of some unknown or partially known parameters such as disease penetrance ratios, mode of inheritance and frequency of disease allele, the calculated contribution of the MHC to the overall disease susceptibility was estimated as substantial (Vorechovsky et al., 2000). Collectively, these data suggest that the MHC is a major locus in determining susceptibility to IgAD/CVID and our genome-wide linkage study in progress is expected to address this issue (I. V et al. in preparation).

2.2 A putative role of non-MHC genes

Several non-MHC genes have been implicated in IgAD/CVID. Chromosome 18 abnormalities were often reported in IgAD (Aksu et al.,

1976), but the linkage analysis did not find any increase in allele sharing across the whole chromosome, arguing against the presence of a strong predisposing locus (Vorechovsky et al., 1999a). In addition to chromosome 18, allelic associations were suggested on chromosomes 14q (Olsson et al., 1992) and 10q11-q21 (Mullighan et al., 2000) and it will be interesting to seek an independent confirmation of these studies in a case-control design in different populations and in family-based allelic association or linkage studies (I.V et al, ms in preparation).

3. IGAD/CVID AND MYTHS ABOUT GENETICS AND ETIOLOGY

Although there is an emerging consensus of impaired T cell activation in CVID (Eibl and Wolf, 1995), no unifying mechanism has been proposed that would explain a number of cellular abnormalities observed in CVID (for review see Strober and Chua, 2000). Instead, it has been argued that CVID represents a heterogenous group of disorders with no common cause, similar to what has been observed for some rare immunodeficiency syndromes such as severe combined immunodeficiency, implying that IgAD/CVID cannot be attributable to a single locus (Schroeder, 2000). Although this looks acceptable, one should remember that the statistically significant evidence for linkage seen in a relatively modest sample size of 83 multiple-case families is unlikely to be observed if IgAD/CVID showed extensive genetic heterogeneity. Likewise, the absence of Mendelian segregation in families with well documented examples of both "recessive" and "dominant" IgAD pedigrees (Koistinen, 1976; Vorechovsky et al., 1995), including a parental bias in the transmission of the defect to the subsequent generation (Vorechovsky et al., 1999b) does not necessarily imply that there is no single major susceptibility locus or even a single genetic determinant. Having the evidence for the susceptibility conferred by the MHC region, which is rich in polymorphic genes involved in antigen processing and presentation, and many examples of similar non-mendelian inheritance in families with autoimmune diseases, with a weak evidence for the involvement of non-MHC susceptibility genes (Concannon et al., 1998), there is still a possibility of a single genetic defect accounting for the majority of IgAD/CVID cases. The stochastic component of MHC-peptide-T cell receptor interactions during thymic development may well explain the irregularities in the family segregation and variability of the IgAD/CVID phenotypes.

The second point of dispute, which originated a decade ago and is increasingly gaining the character of textbook knowledge (Cucca et al., 1998; Schaffer et al., 1989; Schroeder et al., 1998; Schroeder, 2000), is a putative location of the susceptibility gene in the telomeric part of the HLA class III region. Although the largest collection of multiple-case families failed to support this location by analysing the HLA-A1, B8, DR3 haplotypes (Vorechovsky et al., 2000), the exclusion power of fine-mapping studies of complex traits is not absolute. Although high linkage disequilibrium of the selection-driven HLA region has been a major obstacle, this may now be overcome by focusing on all susceptibility haplotypes instead of the haplotype that provides most susceptibility and is associated with high linkage disequilibrium and low informative value for fine mapping studies. This will undoubtedly require collaborative studies and international efforts of clinical immunologists to obtain suitable families, including continued collection of samples from informative individuals.

REFERENCES

1. Aksu, F., Mietens, C. and Scholz, W. (1976). Klin Padiat 188, 220-32.
2. Ambrus, M., Hernadi, E. and Bajtai, G. (1977). Clin Immunol Immunopathol 7, 311-314.
3. Burrows, P. D. and Cooper, M. D. (1997). Adv Immunol 65, 245-276.
4. Collins, A. (2000). Pac Symp Biocomput , 651-62.
5. Concannon, P., Gogolin-Ewens, K. J., Hinds, D. A., Wapelhorst, B., Morrison, V. A., Stirling, B., Mitra, M., Farmer, J., Williams, S. R., Cox, N. J., Bell, G. I., Risch, N. and Spielman, R. S. (1998). Nat Genet 19, 292-6.
6. Consortium. (1999). Nature 401, 921-923.
7. Cucca, F., Zhu, Z. B., Khanna, A., Cossu, F., Congia, M., Badiali, M., Lampis, R., Frau, F., De Virgiliis, S., Cao, A., Arnone, M., Piras, P., Campbell, R. D., Cooper, M. D., Volanakis, J. E. and Powis, S. H. (1998). Clin Exp Immunol 111, 76-80.
8. De La Concha, E. G., Fernandez-Arquero, M., Martinez, A., Vidal, F., Vigil, P., Conejero, L., Garcia-Rodriguez, M. C. and Fontan, G. (1999). Clin Exp Immunol 116, 516-20.
9. Eaves, I. A., Merriman, T. R., Barber, R. A., Nutland, S., Tuomilehto-Wolf, E., Tuomilehto, J., Cucca, F. and Todd, J. A. (2000). Nat Genet 25, 320-3.
10. Eibl, M. M. and Wolf, H. M. (1995). Folia Microbiol 40, 360-6.
11. Espanol, T., Catala, M., Hernandez, M., Caragol, I. and Bertran, J. M. (1996). Clin Immunol Immunopathol 80, 333-335.
12. French, M., Dawkins, R., Christiansen, F. T., Zhang, W., Degli-Esposti, M. A. and Saueracker, G. (1991). Immunology Today 12, 135-136.
13. French, M. A. and Dawkins, R. L. (1990). Immunology Today 11, 271-4.
14. Hammarstrom, L., Persson, M. A. and Smith, C. I. (1983). Scand J Immunol 18, 509-513.
15. Hammarstrom, L., Vorechovsky, I. and Webster, D. (2000). Clin Exp Immunol 120, 225-31.
16. Herr, M., Dudbridge, F., Zavattari, P., Cucca, F., Guja, C., March, R., Campbell, R. D., Barnett, A. H., Bain, S. C., Todd, J. A. and Koeleman, B. P. (2000). Hum Mol Genet 9, 1291-301.
17. Hsieh, S.-L., March, R., Khanna, A., Cross, S. J. and Campbell, R. D. (1997). J Rheumatol 24, 220-222.

18. Ishizaka, A., Nakanishi, M., Yamada, S., Sakiyama, Y. and Matsumoto, S. (1989). Eur J Pediatl149, 175-176.
19. Johnson, M. L., Keeton, L. G., Zhu, Z.-B., Volanakis, J. E., Cooper, M. D. and Schroeder, H. W., Jr. (1997). Clin Exp Immunol 108, 477-483.
20. Koistinen, J. (1976). Vox Sanguinis 30, 181-190.
21. Koskinen, S., Tolo, H., Hirvonen, M. and Koistinen, J. (1994). J Clin Immunol 14, 116-119.
22. Machulla, H. K., Schonermarck, U., Schaaf, A., Muller, L. P., Kloss, C., Kruger, J., Kunze, G., Schonermarck, G. and Langner, J. (2000). Scand J Immunol 52, 207-11.
23. MacLean, C. J., Martin, R. B., Sham, P. C., Wang, H., Straub, R. E. and Kendler, K. S. (2000). Am J Hum Genet 66, 1062-1075.
24. Mullighan, C. G., Marshall, S. E. and Welsh, K. I. (2000). Scand J Immunol 51, 111-22.
25. Olerup, O., Smith, C. I., Bjorkander, J. and Hammarstrom, L. (1992). Proc Natl Acad SciUSA 89, 10653-10657.
26. Olerup, O., Smith, C. I. and Hammarstrom, L. (1990). Nature 347, 289-290.
27. Olerup, O., Smith, C. I. and Hammarstrom, L. (1991). Immunology Today 12, 134-6.
28. Olsson, P. G., Hammarstrom, L., Cox, D. W. and Smith, C. I. (1992). Immunogenetics 36, 389-95.
29. Oxelius, V.-A., Laurell, A. B., Lindqvist, B., Henrika, G., Axelsson, U., Bjorkander, J. and Hanson, L. A. (1981). N Engl J Med 304, 1476-1477.
30. Schaffer, F. M., Palermos, J., Zhu, Z. B., Barger, B. O., Cooper, M. D. and Volanakis, J. E. (1989). Proc Natl Acad SciUSA 86, 8015-8019.
31. Schroeder, H. W., Jr., Zhu, Z. B., March, R. E., Campbell, R. D., Berney, S. M., Nedospasov, S. A., Turetskaya, R. L., Atkinson, T. P., Go, R. C., Cooper, M. D. and Volanakis, J. E. (1998). Mol Med 4, 72-86.
32. Schroeder, H. W. J. (2000). Clin Rev Allergy Immuno. 19, 127-140.
33. Spickett, G. P., Farrant, J., North, M. E., Zhang, J. G., Morgan, L. and Webster, A. D. (1997). Immunology Today 18, 325-8.
34. Strober, W. and Chua, K. (2000). Clin Rev Allergy Immunol 19, 157-181.
35. Volanakis, J. E., Zhu, Z.-B., Schaffer, F. M., Macon, K. J., Palermos, J., Berger, B. O., Go, R., Campbell, R. D., Schroeder, H. W. J. and Cooper, M. D. (1992). J Clin Invest 89, 1914-1922.
36. Vorechovsky, I., Blennow, E., Nordenskjold, M., Webster, A. D. and Hammarstrom, L. (1999a). J Immunol 163, 2236-42.
37. Vorechovsky, I., Cullen, M., Carrington, M., Hammarstrom, L. and Webster, A. D. (2000). J Immunol 164, 4408-16.
38. Vorechovsky, I., Webster, A. D., Plebani, A. and Hammarstrom, L. (1999b). Am J Hum Genet 64, 1096-109.
39. Vorechovsky, I., Zetterquist, H., Paganelli, R., Koskinen, S., Webster, A. D., Bjorkander, J., Smith, C. I. and Hammarstrom, L. (1995). Clin Immunol Immunopathol 77, 185-92.
40. Wilton, A. N., Cobain, T. J. and Dawkins, R. L. (1985). Immunogenetics 21, 333-342.

Ataxia-Telangiectasia

SARA G. BECKER-CATANIA* and RICHARD A. GATTI#
*Department of Psychiatry and Biobehavioral Science and #Department of Pathology and Laboratory Medicine, UCLA School of Medicine, Los Angeles, CA 90095

1. INTRODUCTION

The first documented cases of ataxia-telangiectasia (A-T) were described by Syllaba and Henner in 1926[1]. They described 3 siblings with a progressive choreoathetosis and ocular telangiectasia who were thought to exhibit a variant form of Hunt's familial double athetosis (a disorder involving the basal ganglia)[1]. It was upon later reanalysis of these three patients by Syllaba[2] and Boder (personal communication) that the diagnosis of A-T was established. The syndrome was again described by Louis-Bar[3] who described a patient with progressive cerebellar ataxia and cutaneous telangiectasia. This patient was thought to be affected with either a variant form of Sturge-Weber syndrome, or an entirely new syndrome; consequently the disease was referred to as Louis-Bar syndrome for a period of time.

The earliest complete description of the disease was provided by Boder and Sedgwick (1957)[4]. These physicians reported multiple siblings with similar clinical findings and later analyzed autopsy material on over 100 cases documenting the loss of Purkinje cells and degeneration of the granule cells and basket cells of the cerebellum[5]. Importantly, these reports recognized the recurrent sinopulmonary infections that had not been previously described in conjunction with this syndrome. The other important contribution of these works was naming the syndrome ataxia-telangiectasia (A-T), after the two most visible features of the disease.

Since these initial reports, many advances have been made in understanding the clinical and molecular characteristics of A-T. The disease is a recessively inherited disorder characterized by a wide range of seemingly unrelated pathologic manifestations: progressive cerebellar ataxia, telangiectasia, sensitivity to ionizing radiation, increased cancer risk, immunodeficiency, thymic atrophy, elevated alpha-fetoprotein (AFP) and, more rarely, hypogonadism[6,7]. Patients are usually diagnosed in early childhood, presenting fist with a progressive ataxia, but occasionally, with a malignancy prior to the occurrence of ataxia. This can present serious secondary consequences since patients are radiosensitive and conventional doses of radiotherapy can prove fatal to A-T patients.

2. NEUROPATHOLOGY

The neurologic phenotype of patients is dominated by the progressive cerebellar ataxia. Cranial MRI clearly shows atrophy of the vermis of the cerebellum. Examination of the CNS at a microscopic level shows sporadic loss of pigmented cells within the substantia nigra, neuronal changes within the striatum, and demyelination/gliosis of the dorsal columns, in addition to the cerebellar abnormalities. The pathology in the spinal cord is similar to, but not as severe as, that seen in Friedreich's ataxia (FRDA)[8,9]. The loss of Purkinje and granule cells as well as shrinkage and loss of the deep cerebellar nuclei in A-T patients is reminiscent of the autosomal dominant forms of ataxia such as the spinocerebellar ataxias (SCAs). The athetosis, which is more prominent in older children, is probably due to lesions in areas of the brain other than the cerebellum. A central question in A-T is whether Purkinje cell degeneration is the primary lesion in the CNS, or if the loss is secondary to defects in afferent or efferent pathways. Certainly the Purkinje cells rely upon stimuli from both the climbing fibers originating in the inferior olive, as well as the mossy fiber-granule cell system. The integrity of the deep cerebellar nuclei, the interneurons, and the Golgi cells are also of importance and depletion of any one of these neuronal populations would be likely to affect other members of the pathway.

Most of the initial characterization of the neuropathology of A-T was performed early on with a limited number of cases. We have examined cerebella from eleven A-T patients, one of which is the youngest ever to be studied. Using a diverse panel of antibodies, we were able to detect morphological changes in single cells as well as differences in populations of cells. We found increased numbers of oligodendrocytes and axonal dysmorphology in nearly all of the patients. These cerebellar changes resembled those documented in other Purkinje cell degeneration disorders. In addition, increased numbers of microglial cells, loss of interneurons in the molecular layer, abnormal bcl-2 expression, and disorganization of the parallel fibers were also found in the patients. Of interest, slightly hypertrophic radial fibers, which may adversely affect granule cell migration, were seen in the youngest A-T case. Our results suggest that the neuropathologic changes seen in A-T patients are the result of a two-step process in which there is an initial developmental defect, followed by a later, still undefined event that ultimately results in cerebellar neurodegeneration.

3. IMMUNODEFICIENCY

A-T patients are typically immunodeficient, and although the severity varies, both B and T cell lineages are affected. Most patients have reduced levels of IgA and IgE and decreased resistance to bacterial and viral infections. A-T lymphocytes exhibit chromosomal instability, often with 7:14 translocations near the loci for the Ig genes and T cell receptor genes, which may affect gene rearrangement and explain the low levels of IgA and IgE. Translocations are not the only chromosomal aberrations; telomeric fusions, as well as shortened telomeres, can also be found in A-T cells[10-12]. The thymus of patients is small and the Hassall's corpuscles are absent, indicative of a developmental defect which is likely related to T-cell development and maturation. Patients have increased numbers of $CD8^+$ cells, but decreased numbers of $CD4^+$ cells, which may indicate that the ATM protein plays a specific role in the development or differentiation of T-cells. A-T patients have absent or deficient responses to pneumococcal polysaccharide antigens[13]. V(D)J rearrangement is normal in A-T cells[14]. Decreased numbers of CD45 (RA) cells and markedly increased levels of NK cells have been described in some patients.

4. DNA DAMAGE

Unlike normal cells, A-T cells are deficient in initiating DNA damage repair, resulting in a radiosensitive phenotype, both *in vitro* and *in vivo* [15,16]. The ATM protein functions upstream of DNA repair proteins; thus, A-T cells fail to sense DNA damage and do not arrest at the G1/S checkpoint to repair damage prior to DNA replication and mitosis. The G2/M checkpoint is also abnormal in A-T cells. Murine *atm* has been shown to localize to the synapsing portion of meiotic chromosomes and is required for Chk1 binding to the unsynapsed portion of chromosomes. The dependence of Chk1 on functional Atm suggests a potential mechanism by which A-T cells fail to arrest at the G2/M checkpoint. Two *in vitro* tests, designed to detect cells that respond abnormally to radiation, have been helpful in diagnosing A-T patients. Using the colony survival assay (CSA), immortalized lymphoblastoid cell lines from patients are exposed to ionizing radiation (1Gy), allowed to recover and then viable colonies are counted to determine the survival[17]. The failure of A-T cells to arrest at the G1/S checkpoint following irradiation can also be measured using Radioresistant DNA Synthesis (RDS)[18].

5. CANCER

A-T patients have an increased incidence of cancer, and about one-third of patients will develop a malignancy during their lifetime, which is approximately 100 times the cancer incidence in a normal population[19]. Leukemias, primarily of T-cell origin, and B-cell lymphomas are the most common forms of cancer affecting patients, although some epithelial cancers such as breast cancer have been documented[20]. Most of the translocations in the leukemic cells involve the *TCL-1* gene and the regions of the T-cell receptor and B-cell receptor loci[21]. Because of the sensitivity to radiation, treatment of such cancers with radiotherapy can produce severe adverse effects[15]. With respect to heterozygous carriers of ATM mutations, several large breast cancer populations have been studied, and susceptibility appears to be more complex than initially thought[22]. It was proposed that heterozygous ATM mutations would result in an increased breast cancer risk in women with early-onset disease but this was not supported by a study of 400 affected women. A normal incidence of ATM mutations was reported in another breast cancer cohort that was selected independently of age of onset. In contrast, a study of 775 relatives of A-T patients has shown an increased incidence of breast cancer especially at older ages. Interestingly, Broeks et al.[23] has shown an increased incidence of ATM mutations in a population of breast cancer patients affected by early onset and bilateral occurrence. Most recently, Su and Swift[24] have reported an increased risk of ischemic heart disease and several types of cancer, supporting the initial finding of a five-fold increased susceptiblitiy to breast cancer in A-T heterozygotes[20,24]. It has been suggested that missense, not truncating, mutations in the ATM gene may be the primary predisposing factor for breast cancer and that this may explain the differing results found in the large breast cancer cohort studies[22].

6. ATM GENE/AND PROTEIN

The gene responsible for A-T, ATM (ataxia-telangiectasia *mutated*), was localized to 11q22-23, using linkage analysis[25,26], and cloned by Savitsky et al.[27]. The ATM gene encodes a 13 kb primary transcript, composed of 66 exons and spanning about 150 kb of gDNA[27-29]. The mRNA is expressed in most tissues, including heart, pancreas, spleen, kidney, skeletal muscle, and liver. More interestingly, ATM expression is also found in tissues that show distinct pathology such as the brain, thymus, testis and ovary.

The ATM protein is a 370-kDa polypeptide of 3056 amino acids with several identifiable domains. The protein contains a phosphatidylinositol 3-kinase (PI 3-kinase) domain near the C-terminus which has homology to other high molecular weight PI 3-kinases, such as DNA-PK_{cs}, Tel1 and Mec1 (*S.cerevesiae*), Rad 3 (S.*pombe*), and MEI-41 (*D.melanogaster*). Most of these proteins are involved in the DNA damage response or telomere maintenance. The protein also contains a leucine zipper domain that may facilitate protein-protein interactions or possibly homodimer or homotetramer formation. Binding domains for p53, c-Abl, and MDM2 have also been identified[30].

In vitro studies strongly suggest that the ATM protein is involved in sensing DNA damage and initiates a response by phosphorylating substrates such as the serine-15 position of p53, the p34 subunit of replication protein A (RPA), PHAS-1 (a translational repressor that plays a key role in insulin receptor signalling), c-Abl, chk2, BRCA1, IκB-α, CtIP, and nibrin[31-34] (Fig 1). The p53 protein is known to be upregulated in response to ionizing radiation in normal cells, and this response is deficient in A-T cells. In support of ATM's role as a DNA damage sensor, it has also been shown to be part of the BRCA1-associated genome surveillance complex (BASC)[35]. This complex of about forty different proteins contains known tumor supressors, mismatch repair proteins, DNA damage sensors, and signal transduction molecules that function as a group to initiate DNA repair.

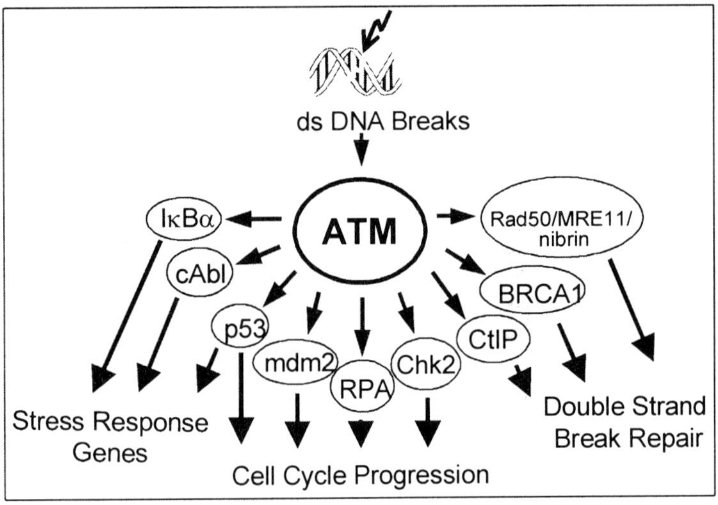

Figure 1. Activation of ATM in response to DNA damage and downstream substrates.

Previous studies on a limited number of ataxia-telangiectasia (A-T) patients with detectable levels of intracellular ATM protein have suggested a genotype/phenotype correlation. We sought to elucidate further this possible correlation by comparing ATM protein levels with mutation types, radiosensitivity, and clinical phenotype. Western blot analysis was used to measure ATM protein in lysates of lymphoblastoid cell lines (LCLs) from 123 unrelated A-T patients[36]. Our western blot protocol detected the presence of ATM protein in as little as 1ug of total protein; at least 25ug of protein was tested for each individual. ATM protein was absent in 105 of the 123 patients (85%); most of these patients had truncating mutations. The remaining subset of 18 patients (15%) had reduced levels of normal-sized ATM protein; missense mutations were more common in this subset. We used the colony survival assay (CSA) to characterize the phenotypic response of the LCLs to radiation exposure[17]; patients with or without detectable ATM protein were typically radiosensitive. These data suggest that although mRNA is abundant in A-T cells, the abnormal ATM protein is probably made but is unstable and is quickly targeted for degradation. We found little correlation between level of ATM protein and the type of underlying mutation, the clinical phenotype, or the radiophenotype.

Mutations in ATM occur along the entire length of the gene and consist of small deletions, insertions, and single nucleotide changes, about half of which lead to splicing defects[37,38]. By far, the most common types of mutations are truncations (~70%). No obvious mutational "hotspot" within the gene has been identified, and over 400 different mutations have been identified to date (http://www.vmresearch.org/atm.htm).

7. MOUSE MODELS

Several different mouse models have been made by knocking out the ATM gene. Fibroblasts taken from these mice were found to exhibit RDS characteristic of A-T[39]. The mice were smaller at birth, were infertile due to the absence of mature male or female gametes, and almost all animals developed thymic lymphomas. Although most A-T patients develop secondary sexual characteristics, hypogonadism does affect a small population of patients. However none of the mouse models exhibit the progressive and incapacitating ataxia seen in patients. Some neurologic abnormalities have been documented such as impaired rota-rod performance, shortened stride length, degeneration of cerebellar neurons and glial activation, loss of dopaminergic nigro-striatal neurons, increased oxidative stress, changes in Purkinje cell dendritic arborization, and an absence of radiation-induced apoptosis in the CNS[39-42]. At a molecular level, $ATM^{-/-}$ cells fail to upregulate p53 in response to ionizing radiation and also have increased constitutive levels of p21. Further work needs to be done to create an ataxic mouse model.

To characterize expression of *Atm* and *Nbs1* message during CNS development, we used *in situ* hybridization in a developing normal mouse. We found that *Atm* and *Nbs1* are highly expressed in germinal zones and proliferating neuroepithelial cells at early stages of development. Both *Atm* and *Nbs1* are widely expressed and in particular, in regions corresponding to those organs affected in A-T patients. Of significance, expression is most prominent during the genesis of the Purkinje cells, the cerebellar nuclei, and the external granule cell layer. Our finding of *Atm* and *Nbs1* co-localization in proliferating neuroepithelial cells supports the known function of ATM in the DNA damage recognition pathway. The expression of *Nbs1* in cell populations exclusive of Atm suggests that nibrin may have other functions not dependent on its interaction with Atm, and may result in the phenotypic differences in A-T and NBS patients.

REFERENCES

1. Syllaba K, Henner K. (1926) Rev Neurol 1:541-62.
2. Henner K. (1968) Rev Neurol 118(1):60-3.
3. Louis-Bar D. (1941) Confin Neurol (Basel) 4:32-42.

4. Boder E, Sedgwick RP. (1957) Univ South California Med Bull 9:15.
5. Boder E, Sedgwick RP. (1958) Pediatrics 21:526-54.
6. Boder E. (1985) In: Gatti RA, Swift M (eds) Ataxia-telangiectasia: An overview. New York, Liss, pp 1-63.
7. Gatti RA, Becker-Catania S, Chun HH et al. (2001) In Clinical Reviews in Allergy & Immunology. M. Ballow (ed).
8. Koeppen AH. (1998) J Neuropath Exp Neuro 57:531-43.
9. Klockgether T, Evert B. (1998) Trends Neuros 21;413-18.
10. Pandita TK, Pathak S, Geard C. (1995) Cytogenet Cell Genet 71:86-3.
11. Metcalfe JA, Parkhill J, Campbell L et al. (1996) Nature Genet 13:350-53.
12. Smilenov LB, Morgan SE, Mellado W et al. (1997) Oncogene 15(22):2659-65.
13. Regueiro F, Arnau A, Perez D et al. (2000) Arch Bronconeumol 36(1):55-7.
14. Hsieh C-L, Lieber MR. (1993) In: Ataxia-Telangiectasia. Eds. RA Gatti and RB Painter. Springer-Verlag, Heidelberg. Pp 143-54.
15. Gotoff SP, Amirmokri E, Liebner EJ. (1967) Am J Dis Child 114:617-25.
16. Taylor AM, Harnden DG, Arlett CF et al. (1975) Nature, 258 (5534):427-29.
17. Huo YK, Wang Z, Hong J-H et al. (1994) Cancer Res 54:2544-47.
18. Painter RB and Young BR. (1980) Proc Natl Acad Sci USA 77:7315-17.
19. Morrell D, Cromartie E, Swift M. (1986) J Natl Cancer Inst 77:89-92.
20. Swift M, Morrell D, Massey RB et al. (1991) N Eng J Med 325:1831-36.
21. Taylor AM, Metcalfe JA, Thick J et al. (1996) Blood 87 (2):423-38.
22. Gatti RA, Tward A, Concannon P. (1999) Molec Genet Metabolism 69:419-23.
23. Broeks A, Floore AN, Urbanus JHM et al. (2000) Amer J Hum Genet 66:494-500.
24. Su Y, Swift M. (2000) Ann Intern Med 133(10):770-78.
25. Gatti RA, Berkel I, Boder E et al. (1988) Nature 336:577-80.
26. Lange E, Corresen A-L, Chen X et al. (1995) Amer J Hum Genet 57:112.
27. Savitsky K, Bar-Shira A, Gilad S et al. (1995) Science 268:1749-53.
28. Savitsky K, Sfez S, Tagle D et al. (1995) Hum Mol Genet 4:2025-32.
29. Uziel T, Savitsky K, Platzer M et al. (1996) Genomics 33:317-20.
30. Khanna KK, Keating KE, Kozlov S et al. (1998) Nature Genet 20:398-400.
31. Zhao S, Yuan FS-S, Weng Y-C et al. (2000) Nature 405: 473-76.
32. Gatei M, Scott SP, Filippovitch I et al. (2000) Cancer Res 60(12):3299-304.
33. Li S, Ting NS, Zheng L et al. (2000) Nature 406: 210-15.
34. Yang DQ, Kastan MB (2000) Nat Cell Biol 12:893-8.
35. Wang Y, Cortez D, Yazdi P et al. (2000) Genes Develop 14:927-39.
36. Becker-Catania S, Chen G, Hwang MJ et al. (2000) Molec Genet Metab 70:122-33.
37. Laake K, Vu P, Andersen TI. (2000) Br J Cancer 83(12):1650-3.
38. Li A, Swift M (2000) Am J Med Genet 92(3):170-7.
39. Barlow C, Hirotsune S, Paylor R et al. (1996) Cell 86:159-71.
40. Herzog K-H, Chong MJ, Kapsetaki M et al. (1998) Science 280:1089-91.
41. Barlow C, Dennery PA, Shigenaga MK et al. (1999) Proc Natl Acad Sci 96: 9915-19.
42. Borghesani PR, Alt FA, Bottaro A et al. (2000) Proc Natl Acad Sci 97:3336

Gene therapy of severe combined immunodeficiencies

ALAIN FISCHER*†, SALIMA HACEIN-BEY*, FRANÇOISE LE DEIST*, GENEVIÈVE DE SAINT BASILE* AND MARINA CAVAZZANA-CALVO*

** INSERM U 429, Hôpital Necker, 149 Rue de Sèvres 75015 Paris, France; †INSERM Unit 429, Hôpital Necker-Enfants Malades, 149 rue de Sèvres, 75730 PARIS CEDEX 15, France, E-mail: fischer@necker.fr*

1. INTRODUCTION

Many of the primary immunodeficiency diseases (PID) are characterized by a susceptibility to recurrent and devastating infections as well as to other severe immunopathological consequences such as autoimmune manifestations. Therefore, these PID can lead to premature death following months or years of debilitating complications. Defects of the T lymphocyte lineage and to some extent of innate immunity represent the most severe forms of PID. Nevertheless, progress has been made in treatment. For more than 30 years, hematopoïetic stem cell transplantation has been successfully utilized to firstly treat severe combined immunodeficiencies (SCID). More recently, a variety of other PID conditions have been treated using this approach. Further progress in the control of infections has resulted in a very high chance of cure for SCID patients who have an HLA identical sibling. Results of T-depleted stem cell transplantation from alternative donors have been used since the early 80's and led to the survival of more than half of the transplanted patients with SCID. The European survey indicates an overall 60 % rate of survival while a recent work from Duke University reported a 78 % survival. These limitations of stem cell transplantation as a treatment of SCID conditions have prompted efforts to establish an alternative option including gene therapy. Because allogeneic stem cell transplantation can cure genetic disorders of the lymphoid system, it is suggested that, in principle, correction of autologous progenitors cells could also work. Correction of an inherited disorder by gene therapy implies firstly gene identification. More than 6 genes, mutations of which are responsible for PID, have been identified including SCID conditions and another 8 severe T cell deficiencies. However, a number of considerations have to be envisaged for each disease. They include disease mechanism, potential selective advantage conferred to transduced cells, temporo-spatial pattern of expression of the gene. Therefore, risks of aberrant transgene expression and possible overexpression as a function of the gene product should be assessed. Finally, the fact that a mutated product could exert a transdominant negative effect should also be tested.

SCID conditions likely represent the most suitable conditions because of intrinsic severity. Moreover, relieving the block in the early lymphoid development should provide a growth advantage to T lymphocyte progenitors since, once differentiated, T cells are long-lived. These characteristics may be sufficient to surmount the present limitation of gene transfer in human hematopoietic stem cells (HSC).

2. XL SCID (SCID-X1)

2.1 Rationale

XL SCID accounts for more than half of SCID cases. It is characterized by faulty development of both T and NK lymphocyte subsets, which are typically absent in the periphery. The thymus gland is hypoplastic and devoid of lymphocyte precursors. Following mapping of the SCID-X1 locus to Xq13, Leonard's group found that the disease is caused by mutations of the gene encoding the γc cytokine receptor subunit. γc plays an essential functional role in the IL-2, IL-4, IL-7, IL-9 and IL-15 receptors. Thus γc deficiency brings about all possible theoretical advantages in a perspective of gene therapy:

1/ γc is a member of cytokine receptors inducing survival, proliferation and possibly differentiation signals for T and NK lymphocyte precursors (IL-7 is required for T cell development and IL-15 for NK cell development). This would predict that γc expression would confer a major selective advantage to transduced cells (see below).

2/ γc gene is constitutively expressed on lymphocytes, although γc membrane expression increases following T lymphocyte activation.

3/ γc is expressed early in the hematopoietic system and by all lineages

4/ γc lacks autonomous function.

The potential selective advantage of γc expressing-lymphoid precursor cells was first demonstrated by the observation of long lasting correction of SCID-X1 phenotype that resulted from a γc gene reverse mutation occurring in a T-cell precursor. This form of a "natural" gene therapy resulted in the development of a peripheral T cell pool that remained stable for five years. Both CD4 and CD8 T cells could be detected with some antigen-specific T responses reflected for instance by the benign course of a varicella zoster infection. The TCRβ repertoire of peripheral T cells was sequentially analyzed by assessing CDR3 size of the various Vβ Jβ family combinations as well as clone sequencing. It was shown that all Vβ and Jβ families were used, albeit diversity of CDR3 length was somewhat reduced. It was estimated that, altogether 1.000 distinct TCRβ chains were utilized, all originating from a single T cell precursor. Although the size of the T cell repertoire in this child was approximately 1 % of controls, these results illustrate the tremendous proliferative potential of a T cell precursor. All T cells in this patient had a memory phenotype indicating that, very likely, only one wave of T cell differentiation occurred in this child. Of note, a similar observation has been made in an ADA deficient child.

2.2 Preclinical studies

These observations constituted the rationale for initiating a γc gene therapy study. A retroviral (MFG) vector was made with the γc cDNA inserted at the exact place of the env gene (16, 17).

It was thought that ex vivo γc gene transfer into hematopoietic precursor cells from a γc deficient animal would be a valuable experience to perform in order to assess 1) feasibility and 2) potential toxicity of γc gene transfer. We and others used γc (-) mice generated by homologous recombination. Following, γc gene transfer into γc(-) bone marrow cells, transplantation led to sustained reconstitution of a functional immune system in the 11 month-follow up. Evidence for antigen-specific B cell responses were also provided. These results indicate that indeed γc gene transfer can indeed restore immune cells development without adverse effects. Meanwhile, similar results were achieved in correcting the closely related JAK-3 deficiency in JAK-3 (-) mice by retrovirally-mediated JAK-3 gene transfer. In addition, it was found that transgene expression was much more frequent in lymphoid than myeloid cells, thus providing in vivo evidence, in that model for a selective advantage conferred to transduced lymphoid cells.

2.3 Clinical Protocol and Results

By using murine CD2 as a marker gene, a clinically applicable protocol for ex vivo gene transfer into CD34 cells was designed. By using a cytokine combination consisting of MGDF, SCF, Flt-3L and IL-3 used in a one day pre-activation step followed by 3 cycles of infection on CH-296 fibronectin (Takara Co, Japan) fragment-coated bags, it was found that 30-40 % CD34 cells were transduced, including some $CD34^{+} CD38^{low}$ immature cells.

Five patients have been enrolled between March 1999 and February 2000. Transduction rate of CD34 (+) cells was 34 to 41 %. The detailed analysis of the results of gene therapy in the first two treated patients (with > 1 year follow up) provides an insight to its potential. Patients were treated at the respective ages of 11 and 8 months. As early as day +15 post treatment, PCR analysis of circulating leukocytes detected the presence of transduced cells. Transduced T cells became detectable 60 to 90 days after treatment while T cell counts are in normal range 6 months and beyond after gene transfer. γc transgene mRNA expression studied by semi quantitative RT-PCR as well as immuofluorescence studies in patient 2 have indicated that virtually all circulating T cells are transduced. T cells were shown to have a diverse repertoire as both determination of Vβ family usage with monoclonal antibodies, and of Vβ/Jβ family usage and distribution of CDR3 length demonstrated an indistinguishable pattern from age matched controls. The different T cell subsets including TCRαβ and γδ+ cells as well as TCRαβ CD4 and CD8 cells could be detected in normal or close to normal proportion. Functional properties of T cells were evidenced by the development of proliferation to mitogens, i.e. PHA and anti CD3 antibody as well as to antigens. The fraction of circulating transduced B lymphocytes is low (≤ 1 %). Nevertheless, B cell immunity has developed in these children. Following immunizations and 12 months after the last IV Ig injection, it was found that patients' sera contained protective titers of antibodies to tetanus toxoid, diphteria toxoid and polio viruses . Serum Ig isotype concentrations have reached normal values in patient 1. Isohemaglutinins can also be detected in both patients' sera. It is actually not known whether antibodies were made by transduced B cells or not.

As a consequence of the development of transduced T and some NK lymphocytes as well as of T and B cell immune responses, a favorable clinical outcome was noticed. In both children, protracted diarrhea ceased, parenteral nutrition could be interrupted while patients have a normal growth. There has been no recurrence of severe infections. In patient 2, GVHD-like skin lesions and eosinophilia thought to have been associated with maternal T cell engraftment disappeared within 3 months. One year after treatment, patients are doing well, they are living at home without any therapy.

These results, together with preliminary results in two additional patients demonstrate that indeed, transduced lymphocyte progenitors were conferred a selective advantage strong enough to enable development of a full blown immune system. They also raise a number of questions.

The main issue deals with the stability of the correction of the immunodeficiency phenotype. It has been previously reported that transgene under LTR transcriptional control could be silenced as observed in ADA deficient treated patients. One can therefore not exclude that this could occur in these patients. One may speculate that γc expression exerts by itself a selection pressure that should favor persistence and/or development of continuously γc-expressive cells.

A decline in transduced lymphocyte populations can also result from the cessation of newly generation of lymphocytes. As the nature of earliest transduced cells is not known, one could envisage that, for instance, the pool of transduced committed lymphocyte progenitors that lack self renewal capacity will progressively disappear. This hypothesis is now unlikely as both patients exhibit, one year after treatment a sizeable thymic gland, while a large majority of T cells in the periphery exhibits a naive phenotype. These data strongly suggest that thymopoiesis is still ongoing, and that, therefore, transduced lymphocyte progenitors do persist. As it has been shown that a proportion (around 1 %) of marrow CD34 + cells analyzed 5 months after treatment in patient 2 were transduced and could give rise to γc (+) CFU-GM colonies in vitro, while, in all patients, a fraction of 0.01 % to 1% of transduced monocytes and granulocytes are detectable 6 months to one year after gene therapy, it is possible that immature pluripotent hematopoietic cells have been transduced. Whether some of the transduced cells exhibit a self-renewal capacity could only be determined by sequential studies over time in these patients. Analysis of provirus integration sites in both lymphocyte and myeloid cells should tell whether this hypothesis is correct. In any case, given the life span of T cells, it is not expected that a significant decline in T cell immunity will occur before several years (unless γc gene expression is extinguished).

3. OTHER SEVERE COMBINED IMMUNO-DEFICIENCIES

The positive results achieved in SCID-X1 suggest that other forms of SCID should also be amenable to ex vivo gene therapy as molecular bases are known and a selective advantage conferred to transduced cells expected.

The closely related IL-R7α and JAK-3 deficiencies represent the most obvious candidates. JAK-3 deficiency in a murine model can be stably corrected by ex vivo gene therapy while a selective advantage for transducing lymphocyte precursors has indeed been demonstrated.

SCID with abnormal V(D)J gene rearrangements caused by Rag-1 and Rag-2 mutations are next on the list. Potential effect of non regulated expression of Rag-1 or Rag-2 protein should be also assessed either in transgenic or in gene transferred mice.

Gene transfer of ADA into CD34 cells isolated from marrow or cord blood gave rather disappointing results without correction of the immunodeficiency. Nevertheless, a fraction, up to 10 %, of T cells were transduced and detected several years after treatment by ex vivo gene transfer into cord blood cells. Several reasons can account for these results: loss of ADA transgene expression, loss of the selective advantage caused by the concomitant treatment with PEG-ADA as well as unmodified consequences of ADA deficiency on non immune cells such as thymic epithelium. It is now possible to envisage that the advances in the technology of gene transfer into human hematopoietic precursors cells will change at least in part the outcome of ADA gene therapy.

4. FUTURE DIRECTIONS

Continuous progress is being made in the technology of gene transfer into hematopoietic progenitor cells. Cytokines combinations can enable cycling of immature CD34+ $CD38^{low}$ cells making them permissive for transgene integration. Improvement in vector production by the design of new packaging cell lines enhanced binding of retrovirus to hematopoietic cells by pseudotyping with the gibbon ape leukemia virus envelope has considerably increase the rate of CD34+ cell transduction.

The design of lentiviral vectors able to infect non-cycling cells, thereby likely hematopoietic stem cells may permit gene therapy for immunodeficiencies in which the gene product does not contribute to cell growth or survival. Results of gene expression in human cells derived from lentivirus infected CD34+ cells grafted in scid/nod mice are indeed promising. They need however confirmation on longer period of time while the safety issues has to be entirely solved. In any case, for several of the immunodeficiency diseases, for which we are considering gene therapy, both efficient and safe processes enabling tight control of gene expression will be also required.

Immune reconstitution after highly active anti-retroviral treatment of HIV infection

BRIGITTE AUTRAN, GUISLAINE CARCELAIN AND PATRICE DEBRE
Laboratoire d'Immunologie Cellulaire et Tissulaire, INSERM U543,
Hôpital Pitié-Salpétrière, Bâtiment CERVI, 83 Bd de l'Hôpital, 75013 Paris, France

1. INTRODUCTION

The introduction of highly active antiretroviral therapy (HAART) combining inhibitors of the HIV-1 reverse transcriptase and protease have dramatically modified the course of the HIV infection during the past four years. Despite some controversies about the extent to which the immune system can normalize, it is generally admitted nowadays that some immune reconstitution can be obtained in both asymptomatic HIV-infected individuals and AIDS patients and can confer host protection against opportunistic events (1-5). The best hallmark of such immune restoration is the massive decline in the mortality and morbidity related to AIDS that have been registered in all industrialized countries (6,7). Although these recent advances warrant optimism, the current HAART regimens are unable to eradicate the virus and to restore an HIV-specific immunity (8,9), except when introduced immediately after virus contamination (10). Nevertheless the immune reconstitution obtained with these antiretroviral drugs alone, even incomplete, has brought definitive evidences for the central role played by HIV itself in the massive immune alterations induced by such infection.

Progress in Basic and Clinical Immunology, Edited by Mackiewicz *et al.*
Kluwer Academic/Plenum Publishers, New York, 2001

2. THE REGENERATION OF A CD4 T CELL COMPARTMENT WITH ANTIRETROVIRAL THERAPIES

Losses in peripheral CD4 T cells are thought to result from cumulative virus cell replication in the CD4 cell subpopulation either by direct virus pathogenicity and/or by CTL-mediated cytolysis, and from activation-induced cell death of non-infected cells. In the meanwhile, compensation by newly produced T cells progressively diminish during the course of the infection. Introduction of new antiretroviral drug regimens combining inhibitors of two HIV enzymes, the reverse transcritase (RTI) and the protease (PI) opened a new era by inducing major and stable reduction in viral load accompanied by sustained CD4 cell increases (11-13) that had never been encountered previously with mono- or bi-therapy with RTI. Such changes immediately raised the question of immune restoration and its mechanisms.

A first study was conducted in 1996 on patients naive of any antiretroviral drugs who were treated with one PI and two nucleoside analogs in late disease stage (CD4 counts below 250/mm3). Our group demonstrated an early increase in CD4 cells mostly composed of transiently activated memory CD4+ cells that lacked markers of cell proliferation (1). Strong expensions of peripheral blood CD4 T cells (1-5 CD4 cell/mm^3/day) were observed during the first two months (5) concurrent as to a rapid and major reduction in virus load of 1 to 2 log magnitude. According to cohort studies the kinetics of the CD4 cell expansion is usually reduced after the 2nd or 3rd month of treatment. Such second phase of immune reconstitution appears to be correlated to the magnitude of the plasma viral load reduction and to its stability over time (14). In contrast, the intensity of CD4 cell depletion at baseline plays only a minor role in such long term kinetics of CD4 cell recovery (14) suggesting that the immune system is repopulated whatever the severity of the immune alterations that had taken place before introduction of HAART.

Considering the mechanisms of such CD4 T cell reconstitution, a biphasic process is usually observed. The first rapid wave of CD4 T cells is mostly composed of memory CD4 T cells bearing the CD45RO isoform. This rapid change is supposed to reflect redistribution of pre-existing residual CD4 T cells from the tissues in which they were sequestered (1,5) rather than proliferation. The second step, observed after 2 or 3 months of virus control, is characterized by a slower rate of memory CD4 T cells (1,5), reflecting a long term T cell production. Indeed in vivo evaluations of T cell proliferation using either deuterated glucose incorporation (15) or Ki67 intra-cellular expression (16) are concordant and suggest a 2 to 3 fold increase in the numbers of proliferating CD4 T cells after 6 months of treatment. Regeneration of naïve T cell is now known to play the major role in the late reconstitution of the whole CD4 subset. Indeed naïve CD4 T cells are significantly increasing both in proportions and absolute numbers after the 3rd month of treatment when introduced at late stages of CD4 cell depletion (1). Such increase in naïve T cells, whatever its kinetics, was surprising. Indeed it contrasted with the very slow and weak regeneration in naïve T cells observed in adults after chemotherapy or bone-marrow transplantation (17) and suggested that HIV-infection had not definitively impaired in adults the capacities of thymic production.

Direct evidence for a thymic participation in T cell regeneration during antiretroviral therapy came only at the end of 1998 in detecting markers of thymic origin (18). Populations of naïve CD4 T cells containing high proportions of T cell receptor rearrangement excision circles or TRECS are called recent thymic emigrants (RTE). TRECs proportions decline with age and HIV infection (18). These defects are corrected under potent antiretroviral therapy, resulting in a rapid and sustained increase in TRECs proportions in the majority of patients that is correlated to the naive T cell subset increase. These findings suggest the contribution of the thymus in the reconstitution of normal CD4 cell numbers and homeostasis, thus ensuring restoration of a naive T-cell repertoire diversity. However thymic regeneration alone might not be responsible for such reconstitution. The decrease in abnormal T cell activation and consumption of memory T cells might also reduce the consumption of the naive cells compartment and help at restoring it in the context of a functional thymus.

The diversity of the T cell repertoire which decreases with age and chronic exposure to antigens is highly perturbated during HIV infection. However the perturbed CD4 T cell repertoire was shown by Gorochov et al. to slowly rediversify after the 6th month of an highly active antiretroviral treatment (2). This process occurred once the activation status of memory CD4 cells had been normalized and after the increase in naive T cells numbers took place. The same phenomenon occurred in the CD8 compartment, though more slowly (2,19). Normalization of T cell repertoires reflects both increased production of a naive diverse T cell repertoire and decreased turn-over of T cell clones that were previously mobilized against various pathogens, once the virus is controlled.

Chronic immune activation is a hallmark of the immune alterations observed during the natural course of the HIV infection. One of our first observations on immune reconstitution was a rapid and remarkable reduction in the cell surface expression of various T cell activation markers such as HLA-DR, CD38 or CD25, the IL-2 receptor, both on CD4 and on CD8 T cells (1). The proportions of activated T cells significantly decreased in parallel to the reduction of the plasma virus load. The strong correlation coefficient (r=0.8) observed between both phenomenous indicate the responsibility of the virus itself in such abnormal activation (1). Other groups reported a similar decrease in soluble markers of immune activation such as inflammatory cytokines TCF-α and IL-6 (4,21). In addition a reduction in the Fas-Fas-ligand cell surface expression was also observed resulting in a decreased T cell sensitivity to apoptosis (20). Both phenomenous, reduced Fas expression and TNF-α levels, certainly help at limiting the abnormal rate of cell death observed in HIV infection and at restoring normal numbers in the T cell compartments. They also have important impacts on other immune cells such as B cells or polymorphonuclear cells.

3. RECONSTITUTION OF HOST DEFENSES DURING HAART

One of the major questions was whether restoring CD4 cell numbers would mean restoration of the host defenses.that had been lost with AIDS. These defects in host defenses were mediated by depletion in naive T cells, anergy of memory T cells reflecting Th1 defects and abnormal activation. The phenotypic improvements reported above strongly suggested that the functional defects in the residual memory T cells would be corrected.

Indeed, such a restoration of CD4 T cell functions was observed after 3 months of HAART in AIDS patients who had previously lost their defenses against CMV and mycobacterium tuberculosis: the memory CD4 cell reactivities against these two opportunistic pathogens were restored and persisted overtime when HAART was successful at controlling the virus load and at increasing CD4 memory cells (1,3). The regeneration of new naive T cells was not required, in such a process, suggesting that the memory defenses against those pathogens had not been completely lost prior to treatment.

These successes have however some limits since no restoration of a CD4 cell reactivity against HIV itself was observed in parallel to the immune reconstitution described above (figure 1) when the tratment was applied in chronically infected patients (1,8,22,23). The CD4 helper cells specific for HIV were restored only when HAART was initiated at time of primary infection (10) and appear to be deleted in chronic disease. A widely accepted hypothesis for such a lack of restoration is the lack of in vivo restimulation in the absence of antigen stimulation due to an efficient virus control with treatment. The regeneration of new naive CD4 cells did not help at restoring such activity even after 2 or 3 years of fully suppressive treatments (9). One of the best hallmark of this unrestored immunity against HIV is the rebound of virus replication observed when HAART is stopped (24,25).

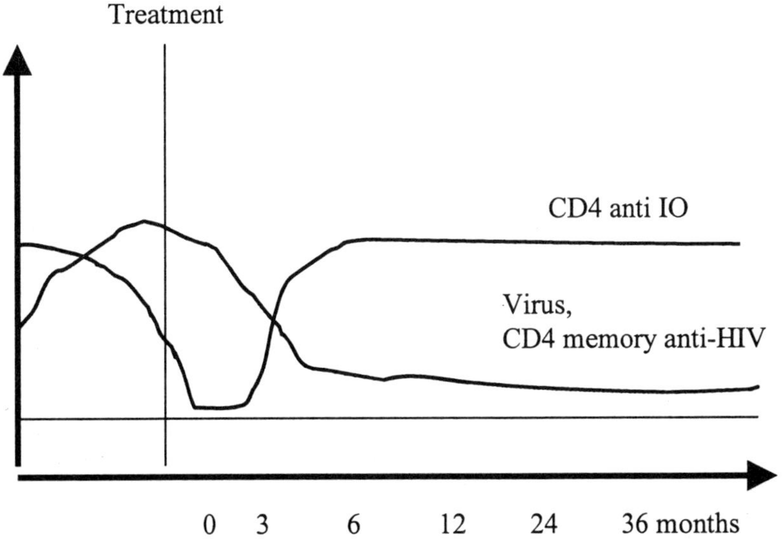

Figure 1. Immune reconstitution obtained when HAART is initiated during late disease. The reappearance of CD4 cell responses to opportunistic antigens contrasts with a lack of restoration of CD4 T cell responses to HIV antigens.

4. CONCLUSION

In conclusion, HAART, whatever the stage of the disease it is initiated, allows immune restoration and protection against opportunistic pathogens. The single condition required for immune reconstitution is an efficient and durable inhibition of virus replication. These positive effects can be obtained at late stages of the disease even when the patients have been heavily pre-treated. These successes demonstrate that HIV does not definitively alter the lymphoïd tissues nor the immune defenses, even after years of infection and severe immune suppression. Initiating HAART in late or in early disease might differ however by 1) the time required to reach normalized immune functions and cell counts and 2) the lack of amplification of HIV-specific T cells in late disease. The delay to recovery or the lack of reconstitution of a solid immunity against HIV itself is currently raising the need for additive therapeutic strategies based upon immune interventions. Several immune therapies are currently being evaluated such as periodic IL-2 infusions in order to accelerate and amplify immune reconstitution or therapeutic vaccinations to resuscitate immune responses to HIV. At a time where virus eradication does not appear plausible with the current drug regimens, the ultimate goal of HAART might be to help at transforming treated patients in long term non progressors.

REFERENCES

1. Autran, B., G. Carcelain, T.S. Li, C. Blanc, D. Mathez, R. Tubiana, C. Katlama, and P. Debre, J. Leibowitch. 1997. Positive effects of combined anti-retroviral therapy on CD4+ T cell homeostasis and function in advanced HIV disease. *Science*. 277:112-116.
2. Gorochov, G., A.U. Neumann, A. Kereveur, C. Parizot, T.S. Li, C. Katlama, M. Karmochkine, G. Raguin, B. Autran, and P. Debre. 1998. Perturbation of CD4 and CD8 T cell repertoires during progression to AIDS and influence of antiviral therapy. *Nature Medicine*. 4(2):215-221.
3. Li, T.S., R. Tubiana, C. Katlama, V. Calvez, H.A. Mohand, and B. Autran. 1998. Long lasting recovery in CD4+ T cell function mirrors viral load reduction after highly active anti-retroviral therapy in patients with advanced HIV disease. *Lancet*. 351:1682-1686.
4. Lederman, M.M., E. Connick, A. Landay, D.R. Kuritzkes, J. Spritzler, M. St Clair, B.L. Kotzin, L. Fox, M.H. Chiozzi, J.M. Leonard, F. Rousseau, M. Wade, J.D. Roe, A. Martinez, and H. Kessler. 1998. Immunologic responses associated with 12 weeks of combination antiretroviral therapy consisting of Zidovudine, Lamivudine and Ritonavir : results of AIDS clinical trials group protocol 315. *J Infect Dis*. 178:70-79.
5. Pakker, N.G., D.W. Notermans, R.J. De Boer, M.T.L. Roos, F. De Wolf, A. Hill, J.M. Leonard, S.A. Danner, F. Miedema, and P.T.A. Schellekens. 1998. Biphasic kinetics of peripheral blood T cells after triple combination therapy in HIV-1 infection: A composite of redistribution and proliferation. *Nat Med*. (4)2:208-214.
6. Hogg, R.S., M.W. O'Shaughnessy, N. Gataric, B. Yip, K. Craib, M.T. Schechter, and J.S. Montaner. 1997. Decline in deaths from AIDS due to new antiretrovirals. *Lancet*. 349:1294.
7. Palella, F.J., K.M. Delaney, A.C. Moorman, M.O. Loveless, J. Fuhrer, G.A. Satten, D.J. Aschman, S.D. Holmberg, and the HIV outpatient study investigators. 1998. Declining Morbidity and mortality among patients with advanced human immunodeficiency virus infection. *N Engl J Med* 338(13):853-60.
8. Plana, M., F. Garcia, T. Gallart, J.M. Miro, and J.M. Gatell. 1998. Lack of T-cell proliferative response to HIV-1 antigens after 1 year of highly active antiretroviral treatment in early HIV-1 disease. *Lancet*. 352:1194-1195.
9. Carcelain, G., R. Tubiana, T.S. Li, V. Calvez, N. Jouy, M. Jouan, M.A. Valantin, C. Olivier, P.M. Girard, P. Debré, C. Katlama, and B. Autran. 1999. Long-Term recovery in CD4+ T cell function with highly efficient antiretroviral therapy. *6th Conference on Retrovirus and Oppotunistic Infections*. Chicago, USA.
10. Rosenberg, E.S, J.M. Billingsley, A.M. Caliendo, S.L. Boswell, P.E. Sax, S.A. Kalams, and B.D. Walker. 1997. Vigorous HIV-1 specific CD4+ T cell responses associated with control of viremie. *Science*. 278:1447.
11. Collier, A.C., R.W. Coombs, D.A. Schoenfeld, R.L. Bassett, J. Timpone, A. Baruch, J.M. Facey, C. Whitacre, V.J. McAuliffe, H.M. Friedman, T.C. Merigan, R.C. Reichman,

C. Hooper, and L. Corey. 1996. Treatment of human immunodeficiency virus infection with saquinavir zidovudine and zalcitabine. *N Engl J Med.* 334:1011-1017.
12. Katzenstein, D.A., S.M. Hammer, M.D. Hugues, et al. 1996. The relation of virologic and immunologic markers to clinical outcomes after nucleoside therapy in HIV-infected adults with 200 to 500 CD4 cells per cubic millimeter. *N Engl J Med.* 335:1091-1098.
13. Hammer, S.M., K.E. Squires, M.D. Hughes, J.M. Grimes, L.M. Demeter, J.S. Currier, J.J. Eron, J.E. Feinberg, H.H. Balfour, L.R. Deyton, J.A. Chodakewitz, M.A. Fischl, and the ACTG 320 study team. 1997. A controlled trial of two nucleoside analogues plus indinavir in persons with human immunodeficiency virus infection and CD4 cell counts of 200 per cubic millimeter or less. *N Engl J Med.* 337(11):725-739.
14. Renaud, M., C. Katlama, A. Mallet, V. Calvez, G. Carcelain, R. Tubiana, M. Jouan, E. Caumes, H. Agut, F. Bricaire, P. Debre, and B. Autran. 1999. Determinants of paradoxical CD4 cell reconstitution after protease inhibitor containing antiretroviral regiment. *AIDS.* 13:669-676.
15. .Hellerstein, M., M.B. Hanley, D. Cesar, S. Siler, C. Papageorgopoulos, E. Wieder, D. Schmidt, R. Hoh, R. Neese, D. Macallan, S. Deeks, and J.M. McCune. 1999. Directly measured kinetics of circulating T lymphocytes in normal and HIV-1 infected humans. *Nat Med.* 5:83-89.
16. Fleury, S., G.P. Rizzardi, A. Chapuis, G. Tambussi, C. Knabenhans, E. Simeoni, J. Meuwly, J. Corpataux, A. Lazzarin, F. Miedema, and G. Pantaleo. 2000. Long-term kinetics of T cell production in HIV-infected subjects treated with highly active antiretroviral therapy. *Proc Natl Acad Sci USA.* 97:5393-5398.
17. Mackall, C.L., L. Granger, M.A. Sheard, R. Cepeda, and R.E. Gress. 1993. T-cell regeneration after bone marrow transplantation: differential CD45 isoform expression on thymic-derived versus thymic-independent progeny. *Blood.* 82:2585-2894.
18. Douek, D.C., R.D. McFarlard, P.H. Keiser, E.A. Gage, J.M. Massey, B.F. Haynes, M.A. Polis, A.T. Haase, M.B. Feinberg, J.L. Sullivan, B.D. Jamieson, J.A. Zack, L.J. Picker, and R.A. Koup. 1998. Changes in thymic function with age and during the treatment of HIV infection. *Nature.* 396:690-695.
19. Gorochov G., Neumann A., Parizot C., Li T.S., Katlama C., Debre P. Down regulation of CD8+ T cell expansions in HIV patients receiving highly active combinaison therapy.. *Blood.* Sous presse 2001.
20. Badley A.D., D.J. Dockrell, A. Algeciras; S. Ziesmer, A. Landay, M.M. Lederman, E. Connick, D. Kuritzkes, D.J. Lynch, P. Roche, H. Yagita, and C.V. Paya. 1998. In vivo analysis of Fas/Fas-L interactions in HIV-infected patients. *J. Clin. Invest.* 102:79-87.
21. Bucy, R.P., R.D. Hockett, C.A. Derdeyn, M.S. Saag, K. Squires, M. Sillers, R.T. Mitsuyasu, and J.M. Kilby. 1999. Initial increase in blood CD4+ lymphocytes after HIV retroviral therapy reflects redistribution form lymphoid tissus. *J. Clin. Invest.* 103:1391-1398.
22. Rinaldo, C.R., J.M. Liebman, X.L. Huang, Z. Fan, A.I. Shboul, D.K. McMahon DK, *et al.* 1999. Prolonged suppression of human immunodeficiency virus type 1 (HIV-1) viremia in persons with advanced disease results in enhancement of CD4 T cell reactivity to microbial antigens but not to HIV-1 antigens. *J Infect Dis.* 179:329-336.
23. Pontselli, O., S. Kerkhof-Garde, D.W. Notermans, N.A. Foudraine, M.T. Roos, M.R. Klein *et al.* 1999. Functional T cell reconstitution and human immunodeficiency virus-1-specific cell-mediated immunity during highly active antiretroviral therapy. *J Infect Dis.* 180:76-86.
24. De Jong, M.D., R.J. De Boeer, and F. De Wolf. 1997. Overshoot of HIV-1 viraemia after early discontinuation of antiretroviral treatment. *AIDS.* 11:F79-F84.

25. Neumann, A.U., R. Tubiana, V. Calvez, C. Robert, T.S. Li, H. Agut, B. Autran, C. Katlama and the Comet study group. 1999. HIV-1 rebound during interruption of HAART has no deleterious effect on reinitiated treatment. *AIDS*. 13:677-683.

Dissimilarity of clinical signs with parameters characterizing immune system

NATALIA K. GORLINA[*], ANATOLY N. CHEREDEEV[*], IVAN G. KOZLOV[*], ALEXANDER R. GUSKOV[#]
[*]*Department of Immunology, Russian State Medical University, Moscow, Russia;* [#]*Scientific Research and Therapeutic Center "Sanos", Moscow, Russia*

1. INTRODUCTION

At present the wide use of quantitative flow cytometry for determination of population and subpopulation composition of lymphocytes (CD markers) in clinical practice has become the main tool for verification of immunodeficiency (ID) diagnosis. As a rule, the practice of the majority of clinical diagnostic laboratories includes the usage of so called "shorten" panel of monoclonal antibodies (mAbs) for the following CD markers (cell types, identified by mAbs, are shown in parentheses): CD3 (T cells), CD4 (T helpers), CD8 (cytotoxic T lymphocytes), CD19/CD72 (B cells), CD16 (NK cells), CD14 (monocytes/macrophages).

The analysis of rather ample experience for the usage of such a panel of mAbs in our country in ID diagnostics has shown that in various immunopathological conditions there are uniform changes of immune status, including the decrease of T cell number, the decline of CD4+ cells, the increase of CD8+ subpopulation, and as a sequence, the elevation of CD4/CD8 ratio. The detection of such changes usually serves as a proof for ID and as an indication to the administration of relevant immunocorrection therapy.

Progress in Basic and Clinical Immunology, Edited by Mackiewicz *et al.*
Kluwer Academic/Plenum Publishers, New York, 2001

Two points should be taken into consideration. Firstly, the detected changes are characterized by the uniformity in many various diseases[1-6], and secondly, the similar changes may be revealed in some physiological conditions, such as pregnancy[7]. The same changes sometimes may be found in practically healthy individuals, whom immunocorrection therapy is administered. Therefore, the aim of our work was to make clinical analysis in patients with ID manifestations and to estimate how the severity of disease may be associated with parameters of immune status.

2. MATERIALS AND METHODS

242 patients with ChP aged 20-55 years old were investigated and received the out-patient treatment at Scientific, Research and Therapeutic Center “Sanos”.

Clinical examination included physical examination and laboratory investigation carried out by standard clinical and laboratory procedures.

The urogenital diagnostics was performed by bacteriological analysis with a use of fluorescent mAbs and polymerase chain reaction. Once clinical signs of ChP exacerbation were revealed antibacterial therapy against the specific bacteria was recommended at the very beginning of the ChP complex treatment.

For immunological investigations patients’ peripheral blood mononuclear cells were isolated by gradient centrifugation on Ficoll-Urographin. The number of lymphocyte populations and subpopulations were assessed with a use of flow cytometry (“Profile”Coultronics, France) and by a method of indirect immunofluorescence with anti-human mouse mAb LT3 (CD3), LT4 (CD4), LT8 (CD8), 3F3 (CD72)) (“Sorbent”, Institute of Immunology, Moscow, Russia) to reveal and discriminate respectively T cells, T helper/inductor, T killers and B cells. Goat anti-mouse Ab labeled by FITC was taken as the secondary Ab.

3. RESULTS

After immunological examination of all patients with ChP (Table 1) we have gotten the values, frequently reported by other authors in various pathological conditions, including chronic prostatitis [see column "Patients (1st + 2nd groups)][6].

Table 2. Immune status parameters in healthy individuals, in patients with chronic prostatitis without (1st group) and with associated chronic inflammatory diseases (2nd group)

Parameters	Measure units	Control (M±m)	Patients (1st +2nd groups) (M±m)	Patients 1st group (M±m)	Patients 2nd group (M±m)
Leukocytes	10^9 cells/l	6.5±1.24	5.89±1.63	5.68±1.49	5.89±1.63
Lymphocytes	%	28.7±3.7	31.65±8.54	32.09±8.4	31.72±6.0
	10^9 cells/l	1.80±0.51	1.82±0.58	1.96±0.66	1.78±0.53
CD3	%	67.8±3.5	67.03±8.58	66.27±9.14	67.42±8.29
	10^9 cells/l	1.825+0.212	**1.218±0.417**	**1.298±0.440**	**1.197±0.410**
CD4	%	40.0±4.4	36.52±7.98	**32.84±7.21***	38,13±7.77*
	10^9 cells/l	1.050±0.210	**0.662±0.249**	**0.642±0.235**	**0.680±0,251**
CD8	%	28.0±3.4	31.78±7.86	**34.87±8.36**	30.41±7.18
	10^9 cells/l	0.505±0.136	0.585±0.249	0.687±0.277	0.550±0.147
CD4/CD8	-	1.75±0.21	**1.24±0.49**	**1.01±0.39***	1.34±0.49*
CD72	%	10.3±1.5	7.95+3.90	8.09±4.39	7.89±3.6
	10^9 cells/l	0,275±0.06	**0.144±0.09**	**0.165±0.13**	**0.137±0.07**
CD16	%	12.0±4.1	10.70±4.81	10.7±4.89	10.67+4.81
	10^9 cells/l	0.224±0.063	0.199±0.137	0.205±1.11	0.197±0.143

Bold values are significantly differed from control

* $P<0.05$ between groups

Further, we divided patients into two groups according to the severity of ID manifestations. The 1st group comprised of 65 patients, having no other signs of secondary ID than ChP. The 2nd group included 177 patients who together with ChP had other expressed signs of ID: chronic inflammatory processes (chronic tonsillitis, bronchitis, sinusitis, pyelonephritis, cystitis, furunculosis and others) and frequently recurrent infections (herpes infections, acute respiratory infections, chlamydiosis, pneumonia, acute tonsillitis and others). About 90% of patients in this group had more than one concomitant disease, associated with manifestations of secondary ID.

No significant differences between groups in relation to infectious agent, caused the inflammatory process were not found after microbiological analysis of prostate secretion.

The data of immunological examination for each group of patients are presented in Table 1. Our attention was drawn to the fact that in the group with more pronounced ID manifestations the deviations from norm were only by 3 parameters, while in the group with minimal ID manifestations - by 6 parameters of immune status. Some examined parameters were differed not only in comparison to healthy donors, but also to different groups. As can be seen from Table 1, the value changes, usually associated with ID, are not the marker of its severity.

In half an year after the conducted examination and the respective treatment, including immunocorrection therapy, we carried out the estimation of immune status in 35 patients with chronic prostatitis. The restoration of normal values and the maintenance of revealed changes were appeared to be not associated with treatment success.

4. CONCLUSION

The data obtained indicate that traditionally diagnosed ID signs (changes in numbers of T cell subsets) do not fully reflect real severity of the associated disease and are likely due to compensatory events in the immune system. These changes can't be the ground to administer immunocorrection therapy, and the indications for it had to be based on the clinical ID manifestations.

REFERENCES

1. Ivanenko T.V., Suchkov C.V., Nazarova L.O. et al., 1999, Diagnostic determination of surface lymphocyte antigens in patients with uveal melanomas and recurrent uveitis. *Russian J. Immunology* 4: (Suppl.1) 185 (in Russian).
2. Markina M.L., Chergeshtov Yu.I., Salmasi Zh.M. et al., 1999, Development of immunodepression in inflammatory processes of maxillofacial area. *Russian J. Immunology* 4: (Suppl.1) 194 (in Russian).
3. Novikova L.M., Starostina N.M., Shirinsky V.S., 1999, Application of immunocorrection preparations in patients with chronic bronchitis. *Russian J. Immunology* 4: (Suppl.1) 243 (in Russian).
4. Ostanin A.A., Khonina N.A., Norkin M.N. et al., 2000, T cell functional disturbances in patients with pulmonary tuberculosis. *Russian J. Immunology* 5: 53-62.
5. Ivanov O.L., Lomonosov K.M., Stenina M.A., 1998, Estimation of immune status in patients with early syphilis and its prognostic importance for negativation of serological reactions. *Russian J. Dermatological and Venereal Diseases* 6: 47-51. (in Russian)
6. Zavarzin A.A., 1999, Therapy of chronic recurrent prostatitis with its course at the background of immunodeficiency. *Russian J. Immunology* 4: (Suppl.1) 193. (in Russian)
7. Castilla I.A., Rueda R., Vargas M.L. et al., 1989, Decreased levels of circulating CD4+ T lymphocytes during normal human pregnancy. *J. Reprod. Immunol.* 15: 103-111.

AUTOIMMUNITY

The role of Fc receptors and complement in autoimmunity

ULRICH BAUMANN AND REINHOLD E. SCHMIDT
Department of Clinical Immunology, Hanover Medical School, D-30623 Hannover, Germay

IgG-autoantibodies are encountered in a number of autoimmune diseases, including rheumatoid arthritis, systemic lupus erythematosus, cryoglobulinaemia, autoimmune haemolytic anaemia, idiopathic thrombocytopenic purpura or hypersensitivity pneumonitis[1-7]. The involvement of autoantibodies in the pathogenesis of autoimmune diseases, however, is far from fully understood.

Noncovalent binding of IgG to souluble or cell surface bound antigens leads to formation of immune complexes (IC) that trigger an immune response if not removed by a specialized clearing system. Two effector pathways are known to be initiated by IC. One is activation of cell surface receptors specific for the Fc subunit of the heavy chain of IgG (FcγR), the other is activation of the classical complement cascade. In recent years, experimental models of autoimmune diseases were applied to mice dysfunctional in distinct mediators of these two pathways which greatly enhanced knowledge on mechanisms by which autoantibodies may propagate disease.

FcγR act at the interface between humoral and cellular immune system. Monomeric or aggregated IgG bound to specific antigen can bind to FcγR and trigger a cellular response. Three distinct classes of FcγR have been defined in human: FcγRI (CD64), FcγRII (CD32), and FcγRIII (CD 16). The FcγR classes differ in cellular distribution, function, and affinity to IgG isotypes. FcγRII and FcγRIII are both constitutively expressed on myeloid cell lines. FcγRI expression is constitutive on monocytic cells and dependent upon activation on granulocytes. Mast cells appear to lack FcγRI. Among lymphocytic cells, B cells express FcγRII and NK cells FcγRIII.

Progress in Basic and Clinical Immunology, Edited by Mackiewicz *et al.*
Kluwer Academic/Plenum Publishers, New York, 2001

Most FγR are transmembrane molecules with an intracellular immunoreceptor tyrosine-based activation motif (ITAM). There are two exceptions, FcγRIIIb, which is a glycosyl-phosphatidyl-inositol (GPI) membrane anchored molecule with activating properties, and FcγRIIb, which has an ihibitory motif (ITIM) in the intracellular domain. In mice, distribution and function of FcγR is largely comparable to human although differences exist in expression of some isoforms and in affinity to IgG isotypes. Murine neutrophils do not express FcγRI and a transmemranous FcγRIII instead of the GPI anchored FcγRIIIb[8].

Activating FcγR induce endocytosis or phagycytosis, antigen presentation, respiratory burst, mediator release, or antibody dependent cytotoxicity (ADCC), while the inhibiting FcγRIIb downregulates B cells and mast cells. FcγRI binds IgG with high affinity for monomeric and aggregated IgG, while FcγRII and FcγRIII are low affinity receptors for complexed IgG. Affinity to IgG isotypes will be discussed below. The diversity of FcγR in cellular expression and function together with IgG isotype specificities underlines that IC FcγR interaction is involved in various ways in the physiological immune response and may, therefore, be also differently contribute to pathophysiology in autoimmune disease.

Activation of the classical complement pathway as well as their sequelae resemble in many ways the FcγR mediated immune response. IC containing IgG can trigger both pathways, even with similar IgG isotype specificity (in human predominantly IgG1 and IgG3). Myeloid cells release oxygen reactive metabolites and proinflammatory cytokines upon activation by either FcγR or G-protein coupled receptors specific for cleavage products of the classical pathway, C3a and C5a. C5a also acts as a potent chemotactic agent for neutrophil migration. The pathophysiologic endpoints of either pathway are increased vascular permeability, infiltration of neutrophils and tissue damage[9].

Both pathways are also thought to be involved in IC clearance. Binding of IC to CR1 present on erythrocytes (in rodents on thrombocytes) is mediated by the complement fragment C3b. Due to this transport mechanism IC can be removed from circulation by specialized macrophages located in the liver, the Kupffer cells, and in the spleen, where C3b facilitates FcγR mediated phagocytosis. The clearance mechanism may be overcharged by persistent autoantibody production as in systemic lupus erythematodes. IC then aggregate and deposit elsewhere in the organism causing undue inflammation. In serum sickness, a repeated application of allogeneic serum protein leads to intravascular IC formation if antibodies directed against this protein have previously been induced.

The classical animal model of an IC reaction was first described by Arthus almost 100 years ago, who observed perivascular oedema, infiltration of neutrophils and tissue damage following repeated injection of antigen intradermally[10]. The most commonly used experimental model is the passive Arthus reverse reaction, owing it's name to the use of preformed IgG antibodies that are deposited in a desired tissue, followed by systemic application of the related antigen. Early experiments with depletion of C3 by an irreversible C3 convertase (cobra venom factor) resulted in marked attenuation of the inflammatory response in this model. Thus it was assumed that IC formation triggers tissue injury mainly by activation of the classical complement pathway[11].

Mice deficient in the γ-chain common to both, FcγRI and FcγRIII (FcRγ chain$^{-/-}$) also exhibited a strongly attenuated passive reverse Arthus reaction in the skin despite the presence of a functional complement system[12]. The authors concluded that FcγR play a dominant role in the initiation of the Arthus reaction. Reconstitution of mast cell deficient $kit^{W}/kit^{W\text{-}v}$ mice with mast cells from FcRγ chain$^{-/-}$ or FcRγ chain$^{+/+}$ demonstrated the critical role of FcγR dependent mast cell activation in the cutaneous Arthus reaction[13]. In contrast to the proposed secondary role of complement, mice deficient in the receptor for C5a, C5aR also exhibited a marked attenuation in the Arthus reaction of lung, peritoneum and skin[14;15].

We now focus on our work on the role of FcγR and complement in models of autoimmune diseases.

The FcγR and complement pathways in the Arthus reaction were characterised in more detail by identification of dominant mediators and tissue dependent reaction patterns. FcγRIII deficiency proved to be as effective in suppressing the cutaneous and pulmonary inflammation as combined FcγRI/FcγRIII deficiency demonstrating FcγRIII to be the dominant FcγR[16]. In IC peritonitis, however, FcγRIII deficiency could not alter the inflammatory response, whereas peritonitis in FcRγ chain$^{-/-}$ mice which lack additionally FcγRI was virtually abolished[17]. The dominant contribution of FcγRI in in IC peritonitis suggested the involvement of a cell line different from mast cells, most likely peritoneal macrophages, had to be involved. Activation of FcγRIII is negatively regulated by another FcγR, FcγRII. Receptor specific blockade or genetic deletion of FcγRII both lowered the threshold by which a substantial cutaneous Arthus reaction could be induced or augmented the cutaneous Arthus reaction at a given dose[18]. As FcγRII and FcγRIII share binding characteristics to IgG, downregulation appeares to prevent an inflammatory reaction at low IC levels.

Repeated complement depletion by cobra venom factor lead to a strong but not complete attenuation in the Arthus reaction of skin and lung. A similar effect was observed following a specific blockade of C5aR. C5a together with the related receptor are therefore key mediators of the complement pathway in the IC Arthus reaction. Interestingly, alveolar infiltration of neutrophils in a model of IC alveolitis was more strongly suppressed by complement dysfunction than by FcγR deficiency. Only the combination of both, deficiency of FcγRIII and blockade of C5aR, however, abrogated cutaneous and pulmonary reactions. Since either FcγR or complement could trigger only a minor response if the other pathway was dysfunctional, both pathways appeared to act synergistically. Our findings demonstrated a codominant role for FcγRIII and C5aR being both neccessary and together sufficient to induce the full strength of the inflammatory response[16].

A critical involvement of FcγR was demonstrated also in autoimmune haemolytic anaemia (AIHA), the oldest recognised autoimmune disease. In the most common form of AIHA, warm IgG-autoantibodies opsonize erythrocytes resulting in extravascular haemolysis. In a murine model of AIHA, monoclonal anti-erythrocytic antibodies of different IgG subclasses induce non-haemolytic anaemia by phagocytosis in liver and spleen. FcγRIII deficiency completely protected mice from anaemia, if a pathogenic IgG1 autoantibody was used, while IgG2a autoantibodies induced a persistent albeit less severe anaemia in FcγRIII $^{-/-}$ mice as in wildtype littermates[19]. Blockade of both FcγRII and FcγRIII could neither prevent IgG2a mediated anaemia, suggesting that IgG2a opsonized phagocytosis can also be mediated by FcγRI. Comparison of IgG class-switch variants of anti-erythrocytic autoantibodies further clarified differential contributions of IgG-FcγR interaction to AIHA. IgG2a had the most potent pathogenicity of all IgG isotypes with a strong affinity to FcγRIII. Interestingly, IgG2a antibodies could induce AIHA also in FcγRIII $^{-/-}$ animals, albeit at higher doses reflecting an only moderate affinity to FcγRI. A low affinity of IgG2b was observed equally to FcγRI and FcγRIII. IgG3 antibodies were unable to induce erythrophagocytosis[20]. In contrast to the findings in the cutaneous Arthus reaction, FcγRII was not a negative regulator of FcγRIII in AIHA *in vivo*, as FcγRIII dependent anaemia was not augmented by specific blockade or deficiency of FcγRII[18]. However, IgG1 opsonized erythrocytes did bind to FcγRII of peritoneal macrophages and enhanced phagocytosis *in vitro.* One hypothesis to explain this apparently different pattern between two monocytic cell lines is that hepatic Kupffer as persistently exposed to IC have upregulated FcγRIII to enable phagocytosis even at low IC levels which otherwise would be downregulated by FcγRII. The contribution of complement in this model seemed to be neglegable or at least substitutable. Depletion of C3 by cobra venom factor could not prevent or attenuate development of anaemia[18].

Deposition of circulating IC that cause vasculitic lesions can be observed in association with collagen diseases and in primary vasculitic disorders such as essential cryoglobulinaemia. We used an animal model with IgG3 anti rheumatoid factor monoclonal antibodies derived from lupus prone (MRL-lpr) mice with cryoglobulin activity. These autoantibodies were able to induce leukocytoklastic skin vasculitis in normal mice. The critical contribution of activating FcγR was demonstrated by use of FcRγ chain$^{-/-}$ mice, which exhibited no vascular lesions despite similar amounts of intravascular IC depositions in this model. Transfer of normal bone marrow derived mast cells (BMMC) to FcRγ chain$^{-/-}$ mice re-established leukocytoklastic vasculitis proving a critical contribution of this cell line to skin vasculitis. In contrast, transfer of macrophages showed no effect. Transfer of BMMC from FcγRIII $^{-/-}$ mice was equally ineffective in triggering vasculitis which excluded the contribution of other FcγR on mast cells. Mast cells appear to mediate skin vasculitis by tumor necrosis factor (TNF) since BMMC from TNFαβ $^{-/-}$ mice failed to induce autoimmune response[21].

The use of FcγR deficient mice provided new insight in the pathogenesis of autoimmune diseases. Due to their critical involvement in these and other models of autoimmune diseases, FcγR are prime targets for therapeutic interventions. Although differences between human and murine FcγR preclude a direct application of experimental findings in human, further research directed to develop mice humanized FcγR may bring bench and bedside more closely together[22].

ACKNOWLEDGEMENTS

The work summarized in this article was supported in part by grants of the Deutsche Forschungsgemeinschaft No. Ge892/2-2, Ge892/5-1, SFB 265/A09, SFB 265/B1, SFB 265 and by the HilF programme of Hanover Medical School.

REFERENCES

1. Korganow, A.S., Ji, H., Mangialaio, S., Duchatelle, V., Pelanda, R., Martin, T., Degott, C., Kikutani, H., Rajewski, K., Pasquali, J.L., Benoist, C., and Mathis, D., 1999, From systemic T cell self-reactivity to organ-specific autoimmune disease via immunoglobulins. *Immunity* 10:451-461
2. Madaio, M.P., 1999, The role of autoantibodies in the pathogenesis of lupus nephritis. *Semin.Nephrol.* 19:48-56
3. Ambrus, J.L.J., and Sridhar, N.R., 1997, Immunologic aspects of renal disease. *JAMA* 278:1938-1945

4. Dispenzieri, A., and Gorevic, P.D., 1999, Cryoglobulinemia. *Hematol.Oncol.Clin North Am* 13:1315-1349
5. Engelfriet, C.P., Overbeeke, M.A., and von dem Borne AE., 1992, Autoimmune hemolytic anemia. *Semin.Hematol.* 29 :3-12
6. Schmidt, R.E., Budde, U., Schafer, G., and Stroehmann, I., 1981, High-dose intravenous gammaglobulin for idiopathic thrombocytopenic purpura. *Lancet* 2:475-476
7. Ando, M., and Suga, M., 1997, Hypersensitivity pneumonitis. *Curr.Opin.Pulm.Med.* 3:391-395
8. Gessner, J.E., Heiken, H., Tamm, A., and Schmidt, R.E., 1998, The IgG Fc receptor family. *Ann.Hematol.* 76:231-248
9. Köhl, J., and Gessner, J.E., 1999, On the role of complement and Fcgamma-receptors in the Arthus reaction. *Mol.Immunol.* 36:893-903
10. Arthus M., 1903, Injections répétées de sérum de cheval chez le lapin. *Soc.Biol.* 55:817-825
11. Janeway, C.A. and P. Travers. 1997. *Immunobiology. The immune system in health and disease*. Current Biology/Garland Publishing, London/New York
12. Sylvestre, D.L., and Ravetch, J.V., 1994, Fc receptors initiate the Arthus reaction: redefining the inflammatory cascade. *Science* 265:1095-1098
13. Sylvestre, D.L., and Ravetch, J.V., 1996, A dominant role for mast cell Fc receptors in the Arthus reaction. *Immunity.* 5:387-390
14. Bozic, C.R., Lu, B., Höpken, U.E., Gerard, C., and Gerard, N.P., 1996, Neurogenic amplification of immune complex inflammation. *Science* 273:1722-1725
15. Höpken, U.E., Lu, B., Gerard, N.P., and Gerard, C., 1997, Impaired inflammatory responses in the reverse arthus reaction through genetic deletion of the C5a receptor. *J Exp Med* 186:749-756
16. Baumann, U., Köhl, J., Tschernig, T., Schwerter-Strumpf, K., Verbeek, J.S., Schmidt, R.E., and Gessner, J.E., 2000, A Codominant Role of FcgammaRI/III and C5aR in the Reverse Arthus Reaction. *J.Immunol.* 164:1065-1070
17. Heller, T., Gessner, J.E., Schmidt, R.E., Klos, A., Bautsch, W., and Köhl, J., 1999, Cutting edge: Fc receptor type I for IgG on macrophages and complement mediate the inflammatory response in immune complex peritonitis. *J.Immunol.* 162:5657-5661
18. Schiller, C., Janssen-Graalfs, I.R., Baumann, U., Schwerter-Strumpf, K., Izui, S., Takai, T., Schmidt, R.E., and Gessner, J.E., 2000, Mouse FcgammaRII is a negative regulator of FcgammaRIII in IgG immune complex triggered inflammation but not in autoantibody induced hemolysis. *Eur.J Immunol.* 30:481-490
19. Meyer, D., Schiller, C., Westermann, J., Izui, S., Hazenbos, W.L., Verbeek, J.S., Schmidt, R.E., and Gessner, J.E., 1998, FcgammaRIII (CD16)-deficient mice show IgG isotype-dependent protection to experimental autoimmune hemolytic anemia. *Blood* 92:3997-4002
20. Fossati-Jimack, L., Ioan-Facsinay, A., Reininger, L., Chicheportiche, Y., Watanabe, N., Saito, T., Hofhuis, F.M., Gessner, J.E., Schiller, C., Schmidt, R.E., Honjo, T., Verbeek, J.S., and Izui, S., 2000, Markedly different pathogenicity of four immunoglobulin G isotype-switch variants of an antierythrocyte autoantibody is based on their capacity to interact in vivo with the low-affinity Fcgamma receptor III. *J Exp.Med.* 191:1293-1302
21. Watanabe, N., Akikusa, B., Park, S.Y., Ohno, H., Fossati, L., Vecchietti, G., Gessner, J.E., Schmidt, R.E., Verbeek, J.S., Ryffel, B., Iwamoto, I., Izui, S., and Saito, T., 1999, Mast Cells Induce Autoantibody-Mediated Vasculitis Syndrome Through Tumor Necrosis Factor Production Upon Triggering Fcgamma Receptors. *Blood* 94:3855-3863

22. Deo, Y.M., Graziano, R.F., Repp, R., and van de Winkel JG., 1997, Clinical significance of IgG Fc receptors and Fc gamma R-directed immunotherapies. *Immunol.Today* 18:127-135

Effect of Hsp70-peptide complexes generated *in vivo* on modulation EAE

GRAZYNA GALAZKA, AGATA WALCZAK, TOMASZ BERKOWICZ and KRZYSZTOF SELMAJ
Department of Neurology, Laboratory of Neuroimmunology, Medical Academy of Lodz, Kopcinskiego Street, Poland.

1. INTRODUCTION

Heat shock proteins (Hsps) are a family of proteins that are constitutively expressed by eukaryotic cells. They act as molecular chaperones, participating in intracellular translocation of proteins and enabling proper folding of polypeptide chains. It is postulated that unique chaperoning properties of Hsps might contribute to generating specific immune responses against peptides bound to them[1, 2]. Many studies have demonstrated that Hsps isolated from cancer or viral infected cells elicit antitumor or antiviral immune response. However, Hsps derived from normal cells did not shown such effect[3, 4.] It has been suggested that peptides associated with Hsps are responsible for this specific immunogenecity[5].

Hsps are expressed in normal central nervous system; its amount is increased in chronic degenerative and inflammatory diseases, what lead to immune response to these proteins. We analyzed the ability of Hsp70-

Progress in Basic and Clinical Immunology, Edited by Mackiewicz *et al.*
Kluwer Academic/Plenum Publishers, New York, 2001

peptide complexes to modulate autoimmune response in a mouse model of human inflammatory demyelinating disease of CNS (multiple sclerosis)-experimental autoimmune encephalomyelitis (EAE).

2. RESULTS

2.1 The effect of preimmunization with Hsp70 on EAE development

The immunogenecity of the Hsp70 preparations were determined by their influence on the development of subsequently induced EAE. Hsp70-peptide complexes generated *in vivo* were isolated from CNS tissues of healthy and EAE mice by ADP- and Hsp70 alone by ATP- affinity chromatography[6].

Hsp70 proteins (12 μg) were used for preimmunization of 6-weeks-old SJL/J female mice twice, at weekly intervals. One week after last proteins injection the EAE was induced with PLP139-151 peptide. The severity of disease as observed and compared to control group (mice with no preimmunization with Hsp70).

Only mice preimmunization with Hsp70-peptide complexes, isolated from EAE mice, protected them from subsequent EAE induction or highly reduced the EAE severity (Fig. 1A). Hsp alone isolated from EAE mice only slightly reduced EAE severity (Fig. 1A). Such effect was not observed after preimmunization with Hsp70 preparations purified from healthy mice (Fig. 1B).

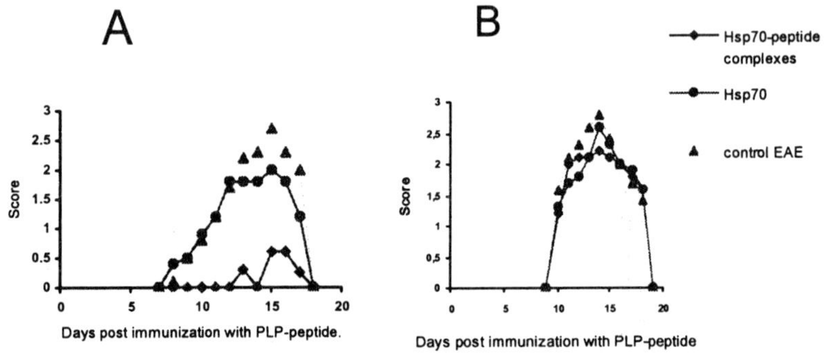

Figure 1. Effect of Hsp70 preparations on development of subsequent induced EAE. Purified Hsp70-peptide complexes and Hsp70 alone isolated from mice with EAE (1A) and healthy mice (1B).

2.2 Dose dependent effect of Hsp70-peptide complexes on EAE development

Mice were preimmunized before induction of EAE with different dose (2, 12, and 24 μg) of Hsp70-peptide complexes purified from EAE mice. The inhibitory effect of Hsp70-peptide complexes increased with higher Hsp70 dose used (Fig. 2A).

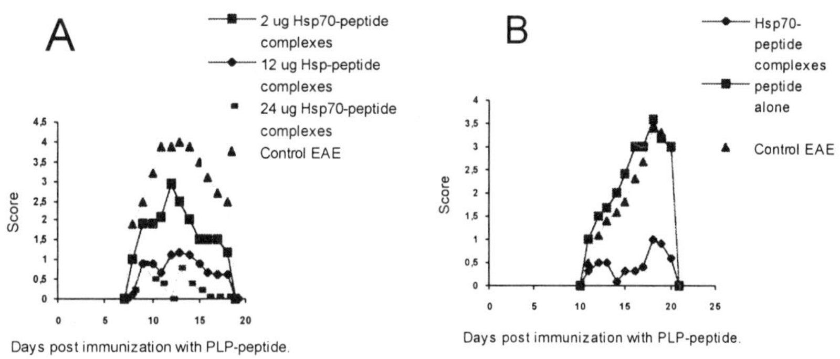

Figure 2. A- Dose dependent effect of Hsp70-peptide complexes on EAE development.
B- Effect of endogenous peptides on development of subsequently induced EAE.

2.3 Effect of endogenous peptides on EAE development

To determine whether EAE resistance dependents on peptides associated with Hsp70, the peptides were stripped from Hsp70-peptide complexes, by incubation with 10 mM ATP and used for preimmunization. There was no effect of preimmunization with peptides alone on EAE (Fig. 2B). These data indicated that peptides alone have no immunogenecity by themselves.

3. CONCLUSION

Previous studies were concentrated on the protective role of Hsps immunization on experimental autoimmune diseases[7]. The preimmunization with mycobacterial Hsp70, Hsp60, Hsp10, human Hsp60 have protective effect on subsequently induced experimental arthritis. The EAE and diabetes in nonobese diabetic mice were also inhibited by preimmunization with mycobacterial Hsp60. However, the protective mechanisms of Hsps in autoimmune diseases remained unclear.

In our study we investigated the role of preimmunization with Hsp-peptide complexes generated *in vivo* on EAE. For the first time, we showed that only Hsp70-peptide complexes derived from CNS tissues of EAE mice have immunological activity. Development of EAE in mice was inhibited by prior immunization with Hsp70-peptide complexes and this effect was dose dependent. Only Hsp70 complexes isolated from EAE mice but not by Hsp70 complexes isolated from healthy mice or any Hsp70 alone or any peptides alone expressed this inhibitory effect. Our data may help to understand the mechanisms of immune responses and may enable to control the autoimmune disease, like multiple sclerosis.

ACKNOWLEDGEMENTS

This work was supported by a KBN Grant 6.PO4A.056.18.

REFERENCES

1. Srivastava, P.K., 1993, Peptide-biding heat shock proteins in the endoplasmic reticulum: role in immune response to cancer and in antigen presentation. Adv. Cancer Res. 62: 153-177.
2. Srivastava, P.K., Meoret, A., Basu, S., Binder, R.J., McQuade, K.L., 1998, Heat shock proteins come of age: primitive function acquire new roles in an adaptive world. Immunity. 8: 657-665.
3. Udono, H., and Srivastava, P.K., 1994, Comparison of tumor-specific immunogenicities of stress-induced proteins gp96, Hsp90, and Hsp70, J. Immunol. 152: 5398-5403.
4. Suto, R., and Srivastava, P.K., 1995, A mechanism for the specific immunogenicity of heat shock protein-chaperoned peptides. Science. 269: 1585-1588.
5. Li, Z., and Srivastava, P.K., 1993, Tumor rejection antigen gp96/grp94 is an ATPase: implications for protein folding and antigen presentation. EMBO J. 12: 3143-3151.
6. Peng, P., Menoret, A., Srivastava, P.K., 1997, Purification of immunogenic heat shock protein 70-peptide complexes by ADP-affinity chromatography. J. Immunolgical Methods. 204: 13-21.
7. van Eden, W., van der Zee, R., Paul, A.G.J., Prakken, B.J., Wendling, U., Anderton, S.M., and Wauben, M.H.M., 1998, Do heat shock proteins control the balance of T-cell regulation in inflammatory diseases?. Immunol. Today. 19: 303-307.
8. Udono, H., and Srivastava P.K., 1993, Heat shock protein 70 – associated peptides elicit specific cancer immunity. J. Exp. Med. 178: 1391-1396. Methods. 204: 13-21.

Gene transfer of protective cytokines in rheumatoid arthritis

OLIVER DISTLER[1], CHRISTIAN A. SEEMAYER[1], THOMAS PAP[1], RENATE E. GAY[1], MICHEL NEIDHART[1], ULF MÜLLER-LADNER[2] AND STEFFEN GAY[1]

[1]*WHO Collaborating Center for Molecular Biology and Novel Therapeutic Strategies for Rheumatic Diseases, University Hospital Zurich, Switzerland;* [2]*Department of Internal Medicine I, University of Regensburg, Germany*

1. INTRODUCTION

Rheumatoid arthritis (RA) is a chronic inflammatory disease primarily affecting the joints resulting in their progressive destruction and in significant morbidity in the individual patient. Although the course of the disease is variable, the cumulative prevalence of work disability is as high as 50% at 10 years after onset of the disease (1). Considering that the prevalence of rheumatoid arthritis among adults has recently been estimated to be 10 per 1000 in the US, and that rheumatoid arthritis affects patients often in their most productive years, the socio-economic consequences for both the individual patient and society are severe (2).

Treatment regimens with disease modifying drugs used in the past were able to slow progression of the disease in some patients, but frequently destruction of the joints could not be prevented. While these treatments were based purely on empiric observations, recent advances in the elucidation of key molecules in the pathogenesis of RA have led to the development of drugs that target more specific pathways. In particular, treatment with anti-TNF and anti-IL-1 reagents resulted in an improvement of a wide range of disease activity parameters in clinical trials. However, the long-term effects on the progressive destruction of articular cartilage and bone that accounts

Progress in Basic and Clinical Immunology, Edited by Mackiewicz *et al.*
Kluwer Academic/Plenum Publishers, New York, 2001

largely for the morbidity of the patients are still unclear. In addition, there are concerns about the development of autoantibodies with the prolonged use of these agents, and the systemic inhibition of these cytokines may have also other yet unknown risks. Thus, the identification of key pathways in the pathogenesis of RA that can be targeted in therapeutic approaches are a major challenge of ongoing research. In the present work, we show that gene transfer into synovial fibroblasts using replication defective retroviral vectors is feasible and may help to elucidate the role of certain molecules in the pathogenesis of RA.

2. SYNOVIAL FIBROBLASTS AND THE SCID MOUSE MODEL OF RA

The main message that has been learned from the discovery and characterization of various pathways during the last years is that the development and progression of RA requires a distinct and highly coordinated interaction of different cell types. T cells are dominant in the inflammatory infiltrates of RA and might regulate the release of IL-1β, TNF-α, IL-15 and other molecules by macrophages and synoviocytes. B cells produce autoantibodies that might have a functional role in the pathogenesis of RA, and endothelial cell proliferation leads to the increased angiogenesis in the rheumatoid synovium that allows the migration of inflammatory cells into the tissue (3).

Along this line, the role of synovial fibroblasts in the pathogenesis of RA has recently been redefined (4). The synovial intimal lining, the interface between the synovium and the intraarticular space, is hyperplastic in RA and consists mainly of macrophages and synovial fibroblasts. Whereas synovial macrophages account for much of the production of IL-1 and TNFα, synovial fibroblasts produce angiogenic factors such as VEGF and, most importantly, large amounts of various matrix-degrading enzymes, including MMP`s, MT-MMP`s, and the cysteine proteinases cathepsin B, L and K (4-7). A crucial question in the pathogenesis of RA is, whether the activated and destructive properties of synovial fibroblasts require the continuous stimulation by mediators released from macrophages and T cells or whether these features are intrinsic for rheumatoid synovial fibroblasts.

To address this question, the SCID mouse model of rheumatoid arthritis was developed in our laboratory (8, 9). In this model, human rheumatoid synovium or cultured fibroblasts are implanted together with normal human cartilage in an inert gel sponge under the renal capsule of SCID mice. Since SCID mice do not reject xenografts due to defects in B- and T-cell functions, the invasion of synovial fibroblasts into the cartilage can be histologically assessed after 60 days. When multiple passaged CD68-negative, prolyl 4-hydroxylase-positive synovial fibroblasts from patients with RA were used in these experiments, an attachment and deep invasive growth into the cartilage was observed (Fig.1), whereas control experiments with foreskin, osteoarthritis and normal synovial fibroblasts showed no or only limited signs of invasion. Matrix degrading enzymes such as cathepsin B and in particular cathepsin L as well as the adhesion molecule VCAM-1 were expressed by rheumatoid synovial fibroblasts at sites of invasion. These data indicate that synovial fibroblasts keep their destructive potential even in the absence of an articular inflammatory milieu. In addition, the expression of VCAM-1 even after long-term culture and an additional 60 days in the SCID mice suggests that there is a stable and intrinsic activation of rheumatoid synovial fibroblasts that does not require additional exogenous stimulation.

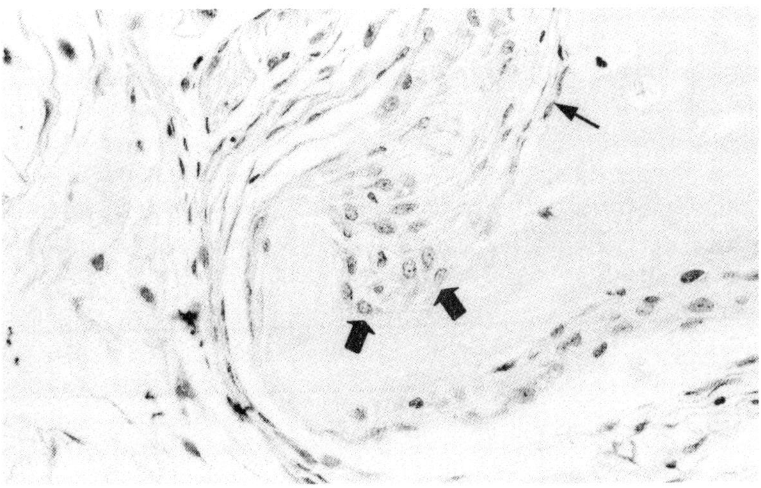

Figure 1. Synovial fibroblasts from a patient with rheumatoid arthritis engrafted together with normal human cartilage under the renal capsule of a SCID mouse. Sixty days after implantation, synovial fibroblasts are attached to the cartilage (small arrow). Large arrows show fibroblasts at sites of invasion into the cartilage. Original magnification x 400.

3. GENE TRANSFER OF PROTECTIVE CYTOKINES IN THE SCID MOUSE MODEL OF RA: IL-1Ra, TNFαR1 AND IL-10

The interleukin-1 (IL-1) gene family consists of three members: IL-1α, IL-1β, and the IL-1 receptor antagonist (IL-1Ra). In the rheumatoid synovium, activated macrophages are the main source of IL-1α and IL-1β, but endothelial cells, chondrocytes as well as synovial fibroblasts have also been shown to express IL-1 (10). Binding of IL-1 to its cell surface receptor (IL-1R) leads to signal transduction and cell activation. IL-1Ra is a naturally occurring inhibitor of IL-1 that is expressed in the rheumatoid synovium and binds competitively to IL-1R, but has no intrinsic activitis. Several studies have suggested that a 10- to 100-fold molar excess of IL-1Ra is needed to inhibit 50% of the IL-1 response that normally occurs in cells expressing IL-R (11, 12). Besides the induction of a wide variety of proinflammatory molecules, the major impact of IL-1 on the pathophysiology of RA might be the stimulation of synovial fibroblasts to produce cartilage degrading enzymes such as collagenases and stromelysin (13). The importance of the IL-1 gene family for the pathogenesis of rheumatoid arthritis is further underlined by studies with IL-1Ra deficient mice (14). IL-1Ra$^{-/-}$ mice on a BALB/cA background develop arthritis spontaneously at 5 weeks of age and at 13 weeks, all of the IL-1Ra$^{-/-}$ mice had developed arthritis. This arthritis resembled rheumatoid arthritis in that synovial inflammation, cartilage and bone erosions as well as activated osteoclasts were found in the affected joints.

To examine the effects of IL-1Ra on the invasive behaviour of synovial fibroblasts, we used a combination of the SCID mouse model and a gene transfer approach with the replication-defective retroviral MFG vector (15). When cultured synovial fibroblasts were transfected with the MFG vector containing the IL-1Ra gene, IL-1Ra protein could be detected in supernatants from these cells by ELISA for as long as 72 days, whereas no IL-1ra was found in supernatants from Mock-transfected and untransfected fibroblasts. Moreover, expression of IL-Ra mRNa was observed by in situ hybridisation in MFG/IL-1Ra transfected synovial fibroblasts that were coimplanted with normal human cartilage into the SCID mouse, but not in mock-transfected fibroblasts in the same setting. These data indicate that the insertion of certain genes of interest into the genome of synovial fibroblasts together with their long-term expression of protein can be achieved using the MFG retroviral vector system.

Synovial fibroblasts that were transfected with the MFG/IL-1Ra vector showed a similar invasion into the coimplanted cartilage as did mock-transfected fibroblasts. In contrast, chondrocyte-mediated cartilage degradation, as measured by the diameter of degradation around individual chondrons in the coimplanted cartilage, was markedly reduced in experiments with MFG/IL-1ra transfected synovial fibroblasts compared to controls. The conclusion that could be drawn from these studies was that the intrinsic potential of synovial fibroblasts to invade human cartilage is independent of IL-1, but that IL-1 is significantly involved in pericullar chondrocyte-meidated cartilage destruction.

Of note, these experiments do not rule out that IL-1 might be a major player in the extrinsic machinery that in addition to the preexisting intrinsic activation can stimulate synovial fibroblasts in RA. This concept is further supported by recent studies in our laboratory, in which a novel in vitro model of cartilage degradation was used (16, 17). In this model, synovial fibroblasts are cocultured with a cartilage like matrix that is ^{35}S labelled and generated by growing isolated chondrocytes in 3-dimensional collagen sponges soaked with bovine extracellular matrix. The release of ^{35}S, subtracted by the spontaneous release, reflects the degradation of the cartilaginous matrix caused by synovial fibroblasts. When IL-1β was added to the cells matrix, matrix degradation by synovial fibroblasts was markedly increased compared to controls as indicated by an increase in the released radioactivity.

Thus, a likely scenario might be that synovial fibroblasts invade human cartilage in RA through intrinsic, IL-1 independent mechanisms. In addition, IL-1 released by synovial macrophages in the rheumatoid synovium stimulates synovial fibroblasts to release MMP's and other matrix degrading enzymes, thereby further enhancing their invasive and degradative behaviour of these cells.

Another cytokine that has been implied in the pathogenesis of RA is the tumor necrosis factor-α (TNF-α). TNF-α is elevated in the serum and synovial fluid of patients with RA and is produced by synovial endothelial cells, lymphocytes and in particular macrophages (18). Transgenic mice expressing a 3`modified human TNF transgene develop a chronic inflammatory polyarthritis that resembles clinically and histologically RA (19). The administration of neutralizing anti-TNF antibodies to mice with type II collagen induced arthritis reduced clinical scores, paw swelling and the histological severity of the disease in various studies (20).

Among other features, TNF mediates a broad range of proinflammatory activities including the induction of proinflammatory cytokines (e.g. IL-1, IL-6) and chemokines (e.g. IL-8, MCP-1, RANTES), the upregulation of adhesion molecules and the stimulation of angiogenesis (21). In addition, TNF-α has been shown to induce proliferation and synthesis of MMP's in rheumatoid synovial fibroblasts (13). The action of TNF-α is mediated via two different receptors, the 55-kd TNF-α receptor p55 and the 75-kd TNF-α receptor p75. The TNF-α receptor p55, also known as TNF-R1, is the high affinity receptor for soluble TNF at 37°C. Thus, cellular responses to the soluble 17-kDa form of TNF seems to be dominated by the interaction with TNF-R1, whereas the TNF-α receptor p75, also known as TNF-R2, appears to be the primary binding receptor for the 26-kd transmembrane form of TNF (22). Both receptors have been found to be expressed by more than 90% of cells in the lining layer in synovial biopsies of patients with RA (23).

Similar to IL-1, the bioavailability of TNF-α is tightly controlled by soluble variants of surface TNF-R1 and TNF-R2. In an attempt to maintain homoeostasis in the inflamed joint, both soluble TNF-receptors are produced spontaneously by synovial cells derived from patients with RA (24).

Due to the prominent role of TNF-α in many pathogenetic features of RA, we attempted next to analyse the role of the TNF pathway in the fibroblast mediated cartilage invasion and degradation using a retrovirus based gene transfer approach similar to the one used for the IL-1Ra studies (25). Due to the higher affinity for TNF at 37°C, and since it had been shown that the cytokine production of synovial fibroblasts is inhibited more effectively by TNF-R1 than TNF-R2, soluble TNF-R1 was chosen as an inhibitor for TNF in these studies (26).

Rheumatoid synovial fibroblasts that were transfected with the retroviral MFG vector containing the human TNF-R1 gene showed a 5-10 fold upregulated level of the soluble TNF-R1 protein in culture supernatants after 48 hours compared to lacZ- and mock-transfected fibroblasts. By in situ RT-PCR, the expression of TNF-R1 mRNA by synovial fibroblasts could still be detected 60 days after implantation into the SCID mouse, thereby proving again that cytokines can be successfully inserted into the genome of human RA synovial fibroblasts using a retroviral vector delivery system. However, when the invasiveness of the TNF-R1 transduced fibroblasts into the human cartilage was compared to the invasiveness of the lacZ- and mock-transduced fibroblasts, no significant differences were found. In contrast to IL-1Ra, the incorporation of TNF-R1 into the genome of RA fibroblasts did not alter perichondrocytic cartilage degradation.

Possible explanations for these findings include that the constitutive expression of TNF-α by RA synovial fibroblasts does not reach the necessary threshold levels to stimulate the expression of cartilage degrading enzymes in an autocrine fashion. To test this hypothesis, recombinant TNF-α was added to the in vitro model of cartilage degradation described above. After stimulation with TNF, cartilage degradation by rheumatoid synovial fibroblasts increased significantly compared to non-stimulated controls (16). However, when the cartilaginous matrix was pretreated with cycloheximide to block protein synthesis from chondrocytes, the addition of TNF-α did not any longer result in an increased cartilage degradation (17). Thus, while IL-1 might be an important trigger in the extrinsic activation of RA synovial fibroblasts, the situation with TNF-α appears to be more complex in that it requires the interaction with chondrocytes to exert its stimulating effects on synovial fibroblasts. The concept of TNF-α as a factor that is primarily involved in perpetuating inflammatory pathways is further supported by experiments from van den Berg and coworkers, who showed in different murine arthritis models that blockade of IL-1 prevents destruction of cartilage and bone, whereas blockade of TNF-α affects mainly joint inflammation (20, 27).

Another interesting candidate for gene transfer studies in rheumatoid arthritis is interleukin-10 (IL-10). Other than TNF-α and IL-1, IL-10 has predominantly anti-inflammatory properties. In particular, IL-10 has been shown to inhibit the synthesis of a wide range of proinflammatory mediators including IL-1, IL-6, IL-8, TNF-α, MIP-1α and prostaglandins. On the other hand, IL-10 has also some stimulatory effects on the immune system in that it enhances the proliferation and differentiation of antibody forming B cells and increases the activity of monocytes by enhancing the expression of Fc receptors. IL-10 is upregulated in RA synovial fluid and serum and has been found to be overexpressed in synovial tissue samples of patients with RA compared to healthy controls. This increase in the production of IL-10 might reflect a physiologic response to the activated immune system in the rheumatoid synovium (28).

For the gene transfer studies in the SCID mouse model of RA, viral and murine IL-10 were each inserted into the MFG vector, replacing the env gene and thereby resulting in an replication defective retrovirus (25). Again, it could be shown that the retrovirus based gene transfer into synovial fibroblasts is feasible, since the IL-10 protein was several fold upregulated after transfection compared to the control experiments. Both the viral and murine IL-10 gene transfer into the RA synovial fibroblasts resulted in a significant reduction of the invasiveness into the adjacent cartilage compared with mock transfected fibroblasts. No effect was seen on the perichondrocytic cartilage degradation. These results were confirmed by a study from Jorgensen et al, in which total human rheumatoid synovium was coimplanted with human cartilage into SCID mice (29). In this study, type 5 E1a E1b-deficient non-replicative adenovirus vector containing the viral IL-10 gene was applied systemically. Similar to our results, cartilage invasion was dramatically inhibited in animals treated with the vector containing the viral IL-10 gene.

The molecular mechanisms that account for the inhibition of the fibroblasts invasion have still to be elucidated in detail. However, IL-10 has been shown to induce TIMP-1 and to inhibit MMP-2 and MMP-9 synthesis in different cell types (30). Further support for a major role of the TIMP/MMP balance in the inhibition of fibroblasts invasion by IL-10 comes from the study from Jorgensen et al. While the number of CD3 positive cells and the expression of IL-1, IL-6, TNF-α and IL-8 was not altered by the gene transfer with viral IL-10, a marked inhibition of the expression of MMP-3 mRNA and an upregulation of TIMP-1 mRNA was observed (29).

Table 1. Gene transfer of protective cytokines into RA synovial fibroblasts using the retroviral MFG vector. Transfected fibroblasts were coimplanted with human cartilage into SCID mice and analyzed after 60 days for their invasion into cartilage and for their effects on the degradation of cartilage by chondrocytes in comparison to mock-transfected controls.

	Feasibility	Invasion	perichondrocytic cartilage degradation
IL-1Ra	++	*no effects*	*inhibited*
TNF-R1	++	*no effects*	*no effects*
IL-10	++	*inhibited*	*no effects*

4. CONCLUSION

The rapid progress in molecular biology techniques has led to the identification of key pathways in the pathogenesis of rheumatoid arthritis during the last decade. The application of molecules that interfere with these pathways might be a novel approach in the therapy of RA. In fact, initial clinical studies with anti-TNF and anti-IL-1 strategies revealed promising results. However, the maintenance of therapeutic levels of these and other molecules that might protect cartilage from degradation is difficult to achieve. Thus, we used the SCID mouse model of RA that was established in our laboratory to evaluate, whether a prolonged expression of genes can be achieved using a retroviral gene delivery approach. Herein, we show that transfection of synovial fibroblasts is feasible using the replication-defective retroviral MFG vector. Transfection resulted in prolonged expression of genes that were inserted into the MFG vector. Moreover, we could show that overexpression of IL-10, but not TNF-R1 and IL-1Ra resulted in an inhibition of fibroblast invasion into human cartilage and that overexpression of IL-1Ra, but not TNF-R1 and IL-10 inhibited cartilage degradation by chondrocytes (Table 1). Thus, the inhibition of only one destructive pathway might not be sufficient to cover all aspects of cartilage degradation, and double gene transfer with IL-10 and IL-1ra might be required to inhibit both invasion of RA synovial fibroblasts and perichondrocytic cartilage degradation as shown recently (31).

ACKNOWLEDGMENTS

The work was supported by a grant from the Leopoldina Foundation (BMBF-LPD 9901/8-7) and the Swiss National Science Foundation.

REFERENCES

1. T.Sokka, H.Kautiainen, T.Mottonen, and P.Hannonen, Work disability in rheumatoid arthritis 10 years after the diagnosis, J Rheumatol. 26:1681 (1999).
2. R.C.Lawrence, C.G.Helmick, F.C.Arnett, R.A.Deyo, D.T.Felson, E.H.Giannini, S.P.Heyse, R.Hirsch, M.C.Hochberg, G.G.Hunder, M.H.Liang, S.R.Pillemer, V.D.Steen, and F.Wolfe, Estimates of the prevalence of arthritis and selected musculoskeletal disorders in the United States, Arthritis Rheum. 41:778 (1998).
3. C.M.Weyand, New insights into the pathogenesis of rheumatoid arthritis, Rheumatology.(Oxford) 39 Suppl 1:3 (2000).
4. G.S.Firestein, Invasive fibroblast-like synoviocytes in rheumatoid arthritis. Passive responders or transformed aggressors?, Arthritis Rheum. 39:1781 (1996).
5. K.M.Hummel, P.K.Petrow, J.K.Franz, U.Muller-Ladner, W.K.Aicher, R.E.Gay, D.Bromme, and S.Gay, Cysteine proteinase cathepsin K mRNA is expressed in synovium of patients with rheumatoid arthritis and is detected at sites of synovial bone destruction, J Rheumatol. 25:1887 (1998).
6. T.Pap, Y.Shigeyama, S.Kuchen, J.K.Fernihough, B.Simmen, R.E.Gay, M.Billingham, and S.Gay, Differential expression pattern of membrane-type matrix metalloproteinases in rheumatoid arthritis, Arthritis Rheum. 43:1226 (2000).
7. G.Cunnane, O.FitzGerald, K.M.Hummel, R.E.Gay, S.Gay, and B.Bresnihan, Collagenase, cathepsin B and cathepsin L gene expression in the synovial membrane of patients with early inflammatory arthritis, Rheumatology.(Oxford) 38:34 (1999).
8. U.Muller-Ladner, J.Kriegsmann, B.N.Franklin, S.Matsumoto, T.Geiler, R.E.Gay, and S.Gay, Synovial fibroblasts of patients with rheumatoid arthritis attach to and invade normal human cartilage when engrafted into SCID mice, Am J Pathol. 149:1607 (1996).
9. T.Geiler, J.Kriegsmann, G.M.Keyszer, R.E.Gay, and S.Gay, A new model for rheumatoid arthritis generated by engraftment of rheumatoid synovial tissue and normal human cartilage into SCID mice, Arthritis Rheum. 37:1664 (1994).
10. C.Q.Chu, M.Field, S.Allard, E.Abney, M.Feldmann, and R.N.Maini, Detection of cytokines at the cartilage/pannus junction in patients with rheumatoid arthritis: implications for the role of cytokines in cartilage destruction and repair, Br.J Rheumatol. 31:653 (1992).
11. B.Bresnihan and G.Cunnane, Interleukin-1 receptor antagonist, Rheum.Dis.Clin.North Am 24:615 (1998).
12. C.A.Dinarello, Biologic basis for interleukin-1 in disease, Blood 87:2095 (1996).
13. B.A.Moore, S.Aznavoorian, J.A.Engler, and L.J.Windsor, Induction of collagenase-3 (MMP-13) in rheumatoid arthritis synovial fibroblasts, Biochim.Biophys.Acta 1502:307 (2000).
14. R.Horai, S.Saijo, H.Tanioka, S.Nakae, K.Sudo, A.Okahara, T.Ikuse, M.Asano, and Y.Iwakura, Development of chronic inflammatory arthropathy resembling rheumatoid arthritis in interleukin 1 receptor antagonist-deficient mice, J Exp.Med. 191:313 (2000).
15. U.Muller-Ladner, C.R.Roberts, B.N.Franklin, R.E.Gay, P.D.Robbins, C.H.Evans, and S.Gay, Human IL-1Ra gene transfer into human synovial fibroblasts is chondroprotective, J Immunol. 158:3492 (1997).
16. M.Neidhart, R.E.Gay, and S.Gay, Anti-interleukin-1 and anti-CD44 interventions producing significant inhibition of cartilage destruction in an in vitro model of cartilage invasion by rheumatoid arthritis synovial fibroblasts, Arthritis Rheum. 43:1719 (2000).

17. T.Pap, W.H.van der Laan, K.R.Aupperle, R.E.Gay, J.H.Verheijen, G.S.Firestein, S.Gay, and M.Neidhart, Modulation of fibroblast-mediated cartilage degradation by articular chondrocytes in rheumatoid arthritis, Arthritis Rheum. 43:2531 (2000).
18. C.Q.Chu, M.Field, M.Feldmann, and R.N.Maini, Localization of tumor necrosis factor alpha in synovial tissues and at the cartilage-pannus junction in patients with rheumatoid arthritis, Arthritis Rheum. 34:1125 (1991).
19. J.Keffer, L.Probert, H.Cazlaris, S.Georgopoulos, E.Kaslaris, D.Kioussis, and G.Kollias, Transgenic mice expressing human tumour necrosis factor: a predictive genetic model of arthritis, EMBO J 10:4025 (1991).
20. L.A.Joosten, M.M.Helsen, F.A.van De Loo, and W.B.van Den Berg, Anticytokine treatment of established type II collagen-induced arthritis in DBA/1 mice. A comparative study using anti-TNF alpha, anti-IL-1 alpha/beta, and IL-1Ra, Arthritis Rheum. 39:797 (1996).
21. A.F.Kavanaugh, Anti-tumor necrosis factor-alpha monoclonal antibody therapy for rheumatoid arthritis, Rheum.Dis.Clin.North Am 24:593 (1998).
22. M.Grell, H.Wajant, G.Zimmermann, and P.Scheurich, The type 1 receptor (CD120a) is the high-affinity receptor for soluble tumor necrosis factor, Proc.Natl.Acad.Sci.U.S.A 95:570 (1998).
23. B.W.Deleuran, C.Q.Chu, M.Field, F.M.Brennan, T.Mitchell, M.Feldmann, and R.N.Maini, Localization of tumor necrosis factor receptors in the synovial tissue and cartilage-pannus junction in patients with rheumatoid arthritis. Implications for local actions of tumor necrosis factor alpha, Arthritis Rheum. 35:1170 (1992).
24. F.M.Brennan, D.L.Gibbons, A.P.Cope, P.Katsikis, R.N.Maini, and M.Feldmann, TNF inhibitors are produced spontaneously by rheumatoid and osteoarthritic synovial joint cell cultures: evidence of feedback control of TNF action, Scand.J Immunol. 42:158 (1995).
25. U.Muller-Ladner, C.H.Evans, B.N.Franklin, C.R.Roberts, R.E.Gay, P.D.Robbins, and S.Gay, Gene transfer of cytokine inhibitors into human synovial fibroblasts in the SCID mouse model, Arthritis Rheum. 42:490 (1999).
26. D.M.Butler, M.Feldmann, F.Di Padova, and F.M.Brennan, p55 and p75 tumor necrosis factor receptors are expressed and mediate common functions in synovial fibroblasts and other fibroblasts, Eur.Cytokine Netw. 5:441 (1994).
27. L.A.Joosten, M.M.Helsen, T.Saxne, F.A.van De Loo, D.Heinegard, and W.B.van Den Berg, IL-1 alpha beta blockade prevents cartilage and bone destruction in murine type II collagen-induced arthritis, whereas TNF-alpha blockade only ameliorates joint inflammation, J Immunol. 163:5049 (1999).
28. E.Keystone, J.Wherry, and P.Grint, IL-10 as a therapeutic strategy in the treatment of rheumatoid arthritis, Rheum.Dis.Clin.North Am 24:629 (1998).
29. C.Jorgensen, F.Apparailly, F.Canovas, C.Verwaerde, C.Auriault, C.Jacquet, and J.Sany, Systemic viral interleukin-10 gene delivery prevents cartilage invasion by human rheumatoid synovial tissue engrafted in SCID mice, Arthritis Rheum. 42:678 (1999).
30. M.E.Stearns, F.U.Garcia, K.Fudge, J.Rhim, and M.Wang, Role of interleukin 10 and transforming growth factor beta1 in the angiogenesis and metastasis of human prostate primary tumor lines from orthotopic implants in severe combined immunodeficiency mice, Clin.Cancer Res. 5:711 (1999).
31. E.Neumann, M.Judex, T.Pap, O.Distler, R.E.Gay, P.D.Robbins, C.H.Evans, J.Schölmerich, S.Gay, and U.Muller-Ladner, Additive cartilage protection by retrovirus-based double gene transfer with IL-1ra and IL-10 in the SCID mouse model for RA, Arthritis Rheum. 43:S170 (2000).

Modification of humoral antisperm response

BEATA GRYGIELSKA, DOROTA FISZER, ALINA DOMAGAŁA, MACIEJ KURPISZ
Institute of Human Genetics, Polish Academy of Sciences, Poznan, Poland

1. INTRODUCTION

Considerable effort has been made to create animal models in which functions of the human immune system can be studied under the experimental *in vivo* conditions. An important step in this direction was demonstrated when the SCID mice were stably grafted with human lymphoid cells. This animal model allows the testing of various antigens and adjuvants in *in situ* conditions inducing human immune effector cells and permitting the optimization of the subsequent response.

1.1 Initial Comments

The surface of sperm is richly glycosylated and ASA induced by glycosylated, native antigen gave a low affinity, poor specificity and low frequency of IgG isotype. We decided to remove the N-linked glycosylated sites and to compare capability of deglycosylated and glycosylated sperm antigen for stimulation of human lymphocytes to produce antisperm antibodies.

2. MATERIALS AND METHODS

Mice C.B-17scid/scid mice, do not exhibit functional immune response, hence they are perfect to host human tissues.

Progress in Basic and Clinical Immunology, Edited by Mackiewicz *et al.*
Kluwer Academic/Plenum Publishers, New York, 2001

Preparation of cells. PBMC were isolated from the blood of vasectomized donors by density gradient centrifugation (d=1.077). Cell suspensions were depleted from $CD8^+$ lymphocytes by using MACS cell separator[2]. For *in vitro* generation of sufficient number of antigen presenting cells ($CD34^+$), we have cultured lymphocytes from the same donor in medium supplemented with GM-CSF and IL-4. Prepared cells were deposited into mice peritoneal cavity (20-30x 10^6 CD8dL/mouse and 1-5x10^6 $CD34^+$ mouse).

Antigen preparation Sperm antigens were prepared from fresh semen donations after treatment with TDOC lysis buffer (TRITON X-100, sodium deoxycholate, NaCl, Tris, benzamidine, leupeptin, pepstain, PMSF-phenylmethylsulfonyl fluoride).

Deglycosylation of sperm extract. Deglycosylation was carried out by using N-glycanase (Genzyme) (4µl/100µg of protein). Efficiency of degycosylation was checked by affinity binding to Concanavalin A. Only fully deglycosylated protein pool was used for immunisation.

Vaccination of human-PBL-SCID mice. The mice were injected three times in two-weeks intervals (with glycosylated and deglycosylated extracts in Freund adjuvant) starting on a day after the reconstitution of mice with human lymphocytes. The mice were bled (1-3 capillary) from tail vein before every injection of antigen.

Determination of human immunoglobulin levels. Serum samples from individual mice were screened for the presence of human immunoglobulins using a quantitative ELISA as previously described[3].

AGA – agglutination assay. After 'swim-up'[4], microwells were filled (4x10^4/well) with motile spermatozoa obtained from healthy donors. Microtest plates were incubated (for one hour in 37°C) with serial 1:2 dilutions of serum samples (from 1:3 to 1:50) from immunized SCID mice. The agglutination of human sperm by ASA was observed under inverted microscope.

3. RESULTS

The influence of removal of N-linked glycosylated sites from sperm antigenic extract on ASA production, was estimated. Hu-PBL-SCID mice were immunized by i.p. injections of deglycosylated and glycosylated sperm extracts. Subsequently, human antisperm antibodies in the serum of these animals were determined by ELISA and agglutination tests. ASA capable for sperm agglutination may impair their motility. Antisperm antibodies induced by the deglycosylated sperm antigen gave stronger agglutination of spermatozoa along the course of immunizations. In such case, the agglutination of spermatozoa was observed beyond 1:50 dilution of tested sera samples (Fig.1a).

Analyzing the response elicited by glycosylated antigen one could notice a strong sperm agglutination after the first immunization, which subsequently decreased after following administrations of antigen. (Fig. 1b).

Comparing different tests in order to determine ASA reactivity, it was evident (Tab. 1) that deglycosylated antigen induced higher levels of antibodies (ELISA) and revealed higher ability for sperm agglutination . However it was observed some discrepancy between results obtained from ELISA/AGA and IBT/fluorescence tests. This situation could arise because in ELISA fixed spermatozoa were used, so slightly modified cell surface can be expected while for IBT/fluorescence motile and live spermatozoa were applied. On the other hand, in AGA also the motile spermatozoa were used but the results differed from those obtained in IBT/fluorescence. We could speculated that agglutination pattern can be observed as the result of different epitope cross-linking while the fluorescence – marked determinants were mainly of carbohydrate origin.

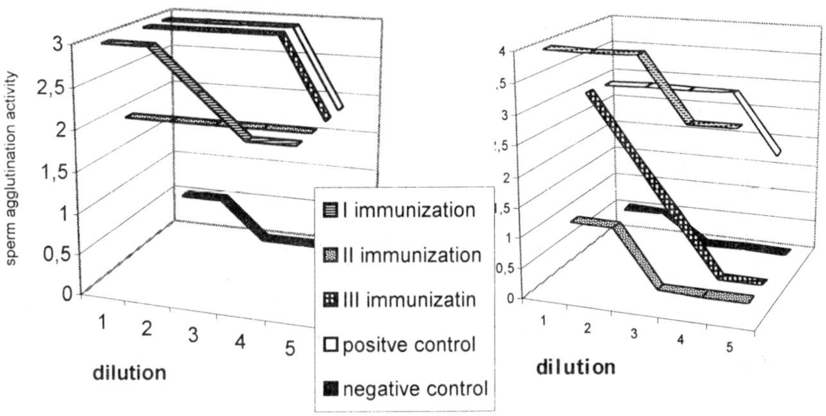

a) b)

Figure 1.a). Agglutination effect of ASA obtained in SCID mice by deglycosylated antigen. b) Agglutination effect of ASA obtained in SCID mice by glycosylated antigen. Axis Y: intensity of agglutination; axis X: the serial 1:2 dilutions from 1- 1:3 to 5- 1:50.
Positive control – serum from vasectomized donor. Negative control – serum from SCID mice.

Table 1. Comparison of ASA activities contained in SCID mice serum tested by different immunological assay. AGA-agglutination assay; IBT- immunobeads test; ELISA-enzyme-linked immunosorbent assay. Positive control – serum from vasectomized donor. Negative control – serum from healthy donor.

	ELISA ng/ml	AGA (dilution 1:50)	IBT	Fluorescence test
Deglycosylated antigen	2433	+++	7%	5.3%
Glycosylated antigen	2233	++	12%	21%
Native control	620	-	1%	6.5%
Positive control	3760	++	49%	37%

4. CONCLUSION

The findings may suggest that the deglycosylated antigen is capable to elicit stronger immune response than the glycosylated sperm extract when deposited into SCID mice lymphocytes were obtained from sensitized donor. Human antibody responses developed to both types of extract (evaluated by ELISA) were maintained on the same level, however, sperm agglutinating activity was significantly stronger when induced by N-glycosylated sperm antigen.

REFERENCES

1. Carlsson R., Martensson C., Kalliomaki S., Ohlin M., Borrebaeck C. 1992, Human peripheral blood lymphocytes transplanted into scid mice consitute an in vivo culture system exhibiting several parameters found in normal humoral immune response and are a source of immunocytes for production of human monoclonal antibodies. J. Immunol. 148:1065-1071
2. Miltenyl S., Muller W., Weichel W.,Radbruch A., 1990, High gradient magnetic cellseparation with MACS. Cytometry 11:231
3. Lynch DM., Leali BA., Howe SE., 1986, A comparison of sperm agglutination assay with a quantitative ELISA for anti-sperm antibodies in serum. Fertil. Steril. 46:285-292
4. Koyama K., Kubota K., Ikuma K., Shigeta M., Isojima S., 1988, Application of the quantitative sperm immobilization test for follow-up study of sperm-immobilizing antibody in sera of serile women. Int. J. Fertil. 33:201-206

ALLERGY/INFLAMMATION

Immunologic mechanisms of allergen-specific immunotherapy

C. A. AKDIS AND K. BLASER
Swiss Institute of Allergy and Asthma Research (SIAF), CH-7270 Davos, Switzerland

1. INTRODUCTION

Allergic diseases basically are immunological disorders, related to activation of a distinct cytokine pattern in T cells, including increased secretion of certain allergic inflammatory cytokines, in particular of IL-4, IL-5 and/or IL-13. (1-3). Whereas the symptoms of immediate and late type allergic reactions can be ameliorated by various pharmacological treatments, the allergen-specific immunotherapy (SIT) represents the only curative approach for specific Type I allergy (4-9). SIT is most efficient in allergy to insect venoms and allergic rhinitis (6,9). However, the mechanism by which SIT achieves clinical improvement remained unclear until recent time. A rise in allergen-blocking IgG antibodies particularly of the IgG4 class (10-12), the generation of IgE-modulating $CD8^+$ T cells and a reduction in the number of mast cells and eosinophils and release of mediators (13-14), were fund to be associated with successful SIT. Furthermore, SIT was found to be associated with a decrease in IL-4 and IL-5 production by $CD4^+$ T cells, and in some cases with a shift towards increased IFN-γ production (9,15-22). However, it appeared, that the induction of an unresponsive or anergic state in peripheral T cells and the reactivation of the response by cytokines from the tissue microenvironment are basic intermediate key steps in the mechanism of SIT (15-17). Thus, conditions of the immunological microenvironment and production of cytokines by tissue cells may finally determine, whether a SIT develops towards a successful or unsuccessful treatment. Therefore, for successful and safe SIT, allergen variants should be

Progress in Basic and Clinical Immunology, Edited by Mackiewicz *et al.*
Kluwer Academic/Plenum Publishers, New York, 2001

created, of which recognition sites for the T cells remained intact, whereas binding sites for IgE antibodies were removed. Intact T cell-epitopes are required in order to enable the induction of specific T cell tolerance or anergy against the antigen/allergen. The antibody- or B cell-epitopes are not only prerequisites for elicitation of adverse reactions, IgE antibodies also focus the allergen efficiently onto antigen-presenting B cells which present it to T cells in a way that favors development of a Th2 dominated cytokine pattern (18,23,24)

An especially suited model for studies of human cellular and molecular mechanisms, regulating specific allergy and normal immunity provides the immune response to bee venom (BV) (15-19,24-26). The BV-phospholipase A_2 (PLA) represents the major antigen and allergen of BV, and SIT with whole BV (BV-SIT) or short PLA peptides representing immunodominant T cell epitopes (PLA-PIT) was applied successfully.

2. MECHANISMS IN SIT

2.1 Allergen concentration and affinity of antigenic peptide to MHC-II and TcR molecules govern the generation of distinct T cell cytokine profiles.

By using a panel of PLA-specific human T cell clones it was demonstrated that the secretion of both absolute and relative amounts of cytokines and distinct cytokine patterns depends on the concentration of the antigen added to the cultures. Typically a 10 to 50 times lower threshold amount of antigen was required for the induction of IL-4 than for IFN-γ. Increasing antigen concentrations favored the IFN-γ production by T cells, whereas IL-4 decreased at high antigen doses (26,27). The same was true for Th2 clones, however, at much higher antigen concentrations. Accordingly, cytokine patterns do not necessarily represent stable phenotypes and can be modulated by the dose of antigen. Low antigen concentration and suboptimal antigenic peptide binding capacity of MHC-II molecules generate weak T cell activation, an IL-4 dominated Th2 cytokine pattern and IgE antibodies. Thus, at the same antigen concentration individuals with high affinity to immunogenic peptides display a higher density of MHC-II/antigen complexes on the APC surface and induce stronger T cell activation, generating sufficient IFN-γ to suppress IgE (23, 26,27). Therefore, the cytokine-regulating forces may be driven by an individual's HLA-class II type and the strength of epitope binding in an APC/peptide/T cell interaction. The modulation of T cell cytokine pattern by the dose of antigen represents a driving force in differential IgE and IgG antibody formation, resulting in either allergy or immunoprotection (23, 26-29).

That the strength of antigen binding by the MHC II-peptide-TcR complex governs the T cell activation and cytokine production is supported by the fact that altered peptide ligands (APL) can modulate specific T cell activation and cytokine production by their diversity in antigen binding to the TcR or MHC class II (23,30). The effect of a particular amino acid substitution on cytokine secretion may result from affinity changes of the peptide ligand to the MHC class II molecule. Exposure of T cells to APL induces a state of specific unresponsiveness or anergy as defined by abrogated proliferation and cytokine synthesis on antigen rechallenge. Indeed, the cytokine changes resulting from a single amino acid mutation in an antigenic PLA peptide increased the IgG4 production significantly and skewed the ratio of specific IgE : IgG4 antibodies towards normal immunity (30). Most remarkably, this demonstrates that physicochemical properties of immunological reactions are fundamental in generation of distinct states of T cell activation, cytokine patterns and finally development of either disease or normal immunity (24,27-30). Such regulatory effects of allergen concentration on cytokine secretion may also reflect a physiological mechanism in allergen-specific immunotherapy in which repeatedly high allergen doses are injected over a longer period of time (24,27,28,29)

The induction of specific anergy in peripheral T cells and reactivation of T cells are intermediate key steps in SIT.

The immunological mechanism of SIT was investigated in BV-SIT (15,16) and further elucidated in PLA-PIT (19) using a mixture of three peptides representing the immunodominant T cell epitopes PLA45-62, PLA82-92, PLA113-124. In both BV-SIT and PLA-PIT, successfully treated patients developed specific T cell unresponsiveness against the entire PLA allergen as well as the three T cell epitope-containing peptides. After 60 days of treatment, the specific proliferative T cell response and secretion of Th2 type cytokines, IL-4, IL-5 and IL-13, as well as the Th1 cytokines IL-2 and IFN-γ were suppressed. The PPD or TT control responses were not affected by these treatments, indicating that the suppressive effect of SIT and PIT was specific to the allergen.

The induction of an anergic state in Th2 cells is an active biochemical process, associated with increased levels of basal tyrosine kinase activity, cytokine production and CD25 upregulation. It is related to alterations in TcR mediated signaling pathway. The anergized Th2 cells failed to respond to anti-CD3 stimulation with increased tyrosine phosphorylation of $p56^{lck}$ and ZAP70 kinases. In addition, intracellular calcium flux, observed in untreated Th2 cells in response to anti-CD3 mAb, was absent in anergic Th2 cells (30, 31).

The abrogated proliferative response was fully restored by antigen stimulation of anergic T cells in the presence of IL-2 or IL-15. Also the full capacity of IL-2 and IFN-γ secretion recovered by this cytokine treatment. In contrast, specific stimulation in the presence of IL-4 induced IL-4, IL-5 and IL-13 and therefore, recovered a Th2 cytokine pattern typical for an allergic response. IL-2 and IL-15 basically display the same immunological properties. However, whereas IL-2 is produced by activated T cells, most immunologically active cells, except T cells, secrete IL-15 (15,17). Thus, microenvironmental cytokines from the tissue recover and regulate T cells from SIT induced anergy (15,17). They can generate distinct Th0/Th1 cytokine patterns associated with successful therapy and normal immunity, or reactivate Th2 cells, supporting the persistence of the respective allergic response. Thus, successful SIT may be difficult to achieve in an established polyspecific allergy and atopy, and such treatment has to be applied at an early stage of the disease.

Decreased T cell proliferative responses in SIT were demonstrated also in allergy to ragweed, cat dander, grass pollen and BV (32-34). In mice antigenic peptides of house dust mite and cat allergen were shown to induce anergy in T cells (35,36), and recent studies with T cell peptides of Fel d 1, clearly indicated peripheral tolerance induction in T cells by PIT also of cat allergy (22,37). In a recent study, T cell epitope peptides of cat allergen were shown to initiate a T cell dependent late asthmatic reaction, without the requirement for an early IgE/mast cell-dependent response, in sensitized asthmatic subjects (38).

2.2 T cell anergy in SIT is induced by IL-10 from specific T cells

The anergized cells showed suppressed PLA-specific T cell proliferative and cytokine responses that could also be reconstituted by *ex vivo* neutralization of endogenous IL-10. This indicates that IL-10 is actively involved in development of anergy in specific T cells. Whereas in both BV-SIT and PLA-PIT the antigen and peptide-induced proliferative responses and Th1 and Th2 cytokine production decreased, the IL-10 production simultaneously increased and reached maximal levels after four weeks, when the specific anergy was fully established. The cellular origin of IL-10 was demonstrated by intracytoplasmic IL-10 staining in PBMC and coexpression of cellular surface markers (16). Intracellular IL-10 significantly increased after seven days of SIT in the antigen-specific T cell population and activated $CD4^+$ T lymphocytes. After four weeks of SIT intra-cytoplasmatic IL-10 was also increased in monocytes and B cells, suggesting an autokrine action of T cell secreted IL-10 as a pivotal step in the induction phase of T cell anergy and its maintenance by IL-10 producing APC and non-specific bystander T cells (16). Interestingly, the same features of anergy were found in T cells of healthy bee keepers, who were previously stung by high numbers of bees. These naturally anergized individuals show increased numbers of IL-10-producing $CD4^{+}CD25^{+}$ T cells and monocytes similar to allergic patients after BV-SIT. Neutralization of endogenous IL-10 in PBMC cultures from these individuals fully reconstituted the proliferative T cell response and cytokine production.

IL-10 is a major regulatory cytokine of inflammatory responses and a general inhibitor of proliferative and cytokine responses in both Th1 and Th2 cells (39-46). IL-10 is released by both Th1 and Th2 type lymphocytes, mononuclear phagocytes and NK cells (40-43). *In vitro* the inhibitory effect of IL-10 in T cells was observed exclusively in APC-dependent systems, but not in T cells stimulated by solid-phase bound anti-CD3 (41,44,45,47).

Beside SIT and PIT of BV allergy, evidence for induction of peripheral T cell anergy was obtained in SIT of wasp venom allergy, grass pollen asthma, conjunctivitis and rhinitis (21,33,34,48,49). Furthermore, downregulated T cell responses were reported in PIT of cat allergy (22). Moreover, IL-10 increase induced by SIT was demonstrated also in wasp allergy, grass pollen asthma and nasal immunotherapy of weed-induced allergic rhinitis (21,48-50). In mice IL-10 administration before allergen treatment induced antigen-specific T cell tolerance and established peripheral T cell anergy (48). Recently, IL-10 derived regulatory $CD4^{+}$ T cells, producing IL-10 but not IL-2 and IL-4, which suppressed antigen-specific T cell response and prevented antigen-induced colitis, were identified in humans and in mice (50). In SIT to aeroallergens, such as birch pollen and house dust mite allergy, also TGF-β could be demonstrated, acting to the same degree as IL-10.

2.3 Specific IgE and IgG4 antibody regulation by SIT and PIT

The serum levels of specific IgE and IgG4 antibodies delineate allergic and normal immunity to allergen. Whereas peripheral anergy was demonstrated in specific T cells, the capacity by B cells to produce specific IgE and IgG4 antibodies was not abolished. In fact, specific serum levels of both isotypes increased during the early phase of treatment. However, the increase in specific IgG4 was more pronounced and the ratio of specific IgE to IgG4 decreased by 10 to 100 fold within a few weeks. Also the *in vitro* production of PLA-specific IgE and IgG4 antibodies by PBMC changed in parallel to the serum levels of specific isotypes. A similar change in specific isotype ratio was observed in SIT of various allergies. Moreover, IL-10 that was induced and increasingly secreted by SIT, appears to counter-regulate antigen-specific IgE and IgG4 antibody synthesis. It is a potent suppresser of both total and PLA-specific IgE, while simultaneously IgG4 formation is increased (16,17). Thus, IL-10 not only generates anergy in T cells; it also regulates specific isotype formation and skews the specific response from an IgE to an IgG4 dominated phenotype.

2.4 The effect of IL-10 on mast cells and eosinophils in allergic inflammation

Despite definite decrease in IgE antibody levels and IgE mediated skin sensitivity normally requires several years of treatment, most patients are protected against bee stings already at an early stage of BV-SIT. Increase of allergen-specific IgG4 antibodies, blocking IgE binding to the allergen, may explain only the late phase of protection by SIT. At the early phase of SIT however, a decrease in histamine and sulfidoleukotrienes release from basophils, may be of more relevance. This decreased basophilic mediator releasability (51) can be attributed to suppression of cytokines in anergic T cells. There is clear evidence that effector cells of the allergic inflammation (mast cells, basophils and eosinophils) require T cell cytokines for priming, survival and activity. In addition, IL-10 was shown to reduce TNF-α, GM-CSF and IL-6 generation from mouse bone marrow and rat peritoneal mast cells (1,51,52-58). Moreover, IL-10 downregulates eosinophil function and activity and suppresses IL-5 production by human resting Th0 and Th2 clones (45,46,54). It inhibits endogenous GM-CSF production and CD40 expression by activated eosinophils and enhances eosinophil cell death (59,60)

2.5 Mechanism of T cell suppression by IL-10

We have demonstrated that IL-10 directly acts on T cells which are stimulated via CD28 by efficiently blocking proliferation and cytokine production. T cells tolerized by IL-10 showed high viability and the unresponsive state was reversed by anti-CD3 stimulation and IL-2, but not by anti-CD28 mAb stimulation. (61-63)

Various experiments demonstrated a direct relationship between IL-10R and CD28. Stimulation by CD28 upregulates the IL-10R expression, which renders the cells more susceptible to IL-10 mediated suppression. It was also demonstrated that the specific inhibitory effect of IL-10 on the CD28 costimulatory signal does not involve direct steric interaction of the two receptors at the cell surface.

Stimulation of CD28 by B7 surface molecules leads to tyrosine phosphorylation of CD28. Ligation of IL-10 receptor (IL-10R) at the time of CD28 stimulation inhibits tyrosine phosphorylation of CD28 within 10 min (61,62). The inhibitory effect of IL-10 on CD28 appeared to be specific for the costimulatory pathway, because IL-10 did not affect CD3-stimulated tyrosine phosphorylation of ZAP-70. As a consecutive event for signal transduction, phosphatidylinositol 3-kinase (PI3-K) should bind to CD28 by its p85 subunit. The association of CD28 with PI3-K p85 was inhibited by IL-10. This inhibition could be blocked specifically by an anti-IL-10R mAb preventing IL-10 binding to its receptor (61-63). PI3-K is a heterodimer that comprises an 85 kD regulatory and a 110 kD catalytic subunit possessing both protein serine-kinase and lipid-kinase activity. The p85 subunit contains a p110 binding site as well as two src-homology-2 (SH2) domains. Binding of PI3-K to CD28 occurs by direct interaction between SH2 domain motifs of p85 PI3-K and a (p)YXXM motif in the cytoplasmic part (64). This requires CD28 tyrosine phosphorylation. There is no indication that the CD28 cytoplasmic tail may display enzymatic activity. However, intervening protein tyrosine kinases, such as $p56^{lck}$ and $p59^{fyn}$ were demonstrated to phosphorylate CD28 at its ^{173}Y position (65,66).

Previous studies have demonstrated that IL-10 not only inhibits T cells, it is also a potent inhibitor of activated monocytes and macrophages (67,68). Since monocytes and macrophages do not express CD28, the inhibitory impact of IL-10 is likely to occur through other mechanisms in these cases. IL-10 exerts its biological functions through the activation of Jak1 and Tyk2, the members of the receptor associated Janus tyrosine kinases family and Stat1 and Stat3 and in certain cells Stat5 (68-69). In monocytes, IL-10 was shown to induce expression of the suppressor of the cytokine signaling 3 (SOCS3) gene that may play a role in inhibition of IFN-induced tyrosine phosphorylation of STAT-1 (70). However, the effect of IL-10 on the inhibition of CD28 tyrosine phosphorylation is visible already after 10 min. Obviously this does not require new protein synthesis and the mechanism of inhibition of CD28 tyrosine phosphorylation remains to be elucidated.

3. CONCLUSION

Induction of specific anergy in peripheral T cells by IL-10 and subsequent reactivation of distinct cytokine patterns by cytokines from the tissue microenvironment are key events in the immunological mechanisms of SIT. These mechanisms have implications, which may reach beyond specific allergy treatment, and induction of specific anergy may be of importance also in autoimmunity and GvH disease. It can facilitate tumor growth, parasite survival and AIDS development. The immunological key steps of SIT and PIT are depicted in (17), Both SIT and PIT generate IL-10, which in an autocrine way of action induces specific anergy in peripheral T cells. Both types of treatment decrease the antigen-specific IgE:IgG4 ratio in peripheral blood. The reactivation and modulation of distinct cytokine patterns in anergic T cells suggests a pivotal role of microenvironmental cytokines development of SIT. T cell secreted cytokines are essential for priming, survival and activity of inflammatory effector cells Therefore, specific T cell reactivity is directly involved in the pathogenesis of allergic inflammation. IL-10 not only induces anergy in T cells; it also inhibits the activation of inflammatory reactions by mast cells and eosinophils. Finally, the generation of new Th2 type cells secreting allergic inflammatory cytokine patterns can be suppressed by administration of high allergen doses inducing IFN-γ dominated cytokine patterns.

The inhibition of the CD28 costimulatory pathway by IL-10 delineates a major mechanism in peripheral T cell tolerance. IL-10 inhibits T cell responses even at high antigen doses and the number of TCR triggered by peptide-MHC complex on the surface of APC appears to be in the range of the requirement for costimulation. IL-10 efficiently increases the threshold for T cell activation rendering optimal conditions provided by professional APC and CD28/B7 interaction. In consequence, IL-10 induces an immunological unresponsive, anergic state in T cells.

Including various molecular mechanisms that generate T cell tolerance, an increase in IL-10 production and suppression of CD28 costimulation mediated T cell proliferative and cytokine responses demonstrate important steps in tolerating high doses of exogenous antigen. These mechanisms have implications, which may reach beyond specific allergy treatment, and induction of specific anergy may be of importance also in autoimmunity and graft versus host disease. It can facilitate tumor growth, parasite survival and AIDS development. The knowledge of this molecular basis is pivotal in understanding the equilibrated regulation of immune response and anergy to immunogenic agents, and their possible therapeutic applications.

Various attempts are undertaken to increase the success of SIT and decrease its risk of side effects. The availability of recombinant allergen technology will permit excellent standardization of allergen preparations for clinical use. The aim of allergen modification is to decrease the allergenicity, while retaining its immunogenicity. This can be achieved by destroying conformational B cell epitopes and simultaneous preserving linear T cell epitopes in allergens.

ACKNOWLEDGEMENTS

This work was supported by the Swiss National Science Foundation nr. 31-50590.97

REFERENCES

1. Mosmann, T.R., and Sad, S., 1996, The expanding universe of T-cell subsets: Th1, Th2 and more. *Immunol Today* 17:142-146.
2. Romagnani, S., 1994, Lymphokine production by human T cells in disease states. *Annu Rev Immunol.* 12:227-257.
3. Paul, W.E., and Seder, R.A., 1994, Lymphocyte responses and cytokines. *Cell* 76:241-251.
4. Bousquet, J., Lockey, R.F., and Malling, H.J., 1998, WHO position paper. Allergen immunotherapy: Therapeutic vaccines for allergic diseases. *Allergy* 53:1-42.
5. Müller, U.R, and Mosbech, H., 1993, Position paper: Immunotherapy with hymenptera venoms. *Allergy* 48:36-46.
6. Müller, U.R, Hebling, A, and Berchtold, E., 1992, Immunotherapy with honeybee venom and yellow jacket venom is different regarding efficacy and safety. *J Allergy Clin Immunol* 89:529-535.
7. Walker, S.M., Varney V.A., Gaga M., Jacobson M.R., and Durham S.R., 1995, Grass pollen immunotherapy: efficacy and safety during a 4 year follow-up study. *Allergy* 50:405-413.
8. Varney, V.A., Gaga, M., and Frew, A.J., 1991, Usefulness of immunotherapy in patients with severe summer hay fever uncontrolled by anti-allergic drugs. *Br Med J* 302:489-500.
9. Durham, S.R., Walker, S.M., Varga E.-V., Jacobson, M.R., O'Brien, F., Noble, W., Till, S.J., Hamid, Q.A., and Nouri-Aria, K.T., 1999, Long-term clinical efficacy of grass-pollen immunotherapy. *New Engl J Med* 341:468-475.
10. Hussain, R., Poindexter, R.W., and Ottesen, E.A., 1992, Control of allergic reactivity in human filariasis. Predominant localization of blocking antibody to the IgG4 subclass. *J Immunol* 48:2731-2739.
11. Reid, M.J., Moss, R.B., Hsu, Y.P., Kwasnicki, J.M., Commerford, T.M., and Nelson, B.L., 1986, Seasonal asthma in northern California: allergic causes and efficacy of immunotherapy. *J Allergy Clin Immunol* 78:590-600.
12. Wetterwald, A., Skvaril, F., Müller, U., and Blaser, K., 1985, Isotypic and idiotypic characterization of anti-bee venom phospholipase A_2 antibodies. *Arch Allergy Appl Immunol* 77:195-197.
13. Creticos, P.S., Franklin Adkinson, Jr. N., Kagey-Sabotka, A., Proud, D., Meier, H.L., Naclerio, R.M., Lichtenstein, L.M., and Norman, P.S., 1983, Nasal challenge with ragweed in hay fever patients: Effect of immunotherapy. *J Clin Invest* 176:2247-2253.
14. Rak, S., Rowhagen, O., and Venge, P., 1988, The effect of immunotherapy on bronchial hyper-responsiveness and eosinophil cationic protein in pollen allergic patients. *J Allergy Clin Immunol* 82:470-480.
15. Akdis, C.A., Akdis, M., Blesken, T., Wymann, D., Alkan, S.S., Müller, U., and Blaser, K., 1996, Epitope specific T cell tolerance to phospholipase A_2 in bee venom immunotherapy and recovery by IL-2 and IL-15 *in vitro*. *J Clin Invest* 98:1676-1683.
16. Akdis, C.A., Blesken, T., Akdis, M., Wüthrich. B., and Blaser, K., 1998, Role of IL-10 in specific immunotherapy. *J Clin Invest* 102:98-106.

17. Akdis, C.A., and Blaser, K., 1999, IL-10 induced anergy in peripheral T cell and reactivation by microenvironmental cytokines: two key steps in specific immunotherapy. *FASEB* 13:603-609.
18. Akdis, C.A., Blesken, T., Wymann, D., Akdis, M., and Blaser, K., 1998, Differential regulation of human T cell cytokine patterns and IgE and IgG4 responses by conformational antigen variants. *Eur J Immunol* 28:914-925.
19. Müller, U.R., Akdis, C.A., Fricker, M., Akdis, M., Bettens, F., Blesken, T., and Blaser, K., 1998, Successful immunotherapy with T cell epitope peptides of bee venom phospholipase A2 induces specific T cell anergy in bee sting allergic patients. *J Allergy Clin Immunol* 101:747-754.
20. Jutel, M., Pichler, W.J., Skrbic, D., Urwyler, A., Dahinden, C., and Müller, U.R., 1995, Bee venom immunotherapy results in decrease of IL-4 and IL-5 and increase of IFN-γ secretion in specific allergen stimulated T cell cultures. *J Immunol* 154:4178-4194.
21. Bellinghausen, I., Metz, G., Enk, A.H., Christmann, S., Knop., J., and Saloga, J., 1997, Insect venom immunotherapy induces interleukin-10 production and a Th2-to-Th1 shift, and changes surface marker expression in venom-allergic subjects. *Eur J Immunol* 27:1131-1139.
22. Marcotte, G.V., Braun, C.M., Norman, P.S., Nicodemus, C.F., Kagey-Sabotka, A., Lichtenstein, L.M., and Essayan, D.M., 1998, Effects of peptide therapy on ex vivo T cell responses. *J Allergy Clin Immunol* 101:506-513.
23. Blaser, K., Carballido, J.M., Faith, A., Crameri, R., and Akdis, C.A., 1998, Determinants and mechanisms of human immune response to bee venom phospholipase A2. *Int Arch Allergy Immunol* 117:1-10.
24. Akdis, C.A., Blesken, T., Akdis, M., Alkan, S.S., Wüthrich, B., Heusser, C.H., and Blaser, K., 1997, Induction and differential regulation of bee venom phospholipase A2-specific human IgE and IgG4 antibodies *in vitro* requires allergen-specific and non-specific activation of T and B cells. *J Allergy Clin Immunol* 99:345-352.
25. Carballido, J.M., Carballido-Perrig, N., Kägi, M.K., Meloen, R.H., Wüthrich, B., Heusser, C.H., and Blaser, K., 1993, T cell epitope specificity in human allergic and non-allergic subjects to bee venom phospholipase A_2. *J Immunol* 150:3582-3591.
26. Carballido, J.M., Faith, A., Carballido-Perrig, N., and Blaser, K., 1997, The intensity of T cell receptor engagement determines the cytokine pattern of human allergen-specific Th cells. *Eur J Immunol* 27:515-521.
27. Carballido, J.M., Carballido-Perrig, N., Oberli-Schraemmli, A., Heusser, C.H., and Blaser, K., 1994, Regulation of IgE and IgG4 responses by allergen-specific T-cell clones to bee venom phospholipase A_2 *in vitro*. *J Allergy Clin Immunol* 93:758-767.
28. Blaser, K., 1996, T cell and B cell epitopes in bee venom phospholipase A_2: Antigen-dose dependent cytokine rations regulate specific IgE and IgG antibody responses. In: Schneider E, ed. Peptides in immunology. New York: Europ. Pep. Soc and John Wiley & Sons. Ltd., 93-101.
29. Blaser, K., 1996, Allergen-dose dependent cytokine production regulates specific IgE and IgG antibody production. In: Sehon A, HayGlass KT, Kraft D, eds. Advances in experimental medicine and biology. Plenum Press, New York. 295-303.
30. Faith, A., Akdis, C.A., Akdis, M., Joss, A., Wymann, D., and Blaser, K., 1999, An altered peptide ligand specifically inhibits Th2 cytokine synthesis by abrogating TCR signaling. *J Immunol* 162:1836-1842.
31. Faith, A., Akdis, C.A., Akdis, M., Simon, H-U., and Blaser, K., 1997, Defective TCR stimulation in anergized type 2 T helper cells correlates with abrogated $p56^{lck}$ and ZAP-70 tyrosine kinase activities. *J Immunol* 159:53-60.

32. Secrist, H., Chelen, C.J., Wen, Y., Marshall, J.D., and Umetsu, D.T., 1993, Allergen immunotherapy decreases interleukin 4 production in CD4 T cells from allergic individuals. *J Exp Med* 178:2123-2130.
33. Creticos, P.S., 1992, Immunological changes associated with immunotherapy. In: Greenberger PA, ed. Immunotherapy of IgE mediated disorders. Philadelphia: W B Saunders, 13-37.
34. Greenstein, J.L., Morgenstern, J.P., LaRaia, J., Counsell, C.M., Goodwin, W.H., Lussier, A., Creticos, P.S., Norman, P.S., and Garman, R.D., 1992, Regweed immunotherapy decreases T cell reactivity to recombinant Amb a I.1. *J Allergy Clin Immunol* 89:322 (abst).
35. Hoyne, G.F., O'Hehir, R., Wraith, D.C., Thomas W.R., and Lamb J.R., 1993, Inhibition of T cell and antibody responses to house dust mite allergen by inhalation of the dominant T cell epitope in naive and sensitized mice. *J Exp Med* 178:1783-1788.
36. Briner, T., Kou, M., Keating, K., Rogers, B., and Greenstein, J., 1993, Peripheral T cell tolerance induced in naive and primed mice by subcutaneous injection of peptides from the major cat allergen Fel *d* I. *Proc Natl Acad Sci USA* 90:7608-7612.
37. Norman, P., Ohmann, Jr. JL., Long, A.A., Creticos, P.S., Gefter, M.A., Shaked, Z., Wood, R., Eggleston, P., Lichtenstein, L.M., and Jones, 1996, N. Treatment of cat allergy with T cell reactive peptides. *Am J Resp Crit Care Med* 154:1623-1628.
38. Haselden, B.M., Kay, A.B., and Larche, M., 1999, Immunoglobulin E-independent major histocompatibility complex-restricted T cell peptide epitope-induced late asthmatic reactions. *J Exp Med* 189:1885-1894.
39. Fiorentino, D.F., Bond, M.W., and Mosmann, T.R., 1989, Two types of mouse T helper cell IV. Th2 clones secrete a factor that inhibits cytokine production by Th1 clones. *J Exp Med* 170:2081-2095.
40. Fiorentino, D.F., Zlotnik, A., Mosmann, T.R., Howard, M., and O'Garra, A., 1991, IL-10 inhibits cytokine production by activated macrophages. *J Immunol* 147:3815-3822.
41. De Waal Malefyt, R., Abrams, J., Bennett , B., Figdor, C.G., and De Vries, J.E., 1991, Interleukin 10 (IL-10) inhibits cytokine synthesis by human monocytes: an autoregulatory role of IL-10 produced by monocytes. *J Exp Med* 174:1209-1220.
42. Hsu, D.H., Moore, K.W., and Spits, H., 1992, Differential effects of interleukin-4 and -10 on interleukin-2 induced interferon-γ synthesis and lymphokine activated killer activity. *Int Immunol* 4:563-569.
43. Del Prete, G., De Carli, M., Almerigogna, F., Giudizi, M.G., Biagiotti, R., and Romagnani, S., 1993, Human IL-10 is produced by both type 1 helper (Th1) and type 2 helper (Th2) T cell clones and inhibits their antigen-specific proliferation and cytokine production. *J Immunol* 150:353-356.
44. Zuany-Amorim, C., Haile, S., Leduc, D., Dumarey, C., Huerre, M., Vergaftig, B.B., and Pretolani, M., et al., 1995, Interleukin-10 inhibits antigen-induced cellular recruitment into the airways of sensitized mice. *J Clin Invest* 95:2644-2651.
45. Zuany-Amorim, C., Creminon, C., Nevers, M.C., Nahori, M-A., Vergaftig, B.B., and Pretolani, M., 1996, Modulation by IL-10 of antigen-induced IL-5 generation, and CD4+ T lymphocyte and eosinophil infiltration into the mouse peritoneal cavity. *J Immunol* 157:377-384.
46. Schandane, L., Alonso-Vega, C., Willems, F., Gerard, C., Delvaux, A., Velu, T., Devos, R., de Boer, M., and Goldman, M., 1994, B7/CD28-dependent IL-5 production by human resting T cells is inhibited by IL-10. *J Immunol* 152:4368-4374.
47. Ding, L., and Shevach, E.M., 1992, IL-10 inhibits mitogen-induced T cell proliferation by selectively inhibiting macrophage co-stimulatory function. *J Immunol* 148:3133-3139.

48. Enk, A.H., Saloga, J., Becker, D., Mohamadzadeh, M., and Knop, J., 1994, Induction of hapten-specific tolerance by interleukin 10 *in vivo*. *J Exp Med* 179:1397-1402.
49. Gaglani, B., Borish, B., Bartelson, B.L., Bucheimer, A., Keller, L., and Nelson, H.S., 1997, Nasal immunotherapy in weed-induced allergic rhinitis. *Annals of Allergy, Asrhma and Immunol* 79:259-265.
50. Groux, H., O'Garra, A., and Bigler M, et al., 1997, A $CD4^+$ T-cell subset inhibits antigen-specific T-cell responses and prevents colitis. *Nature* 389:737-742.
51. Jutel, M., Müller, U.M., Fricker, M., Rihs, S., Pichler, W., and Dahinden, C., 1996, Influence of bee venom immunotherapy on degranulation and leukotriene generation in human blood basophils. *Clin Exp Allergy* 26:112-118.
52. Takanaski, S., Nonaka, R., Xing, Z., O'Byrne, P., Dolovich, J., and Jordana, M., 1994, Interleukin 10 inhibits lipopolysaccharide-induced survival and cytokine production by human peripheral blood eosinophils. *J Exp Med* 180:711-715.
53. Marshall, J.S., Leal-Berumen, I., Nielsen, L., Glibetic, M., and Jordana, M., 1996, Interleukin (IL)-10 Inhibits long-term IL-6 production but not preformed mediator release from rat peritoneal mast cells. *J Clin Invest* 97:1122-1128.
54. Wang, P., Wu, P., Siegel, M.I., Egan, R.W., and Billah, M.M., 1994, IL-10 inhibits transcription of cytokine genes in human peripheral blood mononuclear cells. *J Immunol* 153:811-816.
55. Bogdan, C., Paik, J., Vodovotz, Y., and Nathan, C., 1992, Contrasting mechanisms for suppression of macrophage cytokine relase by transforming growth factor–β and interleukin-10. *J Biol Chem* 267:23301-23310.
56. Ippoliti, F., Ragno, V., Del Nero, A., Mc Ewen, N., Ms Ewen, H., and Businco, L., 1997, Effect of preseasonal enzyme potentiated desensitization on plasma IL-6 and IL-10 of grass pollen-sensitive asthmatic children. *Allergie et Immunologie* 29:123-125.
57. Pretolani, M., and Goldman, M., 1997, IL-10: a potential therapy for allergic inflammation? *Immunol Today* 18:277-280.
58. Ohkawara, Y., Lim, K.G., and Glibetic, M., et al., 1996, CD40 expression by human peripheral blood eosinophils. *J Clin Invest* 97:1761-1766.
59. Wedi, B., Raap, U., Lewrick, H., and Kapp, A., 1997, Delayed eosinophil programmed cell death in vitro: A common feature of inhalant allergy and extrinsic or intrinsic atopic dermatitis. *J.Allergy Clin.Immunol.* 100:536-543.
61. Joss, A., Akdis, M., Faith, A., Blaser, K. and Akdis, C.A., 2000, IL-10 directly acts on T cells by specifically altering the CD28 co-stimulation pathway. *Eur.J.Immunol.* 30:1683-1690.
62. Akdis, C.A., Joss, A., Akdis, M., Faith, A. and Blaser, K., 2000, A molecular basis for T cell suppression by IL-10: CD28-associated IL-10 receptor inhibits CD28 tyrosine phosphorylation and phosphatidylinositol 3-kinase binding. *FASEB J.* 14:1666-1669.
63. Lee, K.P., Taylor, C., Petryniak, B., Turka, L.A., June, C.H. and Thompson, C.B., 1990, The genomic organization of the CD28 gene: Implications for the regulation of CD28 mRNA expression and heterogeneity. *J.Immunol.* 145:344-352.
64. Prasad, K.V.S., Cai, Y-C., Raab, M., Duckworth, B., Cantley, L., Shoelson, S.E., and Rudd, C.E., 1994, T-cell antigen CD28 interacts with the lipid kinase phosphatidylinositol 3-kinase by a cytoplasmic Tyr(*P*)-Met-Xaa-Met motif. *Proc.Natl.Acad.Sci.USA* 91:2834-2838.
65. Raab, M., Cai, Y-C., Bunnell, S.C., Heyeck, S.D., Berg, L.J., and Rudd, C.E., 1995, $p56^{Lck}$ and $p59^{Fyn}$ regulate CD28 binding to phosphatidiylinositol 3- kinase, growth factor receptor-bound protein GRB-2, and T cell-specific protein -tyrosine kinase ITK: Implications for T-cell costimulation. *Proc.Natl.Acad.Sci.USA* 92:8891-8895.

66. Ho, A.S.Y., Wei, S.H.Y., Mui, A.L.-F., Miyajima, A., and Moore, K.W., 1995, Functional regions of the mouse interleukin-10 receptor cytoplasmic domain. *Mol.Cell.Biol.* 15:5043-5053.
67. Del Prete, G., De Carli, M., Almerigogna, F., Giudizi, M.G., Biagiotti, R., and Romagnani, S., 1993, Human IL-10 is produced by both type 1 helper (Th1) and type 2 helper (Th2) T cell clones and inhibits their antigen-specific proliferation and cytokine production. *J.Immunol.* 150:353-356.
68. De Waal Malefyt, R., Abrams, J., Bennett, B., Figdor, C.G., and De Vries, J.E., 1991, Interleukin 10 (IL-10) inhibits cytokine synthesis by human monocytes: an autoregulatory role of IL-10 produced by monocytes. *J.Exp.Med.* 174:1209-1220.
69. Finbloom, D.S., and Winestock, K.D., 1995, IL-10 induces the tyrosine phosphorylation of Tyk2 and Jak1 and the differential assembly of STAT1α and STAT3 complexes in human T cells and monocytes. *J.Immunol.* 155:1979-1090.
70. Ito, S., Ansari, P., Sakatsume, M., Dickensheets, H., Vasquez, N., Donnelly, R.P., Larner, A.C., and Finbloom, D.S., 1999, Interleukin-10 inhibits expression of both interferon □ and interferon γ-induced genes by suppressing tyrosine phosphorylation of STAT1. *Blood* 93:1456-1463.

Phosphorothioate oligonucleotides: looking for the motif(s) possessing immunostimulatory activities in humans

FRANCESCA BRUGNOLO, FRANCESCO ANNUNZIATO, SALVATORE SAMPOGNARO, CINZIA MANUELLI, LORENZO COSMI, SERGIO ROMAGNANI, ENRICO MAGGI and PAOLA PARRONCHI
Department of Internal Medicine, Section of Immunoallergology and Respiratory Diseases, University of Florence, Florence, Italy

1. INTRODUCTION

DNA vaccination is an effective approach in inducing the switch of murine immune responses from a Th2 to a Th1 profile of cytokine production. This activity has been related to the presence of particular immunostimulatory sequences (ISS), represented by an unmethylated hexamer 5'-pur-pur-CpG-pyr-pyr-3', the so called 'CpG motif'[1]. In mouse, CpG motif-containing oligonucleotides (ODNs), probably through the binding to TLR9 receptor[2], are able to induce a Th1 response towards allergens, by the stimulation of IL-12, IFNs and IL-18 production by APC, which in turn activate NK cells. They are also able to induce significant B cell proliferation and differentiation[3]. Despite a large body of evidences suggesting the efficacy of CpG motif-containing ODNs in animals, the activities of these compounds in humans have been less clarified. Moreover, no clear results concerning the sequence(s) actually important in humans have been obtained so far, but it has been postulated that ISS active in mouse and humans are, at least partially, different[4].

Progress in Basic and Clinical Immunology, Edited by Mackiewicz *et al.*
Kluwer Academic/Plenum Publishers, New York, 2001

2. RESULTS

2.1 B cell proliferation can be induced by phosphorothioate ODNs

We have first assessed the ability of a series of CpG dinucleotide-containing ODNs to induce a proliferative response in human B cells. Only phosphorothioate- (PS-) ODNs were powerful activators of B cells, whereas phosphodiester- (PE-), as well as PS-ODNs with methylated cytosines, were completely ineffective. This ability was independent of the presence in the sequence of classic CpG motifs already described in mouse, as CpG motif-lacking ODNs also exerted a maximal effect. On the other hand, the inversion of the CpG dinucleotide into GpC resulted in a remarkable, even if partial, reduction of B cell activation. The proliferative response of B cells was not merely due to the unspecific activity of the PS backbone, as a repetitive sequence of PS-CpG was completely ineffective. The presence of TCG groups could be indeed important for the ODN activity in humans. In fact, a repetitive sequence of TCG, but not ACG, exhibited a remarkable effect on B cells. Moreover, when only two TCG triplettes were present at the beginning of the sequence with a poly-C tail, a significant proliferation of B cells was observed but this effect was further increased when a TT dinucleotide followed this initial hexamer. However, the replacement of the poly-C tail with poly-G rendered this sequence completely ineffective.

2.2 ODNs can modulate the profile of allergen-specific T cells favouring the development of Th1-like effectors

In order to investigate the effects of ODNs on the vitro development of allergen-specific human T cells, Der p 1-specific short term T cell-lines were derived from atopic donors in the presence or absence of different ODNs. PS-, but not PE-, ODNs were able to increase the proportion of IFN-γ-expressing cells and to significantly decrease the proportion of IL-4-expressing cells, in stimulated allergen-specific T cell-lines, as assessed by flow cytometry for intracellular synthesis of cytokines. The Th1-shifting activity of PS-ODNs was due to their ability to induce the production of IL-12 and IFNs (α and γ) by cells of the innate immunity, as the addition of neutralizing antibodies completely abolished the modulation of allergen-specific T cells induced by PS-ODNs. Moreover, a significant increase in the percentage of CD16+ CD56+ (NK) cells with increased expression of IFN-γ was observed in PS-ODN modulated allergen-specific T cell-lines.

Differently from what already described in mouse, the Th1-inducing effect was independent of the presence of classic CpG motifs, as CpG motif-lacking, but CpG dinucleotide-containing, ODNs exerted a maximal effect. Also GpC-inverted PS-ODNs retained the ability to shift allergen-specific T cells towards a prevalent Th1 profile, even if to a lower extent.

Sequences showing a Th1-shifting activity are indeed different from those inducing B cell proliferation. In fact, it was clear that a PS-repetitive TCG sequence was a powerful stimulator of B cells but it could not up-regulate the expression of IFN-γ in allergen-specific T cell-lines, exerting only a mild effect on IL-4 expression.

3. CONCLUSION

From our studies it can be concluded that PS-ODNs can exert various effects on human cells, inducing B cell proliferation, production of 'alert' cytokines from cells of innate immunity, and shifting the functional profile of allergen-specific T cells from a prevalent Th2 towards a prevalent Th1-like phenotype.

These effects are independent of the absence or presence of classic 'CpG motifs', suggesting that ISS active in humans are, at least partially, different from the ones already described in mice. Moreover, CpG dinucleotides are important to obtain the maximal effect, but they are not necessarily required, as PS-ODNs in which CpG dinucleotides were inverted into GpC still retained a remarkable, even if lower, effect on both B and T cells. TCG at initial position may be of importance, but other nucleotides are probably necessary following the initial TCG sequence.

However, in the absence of a well recognized sequence, such as the CpG motif in mice, further studies are required to disclose the 'motif' responsible of the immunostimulatory activity on human cells. Despite this still unsolved problem, the results of this study support the possibility that the injection of allergens mixed to, or conjugated with, 'human ISS'-containing ODNs, may provide a new immunotherapeutic strategy for the treatment of allergic disorders.

ACKNOWLEDGMENTS

This work was supported by grants provided by Associazione Italiana Ricerca sul Cancro, the Italian Ministery of Health (project AIDS 2000) and European Community (project BIO4-98-0458).

REFERENCES

1. Sato, Y., Roman, M., Tighe, H., Lee, D., Corr, M., Nguyen, M-D., Silverman, G.J., Lotz, M., Carson, D.A., and Raz, E. 1996, Immunostimulatory DNA sequences necessary for effective intradermal gene immunization. *Science* 73: 352-357.
2. Hemmi, H., Takeuchi, O., Kawai, T., Kaisho, T., Sato, S., Sanjo, H., Matsumoto, M., Hoshino, K., Wagner, H., Takeda, K., and Akira, S. 2000, A Toll-like receptor recognizes bacterial DNA. *Nature* 408: 740-745.
3. Klinman, D.M., Yi, A.K., Beaucage, S.L., Conover, J., and Krieg, A.M. 1996, CpG motifs present in bacterial DNA rapidly induce lymphocytes to secrete interleukin 6, interleukin 12 and Interferon γ. *Proc. Natl. Acad. Sci. USA*. 93: 2879-2885.
4. Parronchi, P., Brugnolo, F., Annunziato, F., Manuelli, C., Sampognaro, S., Mavilia, C., Romagnani, S., and Maggi, E. 1999, Phosphorothioate oligodeoxynucleotides promote the in vitro development of human allergen-specific CD4+ T cells into Th1 effectors. *J. Immunol.* 163: 5946-5953.

Disorders in mononuclear phagocytes and reduced glutathione and their correction in Chernobyl children with recurrent respiratory infections and chronic inflammatory focal lesions

VIKTOR CHERNYSHOV,[1] LYUDMILA OMELCHENKO[2], GERNOT TREUSCH[3], MAXIM VODYANIK[1], TATYANA POCHINOK[2], MARINA GUMENYUK[1], GENNADY ZELINSKY[1]

[1]Laboratory of Immunology and [2]Pediatric Department, Institute of Pediatrics, Obstetrics and Gynecology, Academy of Medical Sciences, Kiev, Ukraine [3]Medical Information and Research Center, Empuriabrava, Spain

1. INTRODUCTION

Increase of respiratory tract diseases and chronic inflammatory foci in children residing at the radionuclides contaminated territories as a result of the Chernobyl nuclear accident were found by epidemiologic studies [1].

2. DISORDERS IN GSH, PHAGOCYTOSIS AND CYTOKINE RELEASE AND THEIR CORRECTION

12 Chernobyl children residing at the radionuclides contaminated territories (contamination density for ^{137}Cs - 5-15 mCi/Km^2) were treated during 30 days by reduced glutathione, L-cysteine and anthocyane (GCA-therapy) (Recancostat Comp., Clear Vision, Heresau, Switzerland). The scheme of GCA therapy was the following: GSH- first 5 days 20mg/kg, then 10mg/kg; anthocyane - 10mg/kg; L-cysteine - first 5 days 4mg/kg, then

2mg/kg daily *per os*. Entry criteria for this group of RRI children (CIFL group) were chronic inflammatory focal lesions (bronchitis, tonsillitis, maxilla sinusitis). Other 6 RRI children residing at the same territory without chronic inflammatory focal lesions served as placebo-control group. The relevant Ethical Committee has given approval. Majority of 12 children of CIFL group had positive dynamics of clinical symptoms after use of GSH, L-cysteine and anthocyane (GCA-therapy). The main criterion of clinical efficacy was number of RRI during one year after treatment. Children of the CIFL group before treatment had 7.6±0.6 acute RRI. after treatment 1.3±0.7 acute RRI per year. In placebo-control group before treatment children had 7.0±0.9 acute RRI per year, after treatment - 3,5±1.3 acute RRI per year.

Before treatment, levels of total plasma glutathione, whole blood total glutathione in CIFL group of children were lower than in placebo-control group. On contrary, intracellular levels of GSH in lymphocytes and especially in monocytes were higher in CIFL group compared with placebo-control group. After GCA-therapy, levels of total plasma glutathione and whole blood glutathione in CIFL group of children increased and reached ranges of placebo-control group. Intracellular levels of GSH in lymphocytes and monocytes in CIFL group after GCA-therapy decreased and reached the ranges of placebo-control group. Placebo had no marked effects.

In CIFL group of children initial percentage of neutrophils having performed phagocytosis (NPP) was higher and their mean fluorescence intensity (MFI) that reflected the number of ingested bacteria by neutrophils was lower than in placebo-control group. After GCA-therapy percentage of NPP decreased and MFI elevated but both reached ranges of placebo-control group. Elevated oxidative burst activity of neutrophils was estimated in children of CIFL group with fMLP, *E.Coli* both percentage and MFI, but with PMA- MFI only. After GCA-therapy these indices were decreased till ranges of placebo-control group.

Percentage of monocytes having performed phagocytosis in children of CIFL group was higher than in placebo-control group. After GCA therapy these indices became lower reaching ranges of placebo-control group. In contrast, indices of MFI were lower before treatment and increased after treatment in CIFL group of children reaching ranges of placebo-control group. Levels of fMLP-induced MFI in monocytes producing reactive oxygen metabolites in CIFL children initially were lower than in children of placebo-control group. The percentage of monocytes having produced reactive oxigen metabolites with *E.Coli* and PMA decreased after GCA-therapy. Cytokine production by monocytes after LPS stimulation in vitro in children showed that CIFL children had low level of TNF production initially. After GCA-therapy production of TNF increased and reached ranges of placebo-control group. Levels of IL-10 and IL-12 increased too reaching ranges of placebo-control group. Ratio TNF:IL10 not changed significantly after treatment. Proliferation response of T-lymphocytes to anti-CD3 monoclonal antibodies increased in CIFL children after GCA-therapy.

3. GROUNDS FOR GCA-THERAPY

The obtained results indicate that CIFL children had differences in antioxidant protective system from RRI children of placebo-control group. In comparison with RRI placebo-control children CIFL children had lower levels of total plasma glutathione, whole blood total glutathione, but high levels of intracellular GSH in lymphocytes and especially in monocytes and tendency to elevation in neutrophils. Optimal levels of intracellular GSH are inherent for normal cell function [2]. It is known that low intracellular levels and even relatively high intracellular glutathione levels reflect glutathione deficiency [3-5]. So, low levels of total glutathione in plasma and whole blood and low levels of plasma GSH and disorders in intracellular GSH confirmed deficiency in glutathione and antioxidant protective system as a whole in CIFL children. Disorders in glutathione system correlated with some functional immune disorders in CIFL children. Elevated levels of GSH in monocytes correlated with their diminished properties to release such cytokines as TNF, IL-10, IL-12.

Tendency only to elevation of GSH intracellular levels in neutrophils was documented in CIFL children. Perhaps absence of significant differences with placebo-control group related with more intensive participation of GSH in oxidative burst, which is higher significantly in CIFL children. Formation of reactive oxygen species and free radicals supported the oxidative burst directed to destruction of bacteria and stopped or prevented the development of acute infection. But high levels of reactive oxygen species and free radicals resulted alteration of host cells. One of the main factor to defend the host cells is elevated intracellular level of GSH.

Monocyte dysfunction in CIFL children was detected by registration of disorders in phagocytosis and cytokine production by monocytes. Disorders in phagocytosis included insufficiency of intracellular ingesting. Decreased levels of production of TNF, IL-10, IL-12 by monocytes confirmed disorders in cytokine production. Monitoring of monocyte function showed immune-modulating, normalizing effect of GCA therapy. Both disorders in phagocytosis and insufficiency of cytokines production by monocytes were modified and corrected by GCA-therapy. Production of TNF and IL-10 elevated without significant changes in ratio TNF:IL-10. We hope that it was not stimulation but reconstitution of monocyte function to release TNF, IL-10 and IL-12 in response to LPS. IL12 is a very important regulator of cell-mediated immune responses supporting Th1 type of T-cell-mediated response and NK cell activity.

4. CONCLUSION

CIFL children living on territory contaminated by radionuclides had deficiency in glutathione system (antioxidant protective system) and immune disorders: deficiency in cytokine release by monocytes, in phagocytic function of neutrophils and monocytes and disorders in burst activity of neutrophils and monocytes. Use of GCA-therapy resulted normalization (reconstitution) of immune status, glutathione balance (plasma and intracellular levels) and improvement in clinical status.

REFERENCES

1. Loukianova OM, Stepanova Ye.I, Antipkin Yu.G et. al.: The health of the children. In: Chornobyl Catastrophe. Ed. V.G.Baryakhtar. Kyiv, 1997, 451-453.
2. White AC, Thannickal VJ, Fanburg BL: Glutathione deficiency in human disease. J Nutr Biochem 1994, 5, 218-226.
3. Buhl R, Jaffe HA, Holroyd KJ et. al.: Systemic glutathione deficiency in symptom-free HIV seropositive individuals. Lancet 1990, 2, 1294-1298.
4. Staal FJT, Roederer M, Israelski DM et. al.: Intracellular glutathione levels in T cell subset decrease in HIV-infected individuals. AIDS Research and Human Retroviruses 1992, 8, 305-311.
5. Kinscherf R, Fischbach T, Mihm S et. al.: Effect of glutathione depletion and oral N-acetyl-cysteine treatment on CD4+ and CD8+ cells. FASEB Journal 1994, 8, 448-451.
6. Coffer PJ, Koenderman L: Granulocyte signal transduction and priming: cause without effect? Immunology Letters 1997, 57, 27-31.

IMMUNOTHERAPY

Adoptive transfer of mucosal T cells or dendritic cells from animals fed with cholera toxin B subunit alloantigen conjugate induces allogeneic T cell tolerance

BIN-LING LI, JIA-BIN SUN, AND JAN HOLMGREN
Department of Medical Microbiology and Immunology, Göteborg University, S-413 46 Göteborg, Sweden

1. INTRODUCTION

Repeated oral administration of allogeneic antigens (allo-Ag) in animals has been shown to delay rejection of cardiac allografts (1). However, oral tolerance induction by feeding allo-Ag is known to be ineffective to prevent rejection of full allogeneic grafts (1). We have previously found that oral administration of various antigens conjugated to the mucosa-binding molecule cholera toxin B subunit (CTB) can most effectively induce antigen-specific peripheral T cell tolerance (2), and also suppress several autoimmune diseases in experimental models (3). More recently, we and others reported that oral administration of a single dose of allogeneic antigens (allo-Ag) conjugated to CTB significantly prolongs murine allograft survival and inhibits the mixed lymphocyte reactions (MLR), allo-Ag-specific delayed-type hypersensitivity (DTH), as well as cell-mediated cytotoxicity (4, 5).

Progress in Basic and Clinical Immunology, Edited by Mackiewicz *et al.*
Kluwer Academic/Plenum Publishers, New York, 2001

2. METHODS AND MATERIALS

2.1 Induction of oral tolerance and MLR, DTH and IL-4 assays

Balb/c mice were fed with a single dose of C57BL/6 (B6) allogeneic thymocytes (ATC) (4×10^7 cells) conjugated with CTB (50 μg) or given alone in 0.5 ml of PBS on the indicated days. The conjugation method has been described (2, 5). MLR, allogeneic DTH reactions and determination of IL-4 producing cells were performed as previously described (5).

2.2 Preparation and adoptive transfer of dendritic cells and T cells

Peyer's patches (PP) and mesenteric lymph nodes (MLN) collected from the intestines of mice were first digested with RPMI medium containing DNAase, collagenase/dispase and EDTA. For enrichment of dendritic cells (DC), single cell suspensions were separated by gradient centrifugation using 14.5g% Metrizamine and 10% fetal calf serum; and then further incubated with beads labelled with anti-mouse pan T antibodies or anti-mouse IgG (DYNAL, Norway) or anti-mouse F4/80 to remove T cells, B cells and macrophages. Purified T cells were prepared as described (5). More than 90% of the purified cells were DC or T cells, respectively, as judged by FACS using FITC-labelled CD11c or CD3 antibodies.

DC (2×10^5 cells) were adoptively transferred by s.c. injection (for transfer of T cells 2×10^7 cells were injected i.p.) into syngeneic recipients 1 or 2 day before priming by s.c. injection of irradiated B6 ATC in the recipients (5). The recipients were then challenged by injecting irradiated ATC 10 days later.

3. RESULTS

3.1 Oral treatment with CTB-ATC reduces mucosal MLR response, but increases IL-4 production in PP

MLR responses to ATC (B6) were performed using T cells from PP isolated 7 days after the Balb/c mice received a single oral dose of either CTB-ATC, ATC alone or PBS. The MLR responses of cells from CTB-ATC treated animals were markedly suppressed in comparison with control animals treated with either PBS or ATC alone (Fig. 1). Instead, oral treatment with CTB-ATC increased the number of IL-4 producing T cells in PP (Fig. 1); whereas treatment with CTB-ATC instead tended to decrease IL-4 production in MLN or spleen (data not shown). No such effects were found after oral treatment with ATC alone (Fig. 1).

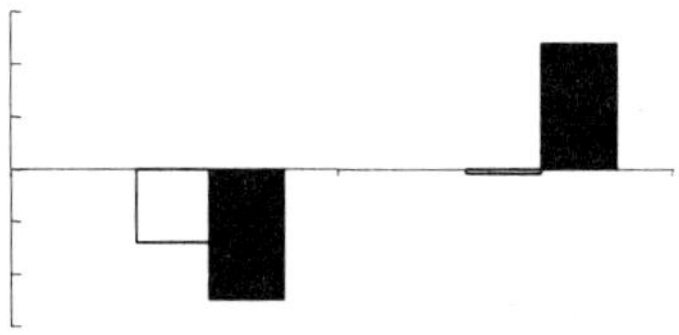

Figure 1. Concurrent decrease in MLR response and increase in IL-4 production by PP T cells from mice treated with oral CTB-alloAg (filled bars) or for comparison with ATC alone (open bars). Results show percentage changes from values obtained with cells from PBS-treated controls.

3.2 Adoptively transferred T cells from PP/MLN of mice fed with CTB-ATC inhibits allogeneic DTH

T cells were isolated from PP/MLN of Balb/c mice given an oral dose of CTB-ATC 7 days earlier. These cells were then transferred into syngeneic recipients by i.p. injection 1 day before these mice were sensitized with a s.c. injection of ATC (B6). Ten days after sensitization, DTH reactivity was measured after *in vivo* challenge by s.c. injection of the irradiated ATC into the left footpad. As shown in Fig. 2A., the transfer of T cells from PP/MLN of animals fed with CTB-ATC strongly suppressed the allogen-specific DTH reactions in recipients compared with T cells from animals treated with PBS or treated with ATC alone.

3.3 Adoptively transferred DC from PP/MLN of animals fed with CTB-ATC can suppress DTH and T cell proliferative responses to allo-Ag

DC were isolated from PP/MLN of Balb/c mice given two oral doses of CTB-ATC 1 and 4 days earlier. These cells were then transferred into syngeneic recipients by s.c. injection 2 day before these mice were sensitized with a s.c. injection of ATC (B6). Ten days after sensitization DTH reactivity and the T cell proliferative response to ATC of T cells from the draining lymph nodes (PLN) (14 days after sensitization) were examined. As shown in Fig. 2B., the transfer of DC from PP/MLN of animals fed with CTB-ATC strongly suppressed both the allogen-specific DTH reactions and T cell proliferative responses to allo-Ag by PLN cells in recipients. In contrast, Transfer of DC from mice treated with ATC alone had much lesser effect. (Fig. 2B).

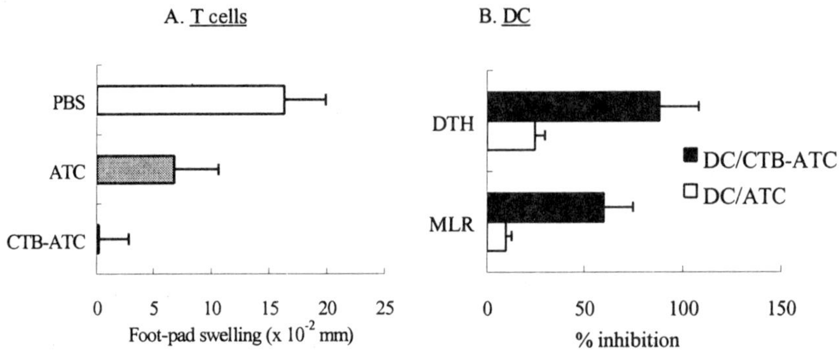

Figure 2. Suppression of allogeneic DTH reactions and/or T cell proliferative responses (MLR) of PLN cells to allo-Ags by adoptive transfer of T cells (i.p.) or DC (s.c.) isolated from PP/MLN of mice who had received earlier oral treatment with CTB-ATC (A) shows DTH results after transfer of T cells; and (B) the effects (% inhibition of DTH or MLR) of DC transfer from differently treated mice compared with DC from PBS-treated controls.

4. CONCLUSION

Oral administration of CTB-ATC can effectively induce allo-Ag specific peripheral tolerance affecting both Th1 and Th2 lymphocytes. The development of tolerance appears to be preceded by a transient Th2-dominant immune response to the fed Ag in the inductive mucosal lymphoid tissues, PP and/or MLN (5). This mucosal Th2 microenvironment may be critical for the development of regulatory TGF-β producing Th3 cells which in their turn appear to mediate the main tolerizing action at peripheral effector sites and/or the draining PLN (5, 6). Such Th3 cells are probably directly responsible for the observed tolerizing effect by transfer of T cells in this study. It is clear from this study that also DC isolated from PP/MLN of CTB-ATC-fed mice can adoptively transfer peripheral tolerance. Since most of the s.c. injected DC appear to localize to the draining PLN it is likely that the main tolerizing effect by these allo-Ag exposed intestinal DC occurs in PLN, whether as a result of a direct tolerogenic signal leading to anergy or apoptosis of pathogenic T cells or through a regulatory Th2/Th3 pathway being under investigation. In other studies we recently found that CD4+ T cells, isolated from animals who had been injected with DC pulsed *in vitro* with CTB-Ag, are capable to suppress immune responses of Ag-specific T cells in adoptive transfer experiments and that these effects were abolished when co-stimulatory molecules (CD80, CD86 and CD40) on DC were blocked or absent (Sun et al, to be published). Practically, the results of this and related studies (4, 5) suggest that oral administration of allogeneic MHC Ag chemically or genetically linked to CTB may be beneficial for the protection of allografts against early rejection.

ACKNOWLEDGMENTS

We thank Annie George and Kristina Eriksson for help with the characterisation of DC by FACS. This work was supported by the Swedish Medical Research Council (project 16x-3382), and the European Union (projects BIO 4-98-0503, BIO 4-CT-96-0374 and BIO 4-CT-97-2818).

REFERENCES

1. Sayegh, M.H., Zhang, Z.J., Hancock, W.W., Kwok, C.A., Carpenter, C.B., and Weiner. H.L., 1992, Down-regulation of the immune response to histocompatibility antigen and prevention of sensitization by skin allografts by orally administrated alloantigens. *Transplantation* 53:163-166.
2. Sun, J.-B., Holmgren, J., and Czerkinsky, C., 1994, Cholera toxin B subunit: An effective transmucosal carrier-delivery system for induction of peripheral immunological tolerance. *Proc. Natl. Acad. Sci. USA.* 91:10795-10799.
3. Sun, J.-B., Rask, C., Olsson, T., Holmgren, J., and Czerkinsky, C., 1996, Treatment of experimental allergic encephalomyelitis by feeding myelin basic protein conjugated to cholera toxin B subunit. *Proc. Natl. Acad. Sci. USA.* 93:196-7201.
4. Ma, D., Mellon, J., and Niederkorn, J. Y., 1997, Oral immunization as a strategy for enhancing corneal allograft survival. *British. J. Ophthalmology.* 81:778-784.
5. Sun, J.-B., Li, B.-L., Czerkinsky, C., and Holmgren, J., 2000, Enhanced immunological tolerance against allograft rejection by oral administration of allogeneic antigen linked to cholera toxin B subunit. *Clin. Immunol.* 97:130-139.
6. Sun, J.-B., Xiao, B.-G., Lindblad, M., Li, B.-L., Link, H., Czerkinsky, C., and Holmgren, J., 2000, Oral administration of cholera toxin B subunit conjugated to myelin basic protein protects against experimental autoimmune encephalomyelitis by inducing TGF-β_1 secreting cells and suppressing chemokine expression. *Int. Immunol.* 12:1449-1457.

Total body irradiation before bone marrow transplantation: aims and results

JULIAN MALICKI[#], JACEK WACHOWIAK[*], GRAŻYNA KOSICKA[#], GRAŻYNA STRYCZYŃSKA[∇], AGNIESZKA NOWAK[#], and JACEK PRACZ[♦]

[#]Medical Physics Department and [∇]Radiotherapy Department, GreatPoland Cancer Centre, Garbary 15 Street, 61-866 Poznań, Poland; [*]BMT Unit, Clinic of Paediatric Oncology and Heamatology, University of Medical Sciences, Szpitalna 29 Street, 60-572 Poznań, Poland; [♦]Soltan Institute for Nuclear Studies, Świerk, 05-400 Otwock, Poland.

1. INTRODUCTION

Total Body Irradiation (TBI) is a procedure performed during the treatment of some disseminated malignancies in patients undergoing bone marrow transplantation[1,2,3,4,5,6,7,8]. TBI has three aims to meet: first, to reduce the population of neoplastic cells, second, to induce immunosupression, and third, to eradicate the recipient's existing marrow cells so as to create room for newly transplanted marrow[1,7,8,9].

Efficacy of killing neoplastic cells depends on the homogeneous radiation dose delivered to the whole body[10,11,12,13]. The aims outlined above were achieved by a method using a combination of lateral and anterior-posterior fields, together with a set of compensators and shields[14,15,16]. Other conditions, important for the treatment included reproducibility and the patient's comfort.

The purpose of this paper was to compare dose homogeneity in two groups of patients, irradiated alternatively with a Cobalt unit or 15 MeV photons from a linear accelerator.

2. PATIENTS AND METHODS

Since 1993 twenty-two patients have been irradiated with a Cobalt-60 unit, and sixteen patients in a linear accelerator with 15 MeV photons, most of them with acute leukaemias (ALL, AML) and non-Hodgkin's lymphomas. All patients, children aged between 5 and 18 years, and from 110 to 186 cm of height, underwent subsequent bone marrow transplantation. The total dose of 12.6 Gy was prescribed for the whole body, and referenced to the point lying in the body midline at the coxa section (central axis–CAX). A dose of 8.2 Gy was delivered from six lateral fields, and a dose of 4.4 Gy from four anterior-posterior fields (AP/PA). The dose to the lungs was reduced to below 10 Gy. The irradiations were performed twice daily during four consecutive days.

Radiation with 6 to 10 MeV electrons (Neptun 10p or other accelerators) was used to irradiate additionally the thorax wall (with the dose of 4 Gy in two fractions), which, despite being shielded together with the lungs, accumulated a dose prescribed for the lungs instead of the necessary dose of 12.6 Gy. The electron energy depended on the thorax wall thickness. Lateral fields were set at a source to the skin distance (SSD) of 275 cm for cobalt irradiations, and that of 306 cm for the linear accelerator, respectively. AP/PA fields were set at SSD of 183 cm and 204 cm, respectively. A set of tissue equivalent compensators (head, neck, lung, knees and feet) was used to improve dose homogeneity inside the body.

The dose was pre-calculated for the midline of the patient, and at the points of the beam's entry to the body, and from the body's exit for ten transversal cross-sections (head, neck, shoulders, lung/mediastinum, elbows, abdomen, coxa-CAX, wrists, knees and feet). The CT scans carried out in these cross-sections made it possible to determine the outer body dimensions and the density of inner organs. The doses were measured *in-vivo* with two types of dosimeters: semiconductor and thermoluminescent devices[17]. The mean dose of their readings at entry and exit points was then recalculated relative to the respective point in the body midline using a known percent depth-dose dependence[18,19,20,21]. The errors in the calculated doses for all points were determined using a total differential method.

3. RESULTS

In table 1 doses calculated for the midline without compensators (with compensators in brackets) are presented for some selected cross-sections of the head, lung, elbows and coxa-CAX in a patient taken as an example. The calculated doses were added up for lateral and AP/PA fields together and shown for a patient treated with Cobalt-60 (column 3). The doses for the same patient but recalculated for 15 MV photons are shown in column 4. The dose calculation errors are given in column 5.

Table 1. Calculated doses (D_c) without compensators (with compensators in brackets) for the points in the midline for cross-sections of the head, lung, elbows and coxa-CAX, for a patient taken as an example. Total doses for lateral and AP/PA fields for a patient treated with Cobalt-60 (column 3) and recalculated for 15 MV photons are shown in column 4. Dose calculation errors are given in column 5.

		Co-60	X 15 MeV	
Section	Critical organ	D_c [Gy]	D_c [Gy]	Error [%]
Head	Lenses	14.2 (13.2)	14.8 (13.2)	5
Lung	Middle of the lungs, top of liver, mediastinum, thorax wall	10.7 (9.6)	11.2 (9.6)	15
Elbows	Bottom of the liver, spleen	12.2	12.5	5
Abdomen	Kidneys	12.8	13.1	5

In tables 2a and 2b, the calculated and measured doses in the midline, added up for lateral and AP/PA fields, with appropriate compensators and lungs' shields are given for the sections of the head, lung, elbows and abdomen. Table 2a presents mean doses determined in a way described above for a group of 22 patients irradiated with Cobalt-60, whereas table 2b shows the respective data for a group of 16 patients irradiated with 15 MV photons. In column 4 differences (ΔD) between the calculated and measured doses are shown as per cent of the calculated doses, respectively.

Table 2. Calculated (D_c) and measured (D_m) doses in the midline, summarised for lateral and AP/PA fields, with appropriate compensators and lungs' shields attached at the sections of the head, lung, elbows and abdomen. $\Delta D = (Dc - Dm)/Dc * 100\%$. Mean doses for a group of 22 patients irradiated with Cobalt-60 (a) and for a group of 16 patients irradiated with 15 MV photons (b).

a)

Section	D_c [Gy]	D_m [Gy]	ΔD [%]
Head	12.9	12.5	+3.1
Lung	8.8	9.9	-12.5
Elbows	11,6	12,6	+7,6
Abdomen	13.4	13.3	+0.7

b)

Section	D_c [Gy]	D_m [Gy]	ΔD [%]
Head	13.1	12.8	+2.2
Lung	8.9	9.9	-11.2
Elbows	12.7	13.3	-4.7
Abdomen	13.2	14.4	-9.1

4. DISCUSSION

In TBI one of the important requirements - the homogeneous dose - is limited by the patient's comfort that enforces the procedure being both therapeutically effective and simple. These two aims have made it necessary to search for various possible procedures, and in consequence have led to the comparison between irradiation performed with cobalt-60 and with 15 MeV photons from a linear accelerator[22]. Such a comparison was found to be difficult to evaluate since doses were related to two cohorts of patients not being randomised or even selected for one of these two specific procedures. The only common denominator was the availability of the equipment at the time when the given procedure was applied.

Firstly, doses without compensators were calculated for cobalt and 15 MeV accelerator for a patient taken as a representative example. The received doses were higher for 15 MeV photons than for cobalt gamma rays in the sections of the head: 14.8 Gy (15 MeV); 14.2 Gy (cobalt) and lung: 11.2 Gy (15 MeV); 10.7 Gy (cobalt) (table 1). This, however, was only a proof of the correctness of the algorithm used, but the data failed to indicate which specific procedure had been superior because for both procedures compensators had had to be added because the doses were found to be too high. With compensators in use, the appropriate thickness had to be determined for each beam separately. Thus the application of compensators reduced the doses to almost the same levels for cobalt and for 15 MeV (13.2 Gy for the head, and 9.6 Gy for the lung), and also reduced deviations from the prescribed 12.6 Gy dose to the values within the limit of +/-10%, respectively.

The differences between the calculated and measured doses (table 2) were more informative because they were averaged for the groups of patients irradiated with cobalt radiation (table 2a) and with 15 MeV photons (table 2b). For cobalt, dose differences varied from -12.5 % at the lung, and +3.1% at the head to +0.7 % at the abdomen. For 15 MeV photons, these values varied respectively from -11.5 % at the lung to +2.2% at the head and –9.1% at abdomen.

Calculation errors (table 1) exceeded the differences between the calculated and measured doses for the sections of the elbows for cobalt, and those of the abdomen for 15 MeV photons, respectively. For the remaining sections the measured doses did not differ from those pre-calculated more than within the error shown in table 1. These results were the best proof of the correctness of our method of calculations and measurements.

The calculated doses (proved to be reliable - see above) for both types of irradiation (cobalt and 15 MeV) did not differ significantly between, if the respective sections had been compared (table 2a and 2b).

In consequence, the analysis carried above showed that neither of the procedures applied proved its superiority when dose deviations inside the body midline were taken into consideration.

5. CONCLUSION

In irradiated patients the doses measured at the most important sections of the head and lung did not differ from those pre-calculated more than by the estimated error for cobalt and 15 MeV photons.

Dose discrepancies for cobalt and 15 MeV photons did not exceed the limits of the prescribed doses to the head and the lungs by more than the recommended 10% .

ACKNOWLEDGMENTS

The work was supported by the KBN grant 8-T11E041 99 C/4351 p.n.

REFERENCES

1 . Barret, A., 1999, Total body irradiation. R. Pract. Oncol. Radiothher 4(3):47-64.
2 . Cosset, J.M., Baume, D., Pico, J.L., Shank, B., Girinski, T., Banhamou, E., Briot. E., Malaise, E., Hayat, M., Dutreix, J., 1989, Single dose versus hyperfractionated total body irradiation before allogeneic bone marrow transplantation: a non-randomized comparative study of 54 patients at the Institute Gustave-Roussy. Radiother. Oncol 15: 151. 60.
3 . Cosset, J.M., Girinski, T., Maloise, E., Chaillet, M.P., Dutreix, J., 1990, Clinical basis for TBI fractionation. Radiother. Oncol. Suppl 18: 60-68.
4 . Inoue, T., Ikeda, H., Yamazaki, H., 1993, Role of total body irradiation as based on comparison of preparation regimens for allogene bone marrow transplantation for acute leukemia in first complete remission. Strahlenther. Onkol 169: 250. 55.
5 . Kolb, H.J., Graitiwohl, A., Zwaan, F.E., 1988, Randomized study comparing busulfan and cyclophosphamide with total body irradiation with cyclophoshamide as conditioning treatment or allogemeic bone marrow transplantation patients with leukemia. Protocol of Acute Leukemia Working Party. European Cooperative Group for Bone Marrow Transplantation (EBMT)
6 . Girinsky, T., Benhamou, E., Bourhis, J.H., Dhermain, F., Guillot-Valls, D., Ganansia, V., Luboinski, M., Perez, A., Cosset, J.M., Socie, G., Baume, D., Bouaouina, N., Briot, E., Beaudre, A., Bridier, A., Pico, J.L., 2000, Prospective randomized comparison of single-dose versus hyperfraction body irradiation in patients with hematologic malignancies. J. Clin. Oncol, 18: 981. 86.
7 . Wachowiak, J., Boruczkowski, D., Malicki, J., Kaczmarek-Kanold, M., Chobot-Musiałkiewicz, U., Radwańska, U., 1999, Allogeneic bone marrow transplantation in

children – eight years experience of paediatric BMT unit in Poznań. Bone Marrow Transplant Suppl: 63.66.

8 . Wachowiak, J., Boruczkowski, J., Malicki, J., Chobot-Musiałkiewicz, U., 1998, Early post-BMT liver function in children with acute leukemia conditioned for allo-BMT with busulfan-containing and with FTBI-containing preparative regimens. Bone Marrow Transplant Suppl: 96. 99.

9 . Sanchez-Doblado, F., Quast, V., Arrians, R., Errazquin, L., Sanchez-Nieto, B., Terron, J.A., 1995, Total body irradiation prior to bone marrow transplantation. EBMT

10 . Quast, U., 1990, Total body irradiation – review of treatment techniques in Europe. Radiother. Oncol Suppl: 158. 62.

11 . Quast, U., 1991, Physical problems of total body irradiation. Strahlenther. Onkol. 167: 135. 57.

12 . Malicki, J., 1998, Doses in critical organs during total body irradiation before bone marrow transplantation. An. Ttransplant 3: 14-19.

13 . American Association of Physicist in Medicine (AAPM). 1986, The physical aspects of total and half body photon irradiation. AAPM Report No. 17

14 . Malicki, J., 1999, The accuracy of dose determination during total body irradiation. Strahlenther. Onkol 175: 492. 96.

15 . Malicki, J., 1998, Doses in critical organs during total body irradiation before bone marrow transplantation. An. Ttransplant 3: 14-19.

16 . Malicki, J., 1997, Beam filter and compensators during total body irradiation on Cobalt-60. R. Pract.Oncol. Radiother 2: 77. 81.

17 . Malicki, J., Kosicka, G., Kierzkowski, J., Górny, A., 1996, An analysis of effectiveness and accuracy of ionization, semiconductor and thermoluminescent detectors used in total body irradiation. J. Med. Phys 21: 10. 13.

18 . International Commission on Radiation Units and Measurements (ICRU). 1993, Prescribing, recording, and reporting photon beam therapy. ICRU Report 50,

19 . International Commission on Radiation Units and Measurement (ICRU). 1976,Determination of absorbed dose in a patient irradiated by beams of X or gamma rays in radiotherapy procedures. ICRU Report 24

20 . Christ, G., Well, F., Nüsslin, F., 1991, In-vivo dosimetry in the thorax region at total body irradiation. Strahlenther. Onkol 167 (3): 148. 50.

21 . Heukelom, S., Lanson, J.H., Mijneer, B.J., 1991, Comparison of entrance and exit dose measurements using ionization chambers and silicon diodes. Phys. Med. Biol 36 (1): 47-59.

22 . Jones, D., Rieke, J.W., Madsen, B.L., Hafermann, M.D., 2000, An isocentrically mounted stand for total body irradiation. Br. J. Radiol 73: 776. 69.

Statins as immunomodulatory drugs

ANDRZEJ GÓRSKI*^, MONIKA KASPRZYCKA^, MARIA NOWACZYK^, PIOTR WIERZBICKI^, GRAŻYNA KORCZAK-KOWALSKA^, PAWEL JEZAK^, DANUTA KŁOSOWSKA^, ANETA EKIERT^, KONRAD KŁODOS^.

*^Department of Clinical Immunology, Transplantation Institute, The Medical University of Warsaw; *L.Hirszfeld Institute of Immunology and Experimental Therapy, Polish Academy of Sciences, Wroclaw, Poland*

1. INTRODUCTION

Statins (inhibitors of HMG-ConA reductase) are widely used as cholesterol-lowering agents and have beneficial action in patients with complications of atherosclerosis (coronary disease). In addition, recent data indicate that they can also modulate a variety of other biological processes inhibiting neointimal proliferation, reducing inflammation and stimulating osteogenesis (1,2,3). Moreover, our preliminary studies point to the role of statins as potential immunosuppressive agents (4). In this report, we confirm and extend those initial observations.

Progress in Basic and Clinical Immunology, Edited by Mackiewicz *et al.*
Kluwer Academic/Plenum Publishers, New York, 2001

2. MATERIALS AND METHODS

Mononuclear and T cell isolation from human peripheral blood and other technics used in our studies reported herein have been described in detail earlier: cell isolation (5); T and B lymphocyte proliferation in response to mitogen and alloantigens using thymidine incorporation assay (5,6); immunoglobulin (Ig) synthesis studied with the aid of reverse plaque forming cell (PFC) assay (PFC)(7); lymphocyte phenotyping and evaluation of cytoplasmatic cytokine synthesis following PMA stimulation using FACS analysis (5,8); cytokine production and secretion in response to alloantigen stimulation using ELISA (9); co-stimulatory and adhesive T cell interactions with the extracellular matrix proteins (elastin, fibronectin)(10); T cell adhesion to inflamed (LPS-activated for 4-24 hrs) human microvascular endothelium and endothelial adhesion molecule expression (11,12).

3. RESULTS

The immunosuppressive action of lovastatin and simvastatin is depicted in Tables 1-3.

Table 1a Immunosuppressive effects of lovastatin /simvastatin
- concentration range: 0.0001-0.1 μg/ml, * denotes $p < 0.05$, data presented as percent control (no statins added)

concentration (μg/ml)	0,0001	0,001	0,01	0,05	0,1
OKT3 induced T cell proliferation				99 (±13)	84 (±7)
				99 (±9)	77 (±8)
Alloantigen induced T cell		104 (±15)	75 (±8)		59 (±6)*
proliferation		84 (±7)	76 (±4)*		78 (±10)*
SAC induced B cell proliferation	73 (±8)*	71 (±8)*	74 (±6)*		81 (±7)*
	86 (±15)	77 (±4)*	73 (±5)*		68 (±7)*
PWM induced Ig synthesis		98 (±6)	75 (±6)*		57 (±5)*
		86 (±10)	62 (±5)*		48 (±4)*
Alloantigen induced Ig synthesis			93 (±5)		86 (±9)*
		83 (±3)	62 (±7)*		52 (±7)*
OKT3 induced CD25 expression					107 (±4)
on T cells					97 (±7)
OKT3 induced CD69 expression					105 (±3)
on T cells					88 (±7)

Table 1b Immunosuppressive effects of lovastatin /simvastatin
- concentration range: 0.5 - 10 μg/ml , * denotes $p < 0.05$, data presented as percent control (no statins added)

concentration (μg/ml)	0,5	1	5	10
OKT3 induced T cell proliferation	93 (±6)	81 (±13)	45 (±9)*	
	77 (±8)*	56 (±7)*	11 (±3)*	
Alloantigen induced T cell		44 (±6)*		
proliferation		6 (±2)*		
SAC induced B cell proliferation		72 (±7)*		
		56 (±6)*		
PWM induced Ig synthesis		55 (±8)*		
		43 (±5)*		
Alloantigen induced Ig synthesis		86 (±19)*		
		51 (±12)*		
OKT3 induced CD25 expression on		88 (±12)		85 (±6)
T cells		90 (±6)		57 (±9)*
OKT3 induced CD69 expression on		82 (±14)		68 (±14)
T cells		78 (±9)*		58 (±13)*
PMA induced synthesis of		95 (±8)		73 (±6)*
cytoplasmatic IL-2 in T cells		80 (±13)		68 (±6)*
Alloantigen induced IL-2		108 (±47)		60 (±17)*
synthesis		103 (±31)		26 (±9)*
Alloantigen induced IFN γ		108 (±39)		51 (±18)*
synthesis		125 (±43)		35 (±9)*
Alloantigen induced TNF α		112 (±27)		87 (±26)
synthesis		106 (±25)		82 (±24)

As may be seen, B cell responses are very sensitive to both lovastatin and simvastatin, as very low statin concentrations inhibit B cell proliferation and Ig synthesis.

T cell proliferative responses are less sensitive, and inhibition of acquisition of activation antigens by T cells can be achieved using higher concentrations. Those higher concentrations also impair cytoplasmatic cytokine synthesis (IL-2) and secretion (IL-2, IFN γ and TNF α).

As described earlier, very low drug concentrations strongly inhibit adhesion of activated T cells to elastin (but not fibronectin) and co-stimulation of T cell activation by those extracellular matrix proteins.

Table 2 Immunosuppressive effects of lovastatin / simvastatin
- * denotes $p < 0.05$, data presented as percent control (no statins added)

Concentration (μg/ml)	0,001	0,01	0,05	0.1	1
Adhesion of PHA activated T cells	99 (±3)	98 (±4)		84 (±9)	91 (±7)
to fibronectin	101 (±4)	102 (±4)			110 (±4)
Adhesion of PHA activated T cells	62 (±5)*	71 (±9)*		69 (±13)*	88 (±7)
to elastin	61 (±8)*	63 (±6)*			91 (±9)
Co-stimulatory effect of elastin on			76 (±3)*	76 (±4)*	79 (±9)
T cell activation			34 (±8)*	48 (±17)*	43 (±1)*
Co-stimulatory effect of fibronectin			100 (±6)	100 (±7)	95 (±5)
on T cell activation			61 (±15)*	55 (±7)*	70 (±7)*

Interestingly, statins can also impair T cell adhesion to microvascular endothelium, as well as endothelial cell activation measured by upregulation and acquisition of adhesion molecules on those cells.

Table 3 Immunosuppressive effects of lovastatin / simvastatin
- * denotes $p < 0.05$, data presented as percent control (no statins added)

concentration (μg/ml)	0,01	0,1	1
T cell adhesion to LPS activated HMEC (4h activation)		111 (±34)	74 (±10)*
		65 (±23)	48 (±5)*
T cell adhesion to LPS activated HMEC (24h activation)	62 (±15)*	89 (±27)	87 (±21)
	50 (±7)*	55 (±13)*	75 (±16)*
T cell adhesion to LPS activated HMEC (4h activation)	63 (±12)*	75 (±9)	95 (±7)
(T cells were preincubated with statin for 1h)	67 (±8)*	64 (±3)*	93 (±8)
T cell adhesion to LPS activated HMEC (24h activation)	60 (±4)*	94 (±10)*	101 (±4)
(T cells were preincubated with statin for 1h)	54 (±2)*	67 (±1)*	87 (±2)*
E-selectin expression on endothelial cells	161 (±6)*	136 (±2)*	95 (±1)
	96 (±1)	94 (±1)*	93 (±1)*
ICAM-1 expression on endothelial cells	110 (±4)	124 (±7)	131 (±8)*
	127 (±8)	122 (±7)	130 (±8)*
VCAM-1 expression on endothelial cells	98 (±5)	89 (±5)*	80 (±4)*
	98 (±3)	90 (±4)	75 (±3)*

4. DISCUSSION

We confirm our earlier report suggesting that statins may have immunosuppressive properties (4). Those findings were recently confirmed by Kwak et al. who showed that statins may act as direct inhibitors of induction of MHC-II antigen expression and thus as suppressors of MHC-II-mediated T-cell activation (13).

Of particular interest are our data indicating that very low concentrations of statins readily attainable in vivo strongly inhibit T cell interactions with the proteins of extracellular matrix (particularly elastin, a major component of adult vessel wall) and microvascular endothelium. Those findings provide a rationale for using statins in clinical immunosuppression in the treatment of vasculitis occurring in autoimmune diseases and graft rejection.

ACKNOWLEDGMENTS

This work was supported by intramural grant 1MG/W1/2000 from the Medical University of Warsaw.

REFERENCES

1. Vaughan, C.J., Murphy, M.B. and Buckley, B.M. 2000, Statins do more than just lower cholesterol. Lancet 348:1079.
2. Senior, K. 2000, The hidden potential for statins. Lancet 356:1905.
3. Rogers, M.J. 2000, Statins: lower lipid and better bones? Nature Medicine 6:21.
4. Górski, A., Orłowska A., Nowaczyk M., et al. 1999, Statins inhibit T-cell interactions with elastin. Transplant.Proc. 31:828-829.
5. Górski, A., Grieb, P., Korczak-Kowalska, G., et al. 1993, Cladribine (2-chloro-deoxyadenosine, CDA): an inhibitor of human B and T cell activation in vitro. Immunopharmacology 26:197-202.
6. Imiela, J., Korczak-Kowalska, G., Małecki R., et al. 1993, Immunomodulatory action of human recombinant erythropoietin in man. Immunology Letters 35:271-276.
7. Górski, A., Wąsik, M., Stępień-Sopniewska, B. et al. 1991, Heparin and platelet interactions influence alloantigen-induced proliferative responses of human T lymphocytes and immunoglobulin synthesis in vitro. Immunology Letters 28:161-166.
8. Ito, M., Watanabe, M., Kamiya H., and Sakurai, M. 1997, Changes in intracellular cytokine levels in lymphocytes induced by measles virus. Clin.Immun.Immunopathol. 83:281-286.
9. Jo, E.K., Kim, J.K. and Lim, J.H. 2000, Dysregulated production of interferon-gamma, interleukin-4 and interleukin-6 in early tuberculosis patients in response to antigen 85B of Mycobacterium tuberculosis. Scand.J.Immunol. 51:209-217.
10. Górski, A., Castronovo, V., Stępień-Sopniewska, B. et al. 1994, Depressed immune surveillance against cancer: role of deficient T cell:extracellular matrix interactions. Cell Adhesion Com. 2:225-233.
11. Korczak-Kowalska, G., Nowaczyk, M., Stępień-Sopniewska, B. et al. 1997, T-cell interactions with the extracellular matrix proteins and endothelium in chronic renal allograft rejection. Transplant.Proc.29:1057-1059.
12. Rokosz, A., Meisel-Mikołajczyk, F., Malchar, C., Nowaczyk, M. And Górski, A. 1999, Adhesion molecule expression stimulated by B.thetaiotaomicron cell-surface antigens. Arch.Immun.Ther.Exp. 47:169-175.

13. Kwak, B., Mulhaupt, F., Myit, S. and Mach, F. 2000, Statins as a newly recognized type of immunomodulator. Nature Medicine 6:1399-1402.

VACCINES

Phage display of epitopes from HIV-1 elicits strong cytolytic responses *in vitro* and *in vivo*

JOHN GUARDIOLA*, PIERGIUSEPPE DE BERARDINIS°, ROSSELLA SARTORIUS °, CRISTINA FANUTTI+, PERHAM RICHARD N.+ and GIOVANNA DEL POZZO*

**International Institute of Genetics and Biophysics, CNR, Naples, Italy; °Institute of Protein Biochemistry Enzymology, CNR, Naples, Italy; +Department of Biochemistry, University of Cambridge, UK*

1. INTRODUCTION

Vaccines based on synthetic peptides representing epitopes recognized by T-helper or cytolytic T-cells have been widely investigated as the basis for effective vaccines. However, their efficacy suffers from a number of important limitations. First, they are poor immunogens and exhibit short life-spans both in serum and within the cell (1). Secondly, the amount of peptide required to bind a threshold number of MHC class II molecules on the surface of an APC is reportedly higher than the minimal amount needed to bind to class II MHC molecules in the intracellular compartment in which the processing of the corresponding parent antigen takes place after internalization (2). Soluble antigens carrying CTL epitopes not only have the same drawbacks, but normally are unable to enter the appropriate intracellular compartment to undergo processing and presentation on class I MHC molecules (3). Thus, delivery systems based on immune-stimulating complexes, liposomes and synthetic lipopeptides have been designed in attempts to circumvent these limitations (1).

In this context, it has been demonstrated that antigenic peptides can be inserted in the N-terminal region of the major coat protein, gVIIIp, of the filamentous bacteriophage fd (4, 5). Because there are 2700 copies of gVIIIp per virion, this system allows for the display of a large number of foreign antigenic peptides. Peptides of 6-8 amino acids can normally be inserted close to the N- terminus of gVIIIp, generating a recombinant virion in which all copies of the major gVIIIp protein display the peptide epitope. However, in order to accommodate larger peptides (6, 7) it has proved necessary to construct a hybrid phage in which the modified gVIIIp proteins are interspersed with wild-type gVIIIp molecules. Given the large number of gVIIIp proteins in the virion, the inserted peptides, even if expressed in a lower copy number on the phage particles, remain densely represented and are strongly immunogenic. Indeed, there is good evidence from immunoassay and NMR spectroscopy that a peptide representing the immunodominant epitope of gp120 from HIV-1, when expressed on filamentous phage virions, can elicit phage-neutralizing antibodies (8) and adopt a persistent three-dimensional structure closely resembling that which it exhibits in the wild-type parent protein (9).

We previously described the capacity of peptides expressed on the pVIII phage major coat protein of eliciting the production of specific antibodies or present a T helper-epitope (10).

2. INDUCTION OF EPITOPE SPECIFIC CYTOTOXIC T CELLS

Here it is described the unexpected ability of bacteriophage virions displaying the antigenic peptide RT2, corresponding to residues 309-317 of the reverse transcriptase (RTase) of HIV-1, to evoke an antigen-specific CTL response both in vitro and in vivo. The peptide epitope RT2 exhibits a high degree of conservation in different viral isolates and, in AIDS patients, induces a specific CTL response which is inversely correlated with virus load (11).

2.1 Construction of hybrid bacteriophage molecules

Because co-expresion of linked helper T-cell and cytotoxic T-cell (CTL) epitopes on the surface of the same antigen-presenting cell (APC) is a strict requirement for priming a CTL response (12-14), we designed hybrid bacteriophages displaying helper and/or cytotoxic epitopes. In particular two hybrid bacteriophage virions were described: one (fd23) in which approximately 10% of the 2700 pVIII subunits in the virion each displayed a single copy of the peptide pep23, an immunodominant T-helper cell epitope (15) of HIV-1 RTase; and another (fdRT2) in which approximately 30% of the pVIII subunits carried the peptide RT2, an HLA-A2 restricted CTL epitope of the same protein (16). We also generated a double-display hybrid virion (fd23RT2) in which both peptides were displayed on the same capsid (7) at approximately the same level as in the single display virions.

2.2 Priming of RT2-specific CTL

We established primary cultures from the peripheral blood mononuclear cells (PBMC) of a healthy individual (LDA). In particular adherent cells, to be used as APCs, were separated by adsorption onto gelatin-coated plates, pulsed variously with the synthetic peptide RT2, with bacteriophage fdRT2, or bacteriophage fd23RT2, and mixed with non adherent cells. The appearance of HLA-A2 restricted cytotoxic T lymphocytes was then tested after 9 days using, as a target, T2 cells (a mutant cell line unable to present endogenously processed peptides because of a deletion of the Tap1 and Tap2 genes) loaded with the peptide RT2. Cultures grown in the presence of peptide RT2 or of bacteriophage virions displaying peptide RT2 alone did not generate RT2-specific CTLs (Fig. 1). In contrast, when cultures were grown in the presence of virions simultaneously displaying peptides RT2 and pep23, CTL activity was induced (Fig. 1). The addition of anti-CD8 mAb to the cytotoxicity assay blocked the lysis of RT2 loaded target cells, indicating that the lytic activity is exerted by CD8+ T cells (data not shown). However, CD4+ T cells play an essential part in the priming of the cytotoxic T-cell activity. In fact, an anti-CD4 mAb, supplied when the primary cultures were being established, blocked the generation of CTLs (data not shown).

We have previously demonstrated that pep23 displayed in the pVIII of filamentous bacteriophage virions is recognized by specific $CD4^+$ HLA-DR5-restricted T-cell clones and that intracellular processing of the virions is required (10). We thus tested PBMC from a HLA-A2 negative and DR5 positive donor. No specific CTL priming with fd23RT2 was observed (insert to Fig.1). These data, and lack of CTL induction in culture primed with single-display fdRT2 phage particles, clearly indicate that bacteriophage virions can deliver both a CTL epitope and T-helper epitope to the appropriate processing compartments of a cell, thus triggering a helper-dependent antigen-specific CTL response in PBMC with appropriate HLA phenotype. In separate experiments, we have also demonstrate that fluorescently tagged fd virions co-localize in APCs with markers of the class II and the class I compartements, and that RT2 specific CTL can lyse APCs, other than T2, pulsed with phage particles displaying the RT2 epitope (M Gaubin et al., unpublished work).

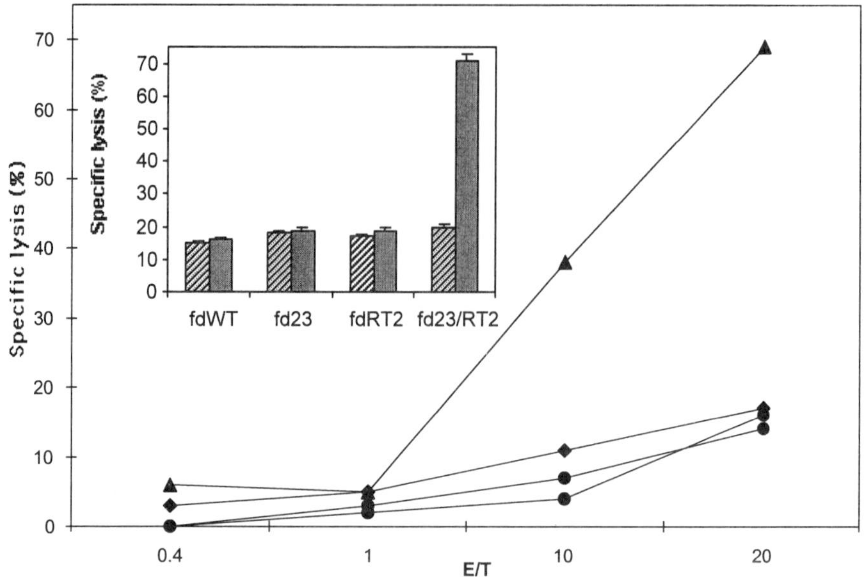

Figure 1. Cytotoxic activity of T-cell lines generated from a (HLA-A2+, DR5+) healthy donor (LDA). $3x10^5$ adherent cells were pulsed for 3 hours with the following antigens: no antigen (■), peptide RT2 (●), single display bacteriophage fdRT2 (♦), double display bacteriophage fd23RT2 (▲). To each of these cultures, $1x10^6$ non-adherent cells were added. Cytotoxicity was assayed after 9 days, using as target cells ^{51}Cr-labelled T2 cells pulsed with peptide RT2. Non-specific lysis was 13% at effector/target (E/T) ratio of 20:1. The insert shows the activity of the T-cell lines generated from the PDB (HLA-A2- DR5+) donor (hatched bars), and from the LDA donor (closed bars). Primary cultures were established in the presence of indicated antigen.

2.3 Production of specific CTLs in vivo

To test whether phages can elicit CTL activity in vivo, HLA-A2 transgenic mice[22,23] were sub-cutaneously immunized with 140 μg of bacteriophage virions displaying relevant antigenic peptides. Splenocytes were isolated after 7 days and re-stimulated in vitro for 5 days with syngenic, LPS-induced, blast cells pulsed with the same virions. The cytotoxic activity of the splenocytes was then tested using as target the RMA-S cells transfected with human HLA-A2.1 (17) and loaded with peptide RT2. As shown in Fig.4, a high antigen-specific cytolytic activity was observed with splenocytes isolated from mice immunized with virions fdRT2 or fd23RT2, carrying the RT2 determinant. Splenocytes isolated from naïve mice and restimulated in vitro with fdRT2 virions exhibited no cytotoxic activity. The splenocytes used in these experiments were isolated from HLA-A2.1 monochain H-2D^b β2m double-knockout transgenic mice[22]; the splenocytes from HLA-A0201 K^b transgenic mice from a different source (18) behaved similarly. The magnitude of lysis obtained was lower than that observed with human PBMC in vitro, which can be attributed to differences in the two systems. In contrast with the results obtained in vitro (Fig. 1), immunization with fdRT2 virions alone in vivo was able to elicit specific CTL activity. This can be attibuted to the existence in the pVIII protein itself of an epitope recognised by murine CD4$^+$ T cells (G. Del Pozzo, unpublished work), which presumably can provide the T-cell help necessary for CTL induction.

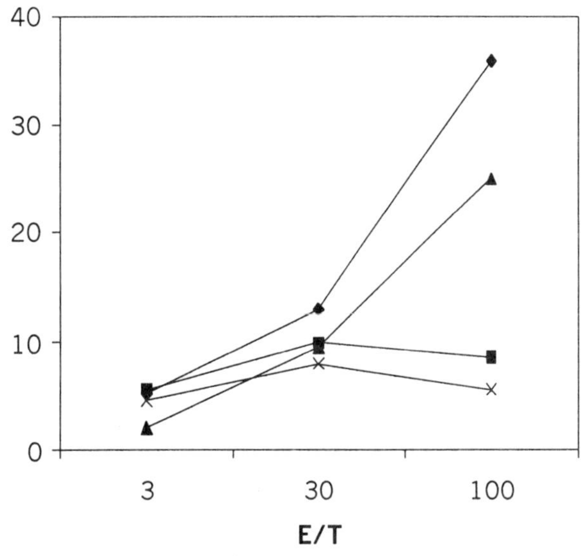

Figure 2. Induction of specific CTL activity in vivo. Specific cytotoxic T cells were induced in twelve HLA-A2 transgenic mice[22] immunized with 140 □g of either fdRT2 (▲) or fd23RT2(♦) virions. Splenocytes isolated 7 days after immunization, and restimulated in vitro with the antigens used for immunization, were employed as effector cells. RMA-S cells transfected with HLA-A2.1 and loaded with peptide RT2 were used as the target of cytotoxicity. The figure illustrates a representative experiment. (■) Lytic activity of splenocytes immunized with wild-type fd virions (not expressing the RT2 epitope), (x) Lytic activity of splenocytes isolated from naïve (unimmunized) mice and restimulated in vitro with fdRT2 virions.

3. CONCLUDING REMARKS

We have clearly demonstrated that non-pathogenic, non-replicating filamentous bacteriophage virions displaying determinants from HIV-1 RTase are able to generate specific cytotoxic T cell responses in a human system in vitro and in transgenic mice in vivo. The size and robostness of the phage scaffold and the high molar ratio of epitopes may be important; the mechanism by which phage virions can target both class I and class II MHC compartements is currently under investigation. No special flanking sequences were inserted either side of the pep23 or RT2 peptides in the pVIII protein, which suggests that the systems of intracellular proteolysis responsible for creating the peptides for subsequent MHC display may be concerned more with the size of the peptides generated (i.e. 9-15 residues) than the sequence context in which they are found. The pep23 and RT2 epitopes derive from the polymerase domain of HIV-1 Rtase (19) and show a high degree of conservation in different viral isolates (16). The pep23 sequence includes a B-cell epitope in addition to a T-helper epitope (10); neutralizing antibodies against this determinant, capable of inhibiting RTase activity, have been found in sera of long-term non-progressor patients infected with HIV-1 and shown to correlate with survival (20). Further, HIV-1^+ patients of the HLA-A2 haplotype have been found to develop at high frequency a circulating CTL activity directed against a few Gag and Pol epitopes (among which is the RT2 determinant used here) and this correlates with protection parameters (11). Thus the bacteriophage constructs described above may be of interest in generating protection against HIV-1. More generally, the ability to elicit in vivo both B and T-cell responses, against specific peptides displayed on benign bacteriophage virions offers a new approach to the design of subunit vaccines capable of evoking both arms of the immune response.

ACKNOWLEDGEMENTS

This research was supported by a grant from the EU to JG and RNP, from ISS II Progetto AIDS to JG, from MURST/CNR L95.95 Biotechnology to JG and from CNR P.F.Biotecnologia to GDP. The core facilities of the Cambridge Centre for Molecular Recognition are supported by the Biotechnology and Biological Sciences Research Council and The Wellcome Trust. We thank P. Barba and C. Sole for excellent technical assistance.

REFERENCES

1. Bona, C. A., S. Casares, T. D. Brumeanu. 1998. Towards development of T-cell vaccines. *Immunol Today*. 19: 126-33
2. Demotz, S., H. M. Grey, A. Sette. 1990. The minimal number of class II MHC-antigen complexes needed for T cell activation. *Science*. 249: 1028-30
3. Bot, A., S. Bot, S. Antohi, K. Karjalainen, C. Bona. 1996. Kinetics of generation and persistence on membrane class II molecules of a viral peptide expressed on foreign and self proteins. *J Immunol*. 157: 3436-42
4. Greenwood, J., A. E. Willis, R. N. Perham. 1991. Multiple display of foreign peptides on a filamentous bacteriophage. Peptides from Plasmodium falciparum circumsporozoite protein as antigens. *J Mol Biol*. 220: 821-7
5. Minenkova, O. O., A. A. Ilyichev, G. P. Kishchenko, V. A. Petrenko. 1993. Design of specific immunogens using filamentous phage as the carrier. *Gene*. 128: 85-8
6. Malik, P., R. N. Perham. 1996. New vectors for peptide display on the surface of filamentous bacteriophage. *Gene*. 171: 49-51
7. Malik, P., R. N. Perham. 1997. Simultaneous display of different peptides on the surface of filamentous bacteriophage. *Nucleic Acids Res*. 25: 915-6
8. di Marzo Veronese, F., A. E. Willis, C. Boyer-Thompson, E. Appella, R. N. Perham. 1994. Structural mimicry and enhanced immunogenicity of peptide epitopes displayed on filamentous bacteriophage. The V3 loop of HIV-1 gp120. *J Mol Biol*. 243: 167-72
9. Jelinek, R., T. D. Terry, J. J. Gesell, P. Malik, R. N. Perham, S. J. Opella. 1997. NMR structure of the principal neutralizing determinant of HIV-1 displayed in filamentous bacteriophage coat protein. *J Mol Biol*. 266: 649-55
10. De Berardinis, P., L. D'Apice, A. Prisco, M. N. Ombra, P. Barba, G. Del Pozzo, S. Petukhov, P. Malik, R. N. Perham, J. Guardiola. 1999. Recognition of HIV-derived B and T cell epitopes displayed on filamentous phages. *Vaccine*. 17: 1434-41
11. Ogg, G. S., X. Jin, S. Bonhoeffer, P. R. Dunbar, M. A. Nowak, S. Monard, J. P. Segal, Y. Cao, S. L. Rowland-Jones, V. Cerundolo, A. Hurley, M. Markowitz, D. D. Ho, D. F. Nixon, A. J. McMichael. 1998. Quantitation of HIV-1-specific cytotoxic T lymphocytes and plasma load of viral RNA. *Science*. 279: 2103-6
12. Stuhler, G., S. F. Schlossman. 1997. Antigen organization regulates cluster formation and induction of cytotoxic T lymphocytes by helper T cell subsets. *Proc Natl Acad Sci U S A*. 94: 622-7
13. Ossendorp, F., E. Mengede, M. Camps, R. Filius, C. J. Melief. 1998. Specific T helper cell requirement for optimal induction of cytotoxic T lymphocytes against major histocompatibility complex class II negative tumors. *J Exp Med*. 187: 693-702
14. Keene, J. A., J. Forman. 1982. Helper activity is required for the in vivo generation of cytotoxic T lymphocytes. *J Exp Med*. 155: 768-82
15. Manca, F., P. De Berardinis, D. Fenoglio, M. N. Ombra, G. Li Pira, D. Saverino, M. Autiero, L. Lozzi, L. Bracci, J. Guardiola. 1996. Antigenicity of HIV-derived T helper determinants in the context of carrier recombinant proteins: effect on T helper cell repertoire selection. *Eur J Immunol*. 26: 2461-9
16. Menendez-Arias, L., A. Mas, E. Domingo. 1998. Cytotoxic T-lymphocyte responses to HIV-1 reverse transcriptase (review). *Viral Immunol*. 11: 167-81
17. Pascolo, S., N. Bervas, J. M. Ure, A. G. Smith, F. A. Lemonnier, B. Perarnau. 1997. HLA-A2.1-restricted education and cytolytic activity of CD8(+) T lymphocytes from beta2 microglobulin (beta2m) HLA-A2.1 monochain transgenic H-2Db beta2m double knockout mice. *J Exp Med*. 185: 2043-51

18. Vitiello, A., D. Marchesini, J. Furze, L. A. Sherman, R. W. Chesnut. 1991. Analysis of the HLA-restricted influenza-specific cytotoxic T lymphocyte response in transgenic mice carrying a chimeric human-mouse class I major histocompatibility complex. *J Exp Med.* 173: 1007-15
19. Ren, J., R. Esnouf, E. Garman, D. Somers, C. Ross, I. Kirby, J. Keeling, G. Darby, Y. Jones, D. Stuart, et al. 1995. High resolution structures of HIV-1 RT from four RT-inhibitor complexes. *Nat Struct Biol.* 2: 293-302
20. Grimison, B., J. Laurence. 1995. Immunodominant epitope regions of HIV-1 reverse transcriptase: correlations with HIV-1+ serum IgG inhibitory to polymerase activity and with disease progression. *J Acquir Immune Defic Syndr Hum Retrovirol.* 9: 58-68

Oral immunization of human with transgenic lettuce expressing hepatitis B surface antigen

JOZEF KAPUSTA*, ANNA MODELSKA*, TOMASZ PNIEWSKI*, MAGDALENA FIGLEROWICZ#, KACPER JANKOWSKI*, OLESIA LISOWA*, ANDRZEJ PLUCIENNICZAK**, HILARY KOPROWSKI***, ANDRZEJ B. LEGOCKI*

**Institute of Bioorganic Chemistry, Polish Academy of Sciences, Noskowskiego 12, 61-704 Poznań, Poland; **Institute of Biotechnology and Antibiotics, Staroscinska 5, Warsaw, Poland, #Marcinkowski Academy of Medical Sciences, Department of Pediatrics, Poznan, Poland, ***Biotechnology Foundation, Thomas Jefferson University, Philadelphia, PA 19107, USA*

1. INTRODUCTION

A number of reports for the past few years have shown that higher plants can be important and useful tools for production and delivery of viral antigens. Oral route represents one of the most efficient and safe ways for administration of therapeutic proteins [1]. Among protein antigens expressed in transgenic plants is hepatitis B surface antigen as reported by several laboratories.

It has already been shown that plant tissue might be a convenient source of recombinant antigen capable of folding within plant cell to a form of highly immunogenic viruslike particles (VLPs) [2]. It has been demonstrated that parenteral immunization of mice with transgenic tobacco expressing HBsAg induces B- and T-cell immune responses comparable to yeast-derived commercial vaccine [3].

In our earlier studies we have shown that antigens expressed in lupine (*Lupinus luteus* L.) callus can induce in mice a specific anti-HBs response when administered orally. Moreover, we have reported for the first time a high immunoglobin G (IgG) response in human volunteers fed with transgenic lettuce (*Lactuca sativa* L.) expressing HBsAg [4,5]. The present studies were undertaken to recognize further time kinetics of anti-HBsAg stimulation in human volunteers after oral delivery of plant tissue producing HBsAg.

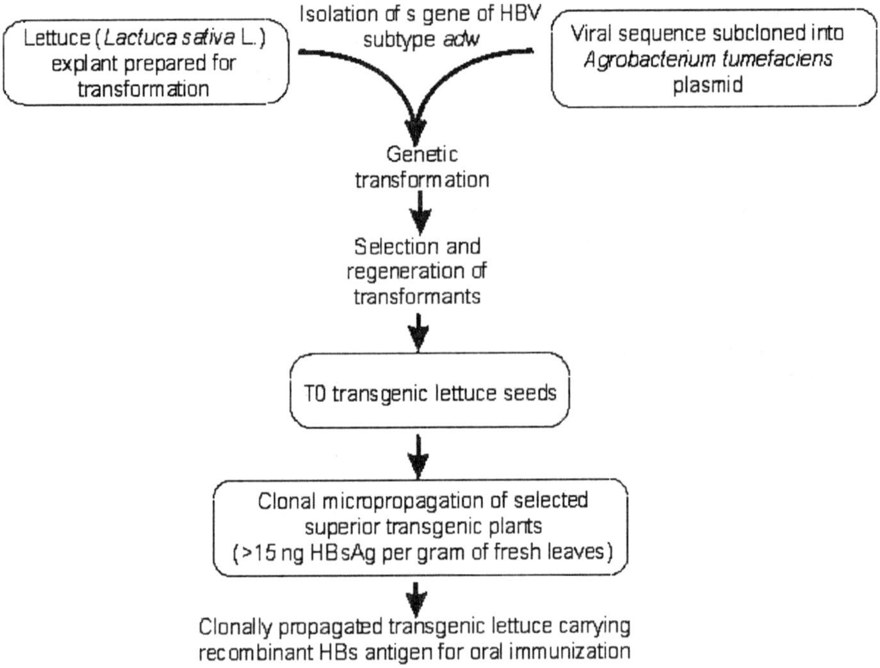

Figure 1. Schematic illustrating preparation of transgenic lettuce carrying of recombinant HBs antigen of hepatitis B virus.

2. TRANSGENIC LETTUCE CARRYING HBsAG

Transgenic lettuce plants carrying HBs antigen of HBV were raised *via A. tumefaciens* transformation as described previously [5]. Since the initial level of HBV surface antigen was low and variable (5-35 ng HBsAg per gram of fresh leaves), further studies on transformants of T1 and T2 generations were undertaken to select and micropropagate individual transgenic lettuce plants with a higher antigen content (*Fig. 1*). Antigen HBs concentration in crude plant protein extracts were assayed with ELISA test and the total amount of HBsAg for each portion of plants was estimated and used as a single dose for oral immunization. In such a way moderately uniform plant material was prepared for each volunteer enrolled in immunization trial. Usually, the leaves of a 2-month-old plant were collected and used for immunization.

3. CLINICAL TRIAL

Twelve healthy volunteers were selected for the trial after analyses showing that their serum is negative for the presence of HBs antigen, anti-HBs and anti-HBc antibodies.

Seven persons of this group (3 women, 4 men, age 18-60, mean 28 years) were immunized three times by eating fresh leaves of genetically modified lettuce carrying HBs antigen. The first and second oral plant administrations were done at one-week interval and the third one four weeks after the second administration. The amount of HBs antigen in 200 g of lettuce which was used for immunization was different in each administration (1st immunization – 510 ng of HBs antigen, 2nd immunization – 780 ng, 3rd immunization – 940 ng). In the control group five volunteers (3 women, 2 men, age 22-66, mean 34 years) were fed with 200 g of fresh leaves of untransformed lettuce according to the same administration schedule as the immunized group.

Blood was collected before trial, two, three, four weeks after the second immunization and two weeks after the third immunization. Serum anti-HBs antibodies were measured using ELISA (Hepanostika anti-HBs Microelisa system, Organon Teknika, Boxtel, Nederland).

4. ANTI-HBS IMMUNE RESPONSE AFTER ORAL IMMUNIZATION

Transgenic lettuce expressing constitutively HBs antigen was delivered orally to selected human volunteers. Two weeks after the second oral immunization a detectable induction of specific anti-HBs antibodies was displayed by 3 test participants (1.6 – 6.0 IU/l). One week later (i.e. three weeks after the second immunization) the antibody presence was detected in all 7 tested volunteers between 1.0 and 3.6 UI/l (*Fig. 2*). At the same time no HBs specific antibodies were detected in the serum of control test participants who received untransformed plant material.

The observed level of serum antibody was initially low. It decreased to the control level on the fourth week after the second immunization. However, a significant rise of antibodies was noted after the third oral immunization. Then, in all test participants an increased level of anti HBs antibodies up to 6.3 IU/l was detected.

It should be mentioned that a relatively low level of the HBs antibody response observed in our study and the fact that the protection level (10 IU/l) has not been reached can be due to sub optimal doses of the applied antigen (totally 2.2 μg HBsAg in 3 oral immunizations) as compared to a protective amount of antigen in commercial vaccine (three doses of each 20 μg of recombinant HBsAg). Moreover, oral administration described in this work did not include the use of any adjuvant which is not the case for commercial vaccine. For that reason the use of adjuvant might be a beneficial approach.

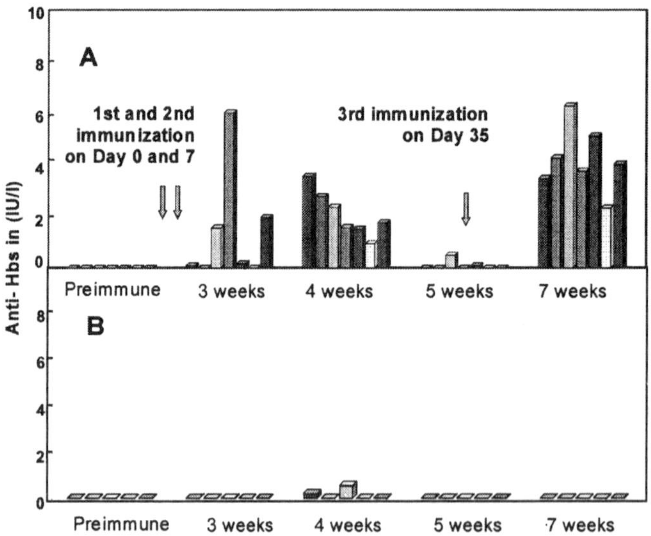

Figure 2. Oral immunization of humans with transgenic lettuce expressing HBsAg. A) Serum immune responses of 7 test participants who were fed 3 times with the HBsAg carrying lettuce. The arrows indicate the immunization schedule: day 0, 7, 35, B) Serum responses of 5 test participants fed 3 times with untransformed lettuce according to administration schedule indicated in A. Each bar represents individual volunteer's serum anti-HBs response.

5. CONCLUSIONS

1. Using transgenic lettuce expressing HBs antigen we are continuing our earlier work on evaluation of oral immunogenicity in humans [5]. Our previous and present observations indicate that oral administration induces specific anti-HBs antibody production in serum.

2. The anti-HBs antibodies induced by primary immunization with antigenic material are shortly prolonged having a tendency to decrease relatively soon after immunization. However, the repeated oral immunization restimulates the antibody production. This observation is important for further preclinical studies which should recognize the level of optimal doses of plant-derived antigens for primary immunization as well as for boosting regimes to ensure a protective level of antibody production in humans.

ACKNOWLEDGMENTS

The work has been supported by State Committee for Scientific Research of Poland (Research project No. 6 P04B 012 16).

REFERENCES

1. Modelska A., Dietzschold B., Sleysh N., Fu Z., Steplewski K., Hooper D., Koprowski H., Yusibov V. (1998) Immunization against rabies with plant-derived antigen. Proc. Natl. Acad. Sci. USA 95, 2481-2485.
2. Mason H. S., Lam D. M.-K., Arntzen c. J. (1992) Expression of hepatitis B surface antigen in transgenic plants. Proc. Natl. Acad. Sci. USA 89, 11745-11749.
3. Thanavakam Y., Yang Y.-F., Lyons P., Mason H. S., Arntzen C. (1995) Immunogenicity of transgenic plant-derived hepatitis B surface antigen. Proc. Natl. Acad. Sci. USA 92, 3358-3361.
4. Kapusta J., Modelska A., Figlerowicz M., Podkowiński J., Pniewski T., Lisowa O., Berbezy P., Helias D., Biesiadka J., Femiak I., Letellier M., Yusibov Y., Plucienniczak A., Koprowski H., Legocki A. B. (1999) Biotechnological approaches to making vaccine in plants. In: Current Plant Science and Biotechnology in Agriculture. Vol. 36. Plant Biotechnology and in vitro Biology in the 21st Century. Proc. IX Intern. Congress of the Intern. Assoc. of Plant Tissue Culture and Biotechnology. Israel, June 14-19, 1998, Kluwer Acad. Publ. 1999, pp. 571-574.
5. Kapusta J., Modelska A.., Figlerowicz M., Pniewski T., Letellier M., Lisowa O. Yusibov Y., Koprowski H., Plucienniczak A., Legocki A. B. (1999) Plant-based edible vaccine against Hepatitis B. FASEB J. 13, 1796-1799.

Nasal administration of *Schistosoma Mansoni* egg antigens-cholera toxin B subunit conjugate to infected mice reduces immunopathology and mortality

JIA-BIN SUN*, BIN-LING LI*, MEKURIA LAKEW*, JEAN-MARIE GRZYCH#, ANDRE CAPRON#, CECIL CZERKINSKY** AND JAN HOLMGREN*

**Department of Medical Microbiology and Immunology, Göteborg University, Sweden; #Centre d'Immunologie et de Biologie Parasitaire, INSERM U167, Institut Pasteur de Lille, **INSERM U364, Nice, France*

1. INTRODUCTION

The immunopathology of schistosomiasis is attributed to the development of granuloma formation around parasite eggs trapped in host liver and intestines resulting from a hypersensitivity reaction mediated by $CD4^+$ T cells sensitized to schistosome egg Ags (SEA) (1). In infected mice, a temporary Th-1-type response usually precedes the development of a Th-2-type milieu during peak granuloma formation (1).

Induction of tolerance of pathogenic T lymphocytes represents an ideal form of specific immunotherapy. Mucosal administration of antigens has been considered as an efficient means to suppress systemic Th1-driven inflammatory responses. Our previous findings have shown that mucosal administration of selected Ags coupled to the mucosa-binding molecule cholera toxin B subunit (CTB) can specifically suppress peripheral Th1-type T cell-mediated DTH reactions (2) and protect from experimental autoimmune diseases in animal models (2). Recently, we have also shown that intranasal (i.n.) administration of the *S. mansoni* vaccine candidate molecule 28 kDa glutathione *S*-transferase (Sm28GST), conjugated to CTB, resulted in a reduction in worm burden as well as in partial inhibition of liver

Progress in Basic and Clinical Immunology, Edited by Mackiewicz *et al.*
Kluwer Academic/Plenum Publishers, New York, 2001

granuloma formation in schistosome-infected mice (3). These findings prompted us to further study the effect of CTB on the experimental schistosome infection in mice, using CTB conjugated to the *S. mansoni* egg Ag (CTB-SEA).

2. MATERIALS AND METHODS

2.1 Induction of infection and measurement of granulomas

Female Balb/c mice (ALAB, Sollentuna, Sweden), aged 6 - 8 wk, were infected percutaneously with 70 or 30 cercariae of *S. mansoni* (Puerto Rico strain). Histopathological measurements of the size of individual granulomas as well as the total liver granuloma area of infected mice were performed as described (3).

2.2 Preparation of CTB conjugates and intranasal immunization

Purified recombinant CTB (2) and SEA (3) were prepared as previously described. For preparation of conjugates, SEA or ovalbumin (OVA) was covalently coupled to CTB using N-succinimidyl 3-(2-pyridyl)-dithio) propionate (SPDP) as bi-functional coupling reagent (3).

Under mild anesthesia, starting two or eight weeks after infection, infected Balb/c mice received 3 weekly 10-μg doses of CTB-SEA or unconjugated SEA or CTB-OVA in 25-μl of PBS given by i.n. instillation.

2.3 Lymphocyte proliferation and cytokine-producing cell assays

Isolation of liver leukocytes and methods used for determination of lymphocyte proliferation and numbers of IL-2-, IL-3-, and IL-4-producing cells were performed as described earlier (3).

3. RESULTS

3.1 Intranasal administration of CTB-SEA reduces liver granuloma formation in S. mansoni infected mice

Balb/c mice were given weekly 3 i.n. administrations of CTB-SEA or SEA alone or no treatment, starting two weeks after infection with 70 *S. mansoni* cercariae. As examined 7 weeks post-infection, i.n. treatment with the CTB-SEA conjugate resulted in a significant (57%) reduction of the mean granuloma size as compared with infected mice without treatment ($p < 0.05$), whereas treatment with unconjugated SEA had no effect (Table 1).

3.2 Nasal CTB-SEA inhibits lymphoproliferation and reduces the numbers of IL-2, IL-3 and IL-4-producing cells

The i.n. treatment with CTB-SEA resulted in a strong inhibition of the proliferative response to SEA in liver leukocytes. By comparison, treatment with SEA alone had no any inhibitory effect (Table 1). There was also a striking inhibition of IL-2 and IL-3-producing cells as well as of IL-4-producing cells responding to SEA in liver leukocytes from CTB-SEA-treated mice (Table 1).

Table 1. Reduction of liver granulomatous inflammation and suppression of T cell proliferative responses as well as cytokine production by liver leukocytes after nasal treatment with CTB-SEA conjugate but not unconjugated SEA in infected animals.

Treatment	Granuloma size (μm^2 x 10^{-3})	Proliferative response (cpm)	Number of liver leukocytes producing (/10^6 cells)		
			IL-2	IL-3	IL-4
Nil	84 ± 14	4071 ± 1500	14 ± 4	30 ± 7	1000 ± 200
SEA alone	90 ± 3.3	4400 ± 1890	16 ± 3	10 ± 5	720 ± 160
CTB-SEA	54 ± 1.5*	749 ± 260**	2 ± 2**	6 ± 3**	320 ± 50**

Statistical significance in comparison with untreated controls is indicated as * $p < 0.05$, ** $p < 0.01$, respectively (Wilcoxon's test); 6 animals per group.

3.3 Treatment with CTB-SEA increases the survival time of infected animals

In other experiments, mice were chronically infected with 30 *S.mansoni* cercariae. Starting 8 weeks after the infection, the animals received i.n. treatments with 3 weekly 10-μg doses of CTB-SEA or CTB-OVA or SEA

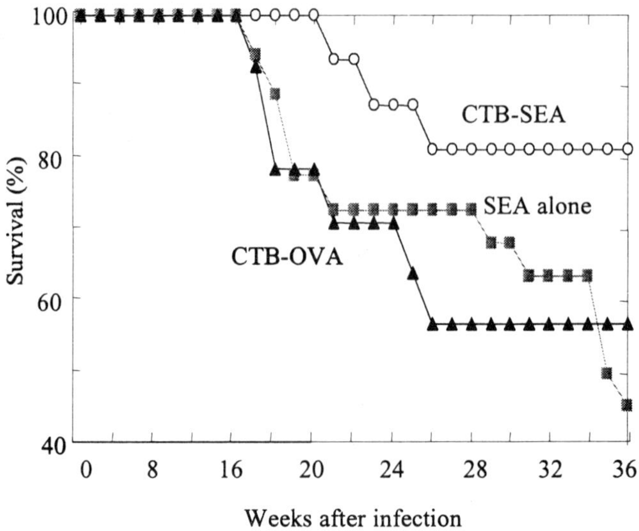

Figure 1. Intranasal treatment with CTB-SEA prolongs survival in mice chronically infected with *S. mansoni*. Balb/c mice were infected with 30 *S. mansoni* cercariae. Groups of 24 mice received 3 i.n. doses of 10-μg CTB-SEA or CTB-OVA or SEA alone eight, nine and ten weeks after infection, and mortality was determined at the indicated times.

alone. Treatment with CTB-SEA significantly prolonged the survival of infected mice as compared with treatment with unconjugated SEA or with CTB-OVA (Fig. 1). The reduction in mortality was associated with suppression of liver granuloma inflammation of mice treated by CTB-SEA as evident by assessment of liver pathology from subgroups of mice examined 12 weeks after infection. In these animals, the extent of granuloma formation was significantly reduced in miçe treated with CTB-SEA as compared with the mice treated with CTB-OVA or SEA alone (data not shown).

4. CONCLUSION

Hepatic and intestinal granuloma formation in *S. mansoni* infection is mediated by $CD4^+$ T lymphocytes sensitized to egg Ags. In this study, we show that i.n. administration of a conjugate of CTB with SEA significantly reduces the hepatic immunopathology as measured by a reduction of granuloma size in *S. mansoni*-infected mice. This protective effect against liver pathology was found to correlate with an inhibition of SEA-specific lymphoproliferation and production of both Th1 and Th2-types of cytokines. Together with the previously reported anti-infectious and anti-immunopathological effects of i.n. treatment with CTB-Sm28GST (3), our findings suggest that CTB-Ag conjugates, either singly or combined, could play a beneficial role in curtailing morbidity in schistosomiasis and possibly in other infectious diseases in which immunopathology is a prominent feature.

ACKNOWLEDGMENTS

We thank Carola Rask and Marianne Lindblad for help with the preparation and characterisation of the CTB-SEA and CTB-OVA conjugates used. This work was supported by the Swedish Medical Research Council (project 16x-3382), and the European Union (projects BIO 4-98-0503, BIO 4-CT-96-0374 and BIO 4-CT-97-2818).

REFERENCES

1. Stadecker, M. J., and Hernandez, H. J., 1998, The immune response and immunopathology in infection with Schistosoma mansoni: a key role of major egg antigen Sm-p40. Parasite Immunol. 20:217-221.
2. Sun, J.-B., Rask, C., Olsson, T., Holmgren, J., and Czerkinsky, C., 1996, , Treatment of experimental allergic encephalomyelitis by feeding myelin basic protein conjugated to cholera toxin B subunit Proc. Natl. Acad. Sci. USA. 93:7196-7201.
3. Sun, J.-B., Mielcarek, N., Lakew, M., Grzych, J. M., Capron, A., Holmgren, J., and Czerkinsky, C., 1999, Intranasal administration of a Schistosoma mansoni glutathione S-transferase-cholera toxoid conjugate vaccine evokes anti-parasitic and anti-pathological immunity in mice. J. Immunol. 163:1045-1052.

Anti-influenza vaccination changes expression of CD45 isoforms on peripheral blood NK cells of the elderly

ANDRZEJ MYŚLIWSKI[*], PIOTR TRZONKOWSKI[*], EWA SZMIT[*], ANITA DOBYSZUK[*], JOLANTA MYŚLIWSKA[*], JERZY FOERSTER[**]
[*]*Department of Histology and Immunology;* [**]*Geriatric Outpatients Department; Medical University of Gdańsk, 80-210 Gdańsk, Poland*

1. INTRODUCTION

Anti-influenza vaccination is strongly recommended for the people above 65 years of life. Unfortunately, the effectiveness of the vaccination in the elderly is not satisfactory for all of them.

Therefore the aim of that study was to assess the effectiveness of anti-influenza seasonal vaccination in the 1999/2000 season in reducing the morbidity among the over 65 years old people and to relate it to an expression of the CD45 isoforms on NK cells. The CD45 molecule appears to play a critical role in regulating the signalling responses of NK cells to target cells[1] and an expression of CD45 isoforms on NK cells is connected with a state of immunological system[2]. In our previous study[3] we found that health status of the elderly correlates with NK cytotoxic activity.

2. MATERIAL AND METHODS

Venous blood was taken from 53 old (74+5 years) people before and one month after vaccination. All individuals selected for the examination were healthy and fulfilled criteria of the SENIOUR Protocol[4]. The inactivated

Progress in Basic and Clinical Immunology, Edited by Mackiewicz *et al.*
Kluwer Academic/Plenum Publishers, New York, 2001

split vaccine (Vaxigrip, Aventis Pasteur, France) containing the antigens: A/Sydney/5/97 (H3N2), A/Beijing/262/95/(H1N1), B/184/93 (HBNB), was given by intramuscular injections. The examined subjects were carefully observed after the vaccine administration during whole epidemic season 1999/2000. Influenza infection was verified by internist using commonly accepted clinical criteria[5].

Whole venous blood samples were stained with anti-CD45RA, anti-CD45RO, anti-CD3, and anti-CD16, FITC, PE and Cy conjugated mAbs (Pharmingen, Becton Dickinson) and subsequently analysed on flow cytometer Epix XL (Coulter). Cytotoxic NK activity was assessed by the Cytotoxicity Detection Kit with LDH (Beringer Mannheim).

The statistical analysis was performed using computer program "Statistica" version 5.1 (Statsoft, Poland). Results were analysed with ANOVA of Kruskal Wallis test. All results are presented as x ± S.D.

3. RESULTS

3.1 Expression of CD45 isoforms on NK (CD16+) cells in the elderly, before and after vaccination

The significant changes in the NK cell phenotype (CD16+) were observed in examined individuals. The percentage of CD16+ CD45RO cells was higher after one month since vaccination. It increased from the 15% to 20% of the CD16+ population after vaccination. However, the absolute number of CD16+ cells did not changed.

3.2 Expression of CD45 isoforms on NK (CD16+) cells, before and after vaccination, in the elderly protected and non-protected against influenza

The subjects protected against influenza, 85% of all vaccinated, had higher level of NK cells than those non-protected. Moreover, the percentage of NK cells with an expression of CD45RA was higher in the protected subjects. One month after vaccination only protected subjects showed an increase of the CD16+CD45RO cells. (Fig 1)

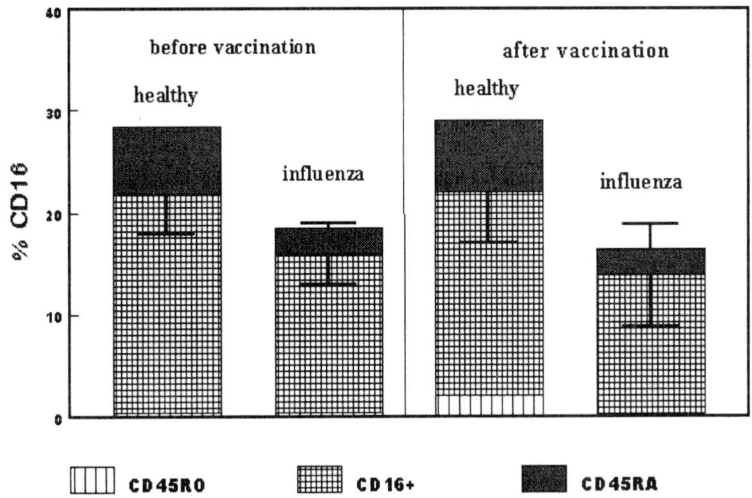

Figure 1. Expression of CD45 isoforms on NK (CD16+) cells, before and after vaccination, in the elderly protected and non-protected against influenza.

3.3 NK cytotoxic activity in protected and non-protected subjects, before and after vaccination

Only the against influenza protected elderly were characterised by an increase of NK cytotoxic activity after vaccination. The results of NK cytotoxic activity are presented in the Table I.

Table I . Level of NK cytotoxic activity in the elderly

	Protected subjects (n=45)	Non-protected (n=8)
Before vaccination	20.97 + 4.24	18.00 + 1.41
One month after vaccination	25.61 + 4.49	22.37 + 1.50
Statistical significance	$\chi 2 = 18.24$; $p = 0.032$	$\chi 2 = 1.2$; $p = 0.54$

4. CONCLUSIONS

In the elderly anti-influenza vaccination can generate changes in an expression of the CD45 isoforms on NK (CD16+) cells.

Protection against influenza infection correlated with higher level of NK cells and with higher cytotoxic activity.

ACKNOWLEDGEMENTS

This work was supported by grant No 4P05A01119 from the State Committee for Scientific Research (to A.M. and P.T.)

REFERENCES

1.Bell, G.M., Dethloff, G.M., and Imboden, J.B., 1993, CD45-negative mutants of a rat Natural Killer cell line fail to lyse tumor target cells, J. Immunology **7**: 3646-3653.
2.Warren, H.S., Kinnear, B.F., Skipsey, L.J., and Pembrey, R.G., 1994, Differential expression of CD45RO on natural killer (NK) cells in patients with an NK lymphocytosis. Immunol. Cell Biol. **72**: 500-507.
3.Myśliwski, A., Myśliwska, J., Chodnik, T., Bigda, J., Bryl, E., and Foerster, J., 1993, Elderly high NK responders are characterised by intensive proliferative response to PHA and Con A and optimal health status, Arch. Gerontol. Geriatr. **16**: 199-205.
4. Lighart, G.J., Corberand, J.X., Fournier, C., Galanaud, P., Hijmans, W., Kennes, B., Muller-Hermelink, H.K., and Steinmann, G.G., 1984, Admission criteria for immunogerontological studies in man: the seniour protocol. Mech. Ageing Dev. **28**: 47-55.
5. Couch, R.B., 1994, Orthomyxovirus infections (Influenza). In *Internal Medicine* (J.H.Stein,ed.), Mosby, St.Louis, pp.1993-2000.

TUMOR IMMUNOLOGY

Presence and functions of immune components in the tumor microenvironment

ISAAC P. WITZ
Department of Cell Research and Immunology, Tel Aviv University, Tel Aviv 69978, Israel

1. INTRODUCTION

There is ample evidence that alterations in oncogenes and tumor suppressor genes are causally involved in malignant transformation (1-3). In addition to alterations in these class I cancer genes (4), changes in the expression of numerous genes whose DNA was not altered i.e. class II cancer genes (4), play crucial roles in tumorigenesis and in tumor progression. Among the important class II cancer genes are proteases, angiogenic factors and angiogenesis inhibitors, cytokines and chemokines and their receptors as well as various adhesion molecules (5-8). It seems that class II cancer genes play a more significant role in the process of tumor progression than in cellular transformation and primary tumorigenesis (4).

In certain cases the aberrant expression of class II cancer genes (e.g. angiogenic factors), can be attributed to the intrinsic properties of progressing cancer cells such as alterations in oncogenes (9). However in addition to intrinsic regulation, factors present in the tumor microenvironment are instrumental in regulating the expression of class II cancer genes and as such control the malignancy phenotype of the cancer cells (10-11). The regulation of class II cancer genes by microenvironmental factors may either confer upon tumor cells a high malignancy phenotype and a metastatic behavior or, in contrast, may restrain tumor progression (10-11). The tumor microenvironment functions, thus, as a double-edged sword: in certain cases it promotes tumor progression in other cases it restricts it.

Progress in Basic and Clinical Immunology, Edited by Mackiewicz *et al.*
Kluwer Academic/Plenum Publishers, New York, 2001

In addition to its gene regulatory functions, the tumor microenvironment may contribute to the genetic instability of cancer cells. Mutagenic factors present in the microenvironment were shown to increase the mutation rate of tumor cells (12).

The relationship between tumor cells and microenvironmental factors is bidirectional. While, as mentioned above, microenvironmental factors may influence cancer cells by regulating their genes or by increasing the rate of mutations in these cells, the tumor cells themselves may influence their own microenvironment (10-11).

Components of the immunity system such as lymphocytes, macrophages, antibodies and cytokines are present in the microenvironment of many types of solid tumors (13-16). These components play important roles in tumor progression. This review will deal with the expression and function of immune components at the tumor site.

1.1 Tumor-associated T cells and macrophages

The presence of tumor-infiltrating immunocytes within the microenvironment of solid tumors is considered to be an indication of an immune response to tumor antigens or of an inflammatory response (17-18). Among tumor-associated lymphocytes, T cells are the most prominent population. B cells, plasma cells and NK cells are sometimes observed in the tumor microenvironment in relatively small numbers (17-19).

The underlying assumption of studies on tumor-associated T cells is that these immunocytes, more than those in the periphery, are a selected population with respect to their ability to recognize putative tumor associated antigens and to exert effector functions against tumor cells expressing such antigens. The role of tumor-associated T cells (TATC) in tumor immunity is of great interest because these cells are employed as effectors in adoptive immunotherapy trials (20-21) and because they are utilized to identify cancer rejection antigens (20-21).

The phenotype of TATC may vary from that of peripheral T cells. For example TATC derived from cervical carcinoma have a down-regulated expression of CD25 which, in turn may impair the proliferative capacity of such cells (22). A low expression or absence of the TCR zeta chain on TATC from stage III or IV head and neck carcinoma renders such cells deficient in signaling functions and a low zeta chain expression on TATC was shown to predict a significantly shorter 5-year survival of the corresponding patients than that of patients with a normal zeta-chain expression on their TATC (23-24). TATC from various types of cancer express Fas. The expression of Fas on TATC was significantly higher than that of peripheral blood lymphocytes from patients carrying the corresponding tumors (25-26). It was postulated that the interaction between Fas on TATC and of Fas-ligand on tumor cells elicits apoptosis of the T cells thus explaining immunosuppression at the tumor site (25-26). Interestingly the Fas-ligand-expressing tumor cells sharing the same microenvironment with the Fas-expressing TATC, expressed very little or no Fas (25).

In spite of these and other deficiencies, TATC may be considered to represent a tumor progression-restraining microenvironmental component. This tentative conclusion was based on studies showing that the adoptive transfer of TATC to tumor bearing mice or to cancer patients with solid tumors caused regressions in certain cases (20-21, 27). It should be mentioned, however, that adoptive immunotherapy utilizing TATC benefited mainly patients with certain solid tumors such as melanoma (28).

In order to increase the efficacy of adoptive cellular immunotherapy, the selective homing of the adoptively transferred lymphocytes to the tumor site should be increased. This could conceivably be achieved by altering the biodistribution of the adoptively transferred cells i.e. reducing their normal tissue retention and enhancing their selective capture at the tumor site (29).

TATC are also used to identify tumor rejection antigens recognized by lymphocytes. Based on strategies developed in mice (30) TATC were utilized to identify melanoma associated antigens such MART-1, Tyrosinase and TRP-1 (20, 31). These antigens were capable of eliciting rejection reactions in certain melanoma patients (20, 31).

Tumor-associated macrophages may be regarded as a typical example for a double edged sword. Due to their tumoricidal potential, activated macrophages may play important anti tumor progression roles (32) However these cells may also exert pro metastatic functions. Macrophages are an important source for angiogenic factors, proteases and cytokines (33-35). Such factors could promote growth, invasiveness and metastasis of the cancer cells.

1.2 Tumor-associated antibodies

Native antibodies, engineered antibodies or antibodies as carriers of radionuclides, or of various sorts of toxins (immunotoxins) and of other therapeutic molecules are used widely in preclinical and clinical cancer immunotherapy trials (36-41). The basic assumption of antibody-based anti tumor immunotherapy is that the delivered antibody will reach the tumor microenvironment and target the cancer cells therein. Several factors such as antibody metabolism, size and affinity; accessibility of tumor antigens; circulating tumor antigens; anti tumor antibodies produced by the patient and Fc receptors expressed by tumor cells may impede efficient tumor localization and anti tumor activity of the administered antibodies. For example it was shown that several types of ex vivo cancer cells from humans or animals are coated in vivo with immunoglobulin mainly of the IgG isotype (42). Whereas some of these molecules may represent antibodies directed against tumor-associated antigens (43), other immunoglobulin molecules may be bound to the cancer cells via receptors to the Fc portion of IgG (44). Moreover Fc gamma receptor expressing mouse tumor cells were more tumorigenic than cells not expressing the receptor (45). The transfer of Fc-gamma receptor cDNA to receptor-negative tumor cells with a low tumorigenicity potential conferred upon the transfectants an increased in vivo tumorigenicity phenotype without altering several malignancy-linked in vitro properties such as proliferation rate (46). The ability of tumor cells to bind IgG in vivo via FcR seems thus to augment their tumorigenicity. Indeed, the administration of IgG eluted from ex vivo tumors to tumor-inoculated mice, enhanced tumor development in these mice (42).

The results summarized in this section demonstrate that the humoral arm of anti tumor immunity can also be characterized as a double-edged sword. Whereas it may negatively influence tumor development it may, under different circumstances, enhance tumorigenicity. This point was proven by the fact that a single monoclonal, tumor reactive naturally-occurring antibody had opposing functions on tumor development (47).

1.3 Cytokines in the tumor microenvironment

Fibroblasts, endothelial cells and various other types of cells residing in the tumor microenvironment, as well as tumor infiltrating cells, secrete a wide spectrum of cytokines. Tumor cells themselves secrete cytokines and may also express receptors to a large variety of cytokines (48). A functional interaction ground between cytokines and cancer cells thus exists in the microenvironment. Indeed various cytokines have been shown to modify the phenotype of cancer cells and vice versa (48). Moreover the presence of cancer cells in a particular site may alter the cytokine representation at this site and even the cytokine profile at distant sites (49).

As major regulators of the immunity system, cytokines are being employed, by direct or indirect approaches, in efforts to boost anti tumor immunity both systemically as well as at the microenvironment (20, 48, 50-51). However, preclinical and clinical trials involving the modulation of anti tumor immune responses by cytokines, should be performed with the realization that the administration of a single cytokine may initiate a complex cascade of events. For example IL-2, a cytokine used widely in the clinic (20), takes part in the activation cascade of both TH1 as well as that of TH2 cells. Activated T cells of both types secrete various cytokines such as interferon γ or IL-4, which in turn activate respectively, macrophages or B cells. Following activation, the latter cells may release IL-12. IL-2 as well as the cytokines it induces may interact with tumor cells with varying results (48).

Cytokines are a good example for a "double-edged" activity of microenvironmental factors. The following examples will illustrate the fact that single cytokines may exert opposing effects with respect to tumor progression. Local TNFα administration (isolated limb perfusion) is being applied as a therapeutic agent in certain malignant diseases (52). On the other hand TNFα may enhance metastasis formation (53). A similar situation exists with TGFβ. This cytokine is a potent growth inhibitor especially during the early phases of progression. As the malignancy of the tumor increases, tumor cells appear to escape TGFβ-mediated growth arrest. Some tumor cells may even use this cytokine as a growth factor (54).

2. CONCLUSION

Interactions between tumor cells and microenvironmental factors (including those of the immune system) play decisive roles in tumor progression and metastasis formation. It is thus imperative to develop novel modalities in which tumor progression-enhancing interactions would be blocked or modulated.

ACKNOWLEDGEMENTS

Isaac P. Witz is the incumbent of the David Furman Chair in Immunobiology of Cancer. Dr. Witz's studies are supported by the Israel Cancer Association; the Gabrielle Rich Leukemia Research Foundation, Lucerne; The Fainbarg Family Fund, Orange County, CA; the Fred August & Adele Wolpers Charitable Foundation, Clifton, NJ and by Mr. amd Mrs. Steven Stern, New York, NY.

REFERENCES

1. Lengauer, C., Kinzler, K.W. and Vogelstein, B. Genetic instabilities in human cancers. Nature, 396: 643-649, 1998.
2. Schwab, M. Oncogene amplification in solid tumors. Semin. Cancer Biol. 9: 319-325, 1999.
3. Macleod, K., Tumor suppressor genes. Curr. Opin. Genetic. Dev. 10: 81-93, 2000.
4. Sager, R. Expression genetics in cancer: shifting the focus from DNA to RNA. Proc. Natl. Acad. Sci. USA 94: 952-955, 1997.

5. Negus, R.P. and Balkwill, F.R. Cytokines in tumour growth, migration and metastasis. World J. Urol. 14: 157-165, 1996.
6. Hanahan, D. and Folkman, J. Patterns and emerging mechanisms of the angiogenic switch during tumorigenesis. Cell 86: 353-364, 1996.
7. Lochter, A., Sternlicht, M.D., Werb, Z. and Bissell, M.J. The significance of matrix metalloproteinases during early stages of tumor progression. Ann. NY Acad. Sci. 857: 180-193, 1998.
8. Ruoslahti, E. Fibronectin and its integrin receptors in cancer. Adv. Cancer Res. 76: 1-20, 1999.
9. Kerbel, R.S., Viloria-Petit, A., Okada, F. and Rak, J. Establishing a link between oncogenes and tumor angiogenesis. Mol. Med. 4: 286-295, 1998.
10. Witz, I.P. Differential expression of genes by tumor cells of a low or a high malignancy phenotype: The case of murine and human Ly-6 proteins. J. Cell. Biochem. (Suppl.) 34: 61-66, 2000.
11. Fidler, I.J. Critical determinants of cancer metastasis: rationale for therapy. Cancer chemother. Pharmacol. 43 (Suppl. 1A)S3-10, 1999.
12. Yuan, J. and Glazer, P.M. Mutagenesis induced by the tumor microenvironment. Mutat. Res. 400: 439-446, 1998.
13. Goedegebuure, P.S. and Eberlein, T.J. The role of CD4+ tumor-infiltrating lymphocytes in human solid tumors. Immunol. Res. 14: 119-131, 1995.
14. Mantovani, A., Bottazzi, B., Sozzani, S., Peri, G,. Allavena, P., Dong, Q.G.,Vecchi, A. and Colotta, F. Cytokine regulation of monocyte recruitment. Arch. Immunol. Ther. Exp. (Warz) 43: 149-152, 1995.
15. Wagner, S.N., Schultewolter, T., Wagner, C., Briedigkeit, L., Becker, J.C., Kawasnicka, H.M. and Goos, M. Immune response against human primary malignant melanoma: a distinct cytokine mRNA profile associated with spontaneous regression. Lab. Invest. 78: 541-550, 1998.
16. Russell, S.W., Witz, I.P. and Herberman, R.B. A review of data, problems, and open questions pertaining to in situ tumor immunity. In: Contemporary Topics in Immunobiology (Witz, I.P. and Hanna, M.G.Jr., Eds) Vol. 10, Plenum Press, New-York, pp. 1-20, 1980.
17. Klein, E., Vánky, F., Galili, U., Vose, B.M. and Fopp, M. Separation and characteristics of tumor-infiltrating lymphocytes in man. In: Contemporary Topics in Immunobiology (Witz, I.P. and Hanna, M.G.Jr., Eds) Vol. 10, Plenum Press, New-York, pp. 79-108, 1980.
18. Ioachim, H.L. Correlations between tumor antigenicity, malignant potential, and local host immune response. In: Contemporary Topics in Immunobiology (Witz, I.P. and Hanna, M.G.Jr., Eds) Vol. 10, Plenum Press, New-York, pp. 213-238, 1980.
19. Yron, I., Wood, T.A.Jr, Spiess, P.J. and Rosenberg, S.A. In vitro growth of murine T cells. V. The isolation and growth of lymphoid cells infiltrating syngeneic solid tumors. J. Immunol. 125: 238- , 1980.
20. Rosenberg, S.A. Cancer vaccines based on the identification of genes encoding cancer regression antigens. Immunology Today 18: 175-182, 1997.
21. Wang, R.F. and Rosenberg, S.A. Human tumor antigens for cancer vaccine development. Immunol. Rev. 170: 85-100, 1999.
22. Sheu, B.C., Lin, R.H., Ho, H.N. and Huang, S.C. Down-regulation of CD25 expression on the surface of activated tumor-infiltrating lymphocytes in human cervical carcinoma. Hum. Immunol. 56: 39-48, 1997.

23. Reichert, T.E., Day, R., Wagner, E.M. and Whitesite, T.L. Absent or low expression of the zeta chain in T cells at the tumor site correlates with poor survival in patients with oral carcinoma. Cancer Res. 58: 5344-5347, 1998.
24. Whiteside, T.L. Signaling defects in T lymphocytes of patients with malignancy. Cancer Immunol. Immunother. 48: 346-352, 1999.
25. Sikora, J., Dworacki, G. and Zeromski, J. Expression of Fas and Fas ligand and apoptosis in tumor-associated lymphocytes and in tumor cells from malignant pleural effusions. Nat. Immun. 16: 244-255, 1998.
26. Cardi, G., Heaney, J.A., Schned, A.R. and Emstoff, M.S. Expression of Fas(APO-1/CD95) in tumor-infiltrating and peripheral blood lymphocytes in patients with renal cell carcinoma. Cancer Res. 58: 2078-2080, 1998.
27. Hoffman, D.M., Gitlitz, B.J., Belldegrun, A. and Figlin, R.A. Adoptive cellular therapy. Semin. Oncol. 27: 221-233, 2000.
28. Bordignon, C., Carlo-Stella, C., Colombo, M.P., De Vincentiis, A., Lanata, L., Lemoli, R.M., Locatelli, F., Olivieri, A., Rondelli, D., Zanon, P. and Tura, S. Cell therapy: achievements and perspectives. Haematologica 84: 1110-1149, 1999.
29. Zhu, H., Melder, R.J., Baxter, L.T. and Jain, R.K. Physiologically based kinetic model of effector cell biodistribution in mammals: implications for adoptive immunotherapy. Cancer Res. 56: 3771-3781, 1996.
30. Sibille, C., Chomez, P., Wildmann, C., Van Pel, A., De Plaen, E., Maryanski, J.L., de Bergeyck, V. and Boon, T. Structure of the gene of tum-transplantation antigen P198: a point mutation generates a new antigenic peptide. J. Exp. Med. 172: 35-45, 1990.
31. Boon, T., Coulie, P.G. and Van den Eynde, B. Tumor antigens recognized by T cells. Immunol. Today 18: 267-268, 1997.
32. Killion, J.J. and Fidler, I.J. Therapy of cancer metastasis by tumoricidal activation of tissue macrophages using liposome-encapsulated immunomodulators. Pharmacol. Ther. 78: 141-154, 1998.
33. Mantovani, A., Bottazzi, B., Colotta, F., Sozzani, S. and Ruco. L. The origin and function of tumor-associated macrophages. Immunol. Today 13: 265-270, 1992.
34. Mantovani, A. Tumor-associated macrophages in neoplastic progression: a paradigm for the in vivo function of chemokines. Lab. Invest. 71: 5-16, 1994.
35. Lewis, C.E., Leek, R., Harris, A. and McGee, J.O. Cytokine regulation of angiogenesis in breast cancer: the role of tumor-associated macrophages. J. Leukoc. Biol. 57: 747-751, 1995.
36. Liu, L., Barth, R.F., Adams, D.M., Soloway, A.H. and Reisfled, R.A. Critical evaluation of bispecific antibodies as targeting agents for boron neutron capture therapy of brain tumors. Anticancer Res. 16: 2581-2587, 1996.
37. Ross, J.S. and Fletcher, J.A. The HER-2/neu oncogene: prognostic factor, predictive factor and target for therapy. Semin. Cancer Biol. 9: 125-138, 1999.
38. Weiner, L.M. Monoclonal antibody therapy of cancer. Semin. Oncol. 26: 43-51, 1999.
39. Welt, S., Ritter, G. Antibodies in the therapy of colon cancer. Semin. Oncol. 26: 683-690, 1999.
40. Brinkmann, U. Recombinant antibody fragment and immunotoxin fusions for cancer therapy. In Vivo 14: 21-27, 2000.
41. Green, M.C., Murray, J.L. and Hortobagyi, G.N. Monoclonal antibody therapy for solid tumors. Cancer Treat. Rev. 26: 269-286, 2000.
42. Witz, I.P. Tumor-bound immunoglobulins: in situ expression of humoral immunity. Adv. Cancer Res. 25: 95-148, 1977.

43. Ran, M., Yaakubowicz, M. and Witz, I.P. Lymphocytotoxic auto antibodies eluted from in-vivo propagating sarcoma cells. J. Natl. Cancer Inst. 60: 1509-1513, 1978.
44. Ran, M., Katz, B., Kimchi, N., Halachmi, E., Teillaud, J-L., Even, J., Berko, Y., Atlas, E., Fridman, W.H. and Witz, I.P. The in-vivo acquisition of Fc gamma RII expression on polyomas virus transformed cells derived from tumors of long latency. Cancer Res. 51: 612-618, 1991.
45. Witz, I.P. and Ran, M. FcR may function as a progression factor of non-lymphoid tumors. Immunol. Res. 11: 283-295. 1992.
46. Zusman, T., Lisansky, E.,Arons, E., Anavi, R.,Bonnerot, C., Sautes, C.,Fridman, W.H., Witz, I.P. and Ran, M. The contribution of the intracellular domain of the murine Fc-gamma receptor type II B1 to its tumor enhancing potential. Int. J. Cancer, 67: 1-9, 1996.
47. Cahalon, L., Korem, S., Puri, Y., Smorodinsky, N.I. and Witz, I.P. Regulation of tumor growth and immunomodulation mediated by naturally-occurring autoantibodies. Ann. N.Y. Acad. Sci. 651: 393-408, 1992.
48. Tartour, E. and Fridman, W.H. Cytokines and Cancer. Int. Rev. Immunol. 16: 683-704, 1998.
49. Goto, S., Sato, M., Kaneko, R., Itoh, M., Sato, S. and Takeuchi, S. Analysis of Th1 and Th2 cytokine production by peripheral blood mononuclear cells as a parameter of immunological dysfunction in advanced cancer patients. Cancer Immunol. Immunother. 48: 435-442, 1999.
50. Lode, H.N. and Reisfeld, R.A. Targeted cytokines for cancer immunotherapy. Immunol. Res. 21: 279-288, 2000.
51. Tagawa, M. Cytokine therapy for cancer. Curr. Pharm. Des. 6: 681-699, 2000.
52. Bickels, J., Manusama, E.R., Gutman, M., Eggermont, A.M., Kollender, Y., Abu-Abid, S., Van Geel, A.N., Lev-Shlush, D., Klausner, J.M. and Meller, I. Isolated limb perfusion with tumour necrosis factor-alpha and melphalan for unresectable bone sarcomas of the lower extremity. Eur. J. Surg. Oncol. 25: 509-514, 1999.
53. Hafner, M., Orosz, P., Kruger, A. and Männel, D.N. TNF promotes metastasis by impairing natural killer cell activity. Int. J. Cancer 66: 388-392, 1996.
54. Gold, L.I. The role of transforming growth factor-beta (TGF-beta) in human cancer. Crit. Rev. Oncog. 10: 303-360, 1999.

Expression of TCR ζ chain of tumor associated lymphocytes from malignant pleural effusions

JAN SIKORA, GRZEGORZ DWORACKI, and JAN ŻEROMSKI
Chair and Department of Immunology Karol Marcinkowski University School of Medical Sciences, 49 Przybyszewski Str., 60-355 Poznan, Poland

1. INTRODUCTION

Recently, the focus of research in tumor induced immunosuppression has centered on alterations in the T-cell-receptor (TCR) complex [1]. The TCR, which plays a central role in antigen-specific activation of the immune system, is composed of an antigen recognition motif formed by the αβ or γδ chains as well as a signal tranduction apparatus made up of the CD3 proteins γ, δ and ε plus the ζ-ζ homodimer. The TCR couples antigen binding to events within the T lymphocyte such as phosphoinositide metabolism, protein phosphorylation, and calcium mobilization, which lead to T-lymphocyte activation. The TCR subunit in particular seems to be resposible for several important signal transduction functions. It also amplifies the activation signal initiated by antigen binding [2]. Several investigators have reported significantly diminished or absent levels of TCRζ and associated protein kinases in T lymphocytes infitrating tumors of human cancer patients. Thus, alteration in TCRζ expression has been proposed as a marker for T cells subject to tumor-induced immunosuppression, although few studies have directly linked the decreased expression of TCRζ with impaired function in vivo [3].

2. MATERIAL AND METHODS

2.1 Patients Characteristics

Among 20 patients with malignant pleural effusions whose lymphoid cells were studied for ζ chain expression, 15 patients were pathologically diagnosed to have stage IIIB disesase and 5 had stage IV disease. Patients with benign pleural effusions had tuberculosis (1 case) and pleuritis exudativa (8 cases).

2.2 Flow Cytometry

Lymphocytes from malignant (MPE) and benign (BPE) pleural effusions (0,5x106 cells) were stained with one of the following FITC-conjugated anti human mAbs for surface proteins: anti CD3 ε (Dako), anti CD4, anti CD8 (Becton Dickinson) at 4^0C for 30 min., and next washed twice in cold PBS. Expression of the ζ chain was investigated in cells using a mAbs to CD3ζ - PE (TIA-2, IgG1; Coulter Immunotech), which recognizes the cytoplasmic domain of the ζ submit of the TCR and a modification of a permeabilization protocol originally described by Anderson et al.[4]. Cells were fixed at 4^0C for 30 min with freshly prepared 1% paraformaldehyde in PBS to permit the cell membrane to stabilize. After washing cells were permeabilized with 0,1% saponin at 4^0C, for 30 min. Anti -ζ- chain antibody were allowed to react with cell preparations for 30 min. at room temperature in the dark. The IgG1-FITC and IgG2-PE isotype controls were included in all experiments. Next, cells were washed in PBS and analysed the same day on a Becton Dickinson FACScan using 488-nm argon laser.

To identify fragmented DNA in lymphocytes from pleural effusions, a terminal deoxynucleotidyl transferase (TdT)-mediated dUTP nick-end labeling (TUNEL; Pharmingen) assay was performed and assessed by either flow cytometry in cell suspensions or by immunofluorescence on cytosmears. Control cells were treated with the TUNEL reaction mixture without TdT [5]

3. RESULTS

3.1 Expression of TCR ζ chain in lymphocytes from malignant and benign pleural effusions

The MFI for the ζ chain staining was significantly reduced in CD3+ cells of patients with malignant pleural effusions compared to patients with benign ones, with a mean +/- SE of 49+\-15 for patients with MPE and 79+\-21 for patients with BPE ($p<0,05$). The MFI walues for ζ in CD4+ cells were 55+\-17 for patients with PE and 79+\-19 for patients with BPE ($p<0.05$), and those for CD8+ cells were 54+\-16 and 80+\-20, $p<0,05$, respectively.

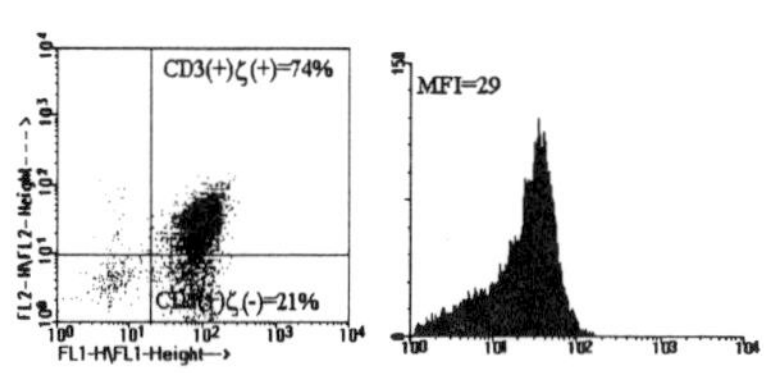

Figure 1. The shift in the MFI and percentage of TCR ζ (+) lymphocytes from representative patients with malignant disease

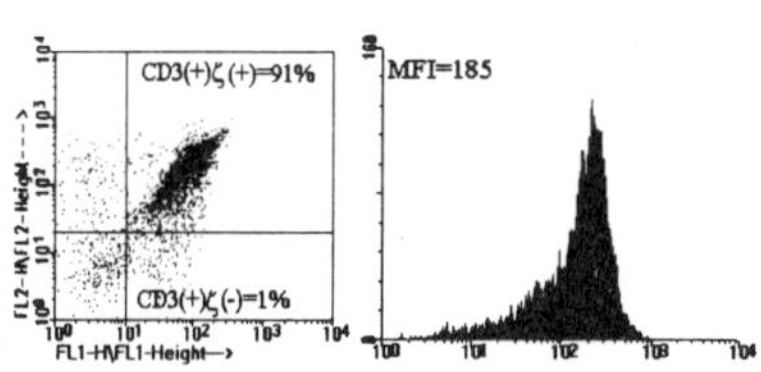

Figure 2. The shift in the MFI and percentage of TCR ζ (+) lymphocytes from representative patients with non-malignant disease

Fig. 1 and 2 illustrates the shift observed in the MFI and percentage of CD3ζ in MPE and BPE of a representative patients. The entire CD3ζ peak is shifted to the left, indicating that in this patients with MPE, expression of the ζ chains is considerably decreased relative to that in the BPE. In the previous study of these same specimens of pleural effusions we have evaluated of spontaneous apoptosis using TUNEL assay. We observed that the proportion of lymphocytes from MPE (Fig. 3) with spontaneous DNA fragmentation was significantly higher than from BPE. In the same effusions, there were also sigificantly more T cells wit low ζ chain in MPE compared with BPE.

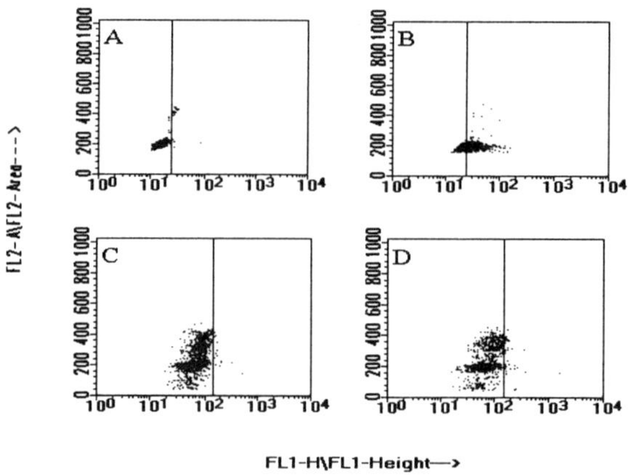

Figure 3. Assessment of apoptosis in cells from malignant pleural effusion. A. apoptosis of lymphocytes (control) – TUNEL assay without terminal transferase; B. apoptosis of lymphocytes, TUNEL assay; C. apoptosis of malignant cells, control; D. only single malignant cells are TUNEL positive

4. DISCUSSION

Since the ζ chain has been shown to play a prominent role in the TcR expression and antigen-driven activation, it is reasonable to assume that deficiency in expression of this protein may be directly related to the cellular dysfuction observed in tumor-bearing host. The absence or reduced expression of the ζ chain impairs T-cell signaling and, thus, contributes to immune cell dysfunction. Our data indicate that low or absent ζ expression in immune cells is biologically significant, and it appears to be a marker of advanced or aggressive disease. Another observation made in this study is the presence of CD3(-) low ζ population in the malignant pleural effusions. Not only T cells but also NK cells showed decreased expression of ζ. Thus, in patients with cancer, the two main effector cell populations that could mount an antitumor immune respose, T and NK cells, show decreased expression of ζ. The mechanisms responsible for the z chain defect are currently unknown but appear to be related to apoptosis, which might be tumor-induced. In the previous study of these same specimens of effusions we have evaluated of spontaneous apoptosis. We observed that the proportion of lymphocytes from malignant pleural effusions with spontaneous apoptosis was significantly higher than from benign ones. In the same material, there were also more T cells with low z chain in MPE compared with BPE. Statistical analysis of these data indicated no correlation between decreased expression of ζ chain in MPE and a higher apoptosis rate. Nevertheless, the concomitant presence of these abnormalities in MPE suggest that they are both cancer related.

REFERENCES

1. Horiguchi, S., Peterson, M., Nakazawa, T., Kanda, M., Zea, A.H., Ochoa, A.C., Kiessling, R., 1999, Primary chemically induced tumors induce profound immunosuppression concomitant with apoptosis and alternations in signal transduction in T cells and NK cells. Cancer Research, 59: 2950-2956.
2. Neumeister Kersh, E., Shaw, A.S., Allen, P.M., 1998, Fidelity of T cell activation trough multistep T cell receptor z phosphorylation. Science, 281: 572-575.
3. Lai, P., Rabinowich, H., Crowley-Nowick, C., Bell, C., Mantovani, M., Whiteside, T.L., 1996, Alterations in expression and function of signal-transducing proteins in tumor-associated T and natural killer cells in patients with ovarian carcinoma. Clin Cancer Res, 2: 161 - 173.
4. Anderson, P., Blue, M.L., O'Brien, C., Schlossman, S., 1989, Monoclonal antibodies reactive with the T cell receptor zeta chain: Production and characterization using a new method. J Immunology, 143: 1899-1904.
5. Gorczyca, W., Gong, J., Darzynkiewicz, Z., 1993, Detection of DNA strand breaks in individual apoptotic cells by the in situ terminal deoxynucleotidyl transferase and nick translocation assays. Cancer Research, 53: 1945-1951.

Cytochrome c is rapidly extruded from apoptotic cells and detectable in serum of anticancer-drug treated tumor patients

ANDREA RENZ, CHRISTOF BUREK, *WALTER MIER, MALGORZATA MOZOLUK, KLAUS SCHULZE-OSTHOFF and MAREK LOS
*Dept. Immunology & Cell Biology, University of Münster, D-48149 Münster, *Institute of Nuclear Medicine, University of Heidelberg, D-69120 Heidelberg, Germany*

1. INTRODUCTION

Two major forms of cell death, necrosis and apoptosis, exist. Apoptosis, also known as programmed cell death (PCD), is the form of cell death that commonly occurs in development and many pathophysiological situations[1,2]. In contrast, necrosis is a more passive process that occurs when cells have been severely damaged by noxious insults. Apoptosis is triggered by two major signaling pathways that are either controlled by death receptors or mitochondria. In the mitochondrial pathway the initial and crucial event is the release of cytochrome c (Cc) from mitochondria into the cytosol, which can be triggered by diverse apoptotic stimuli including anticancer drugs. Cytosolic Cc together with dATP binds to the apoptosis regulator Apaf-1[3,4], thus leading to the formation of the apoptosome and the initiation of the proteolytic death cascade. Antiapoptotic Bcl-2 family members suppress Cc release[3,4], whereas proapototic members such as Bax promote its liberation[5,6]. However, the exact mechanism of Cc release remains unknown.

In the present study, we communicate that Cc does not only enter the cytoplasm during apoptosis, but furthermore leaves the "committed to die" cell. Cc can be specifically detected in the extracellular medium of apoptotic cells and, moreover, in serum of cancer patients. Interestingly, the serum Cc

Progress in Basic and Clinical Immunology, Edited by Mackiewicz *et al.*
Kluwer Academic/Plenum Publishers, New York, 2001

levels increased strongly upon the onset of chemotherapy and decreased gradually upon remission induction.

2. RESULTS AND DISCUSSION

An early event in apoptosis is the translocation of Cc into the cytosol[3,4]. This process activates the apoptosome-dependent death machinery by binding of Cc to Apaf-1 and the subsequent activation of caspase-9[7]. In our effort to develop an assay for monitoring cell death *in vivo*, we investigated which cellular proteins can be detected in the extracellular medium upon induction of cell death. Among others, we could detect a large amount of Cc in the medium of Jurkat T-cells upon apoptosis induction by different stimuli including staurosporine, agonistic anti-CD95 antibody or anticancer drugs (Fig. 1A). This event paralleled the decrease of Cc in the cellular fractions.

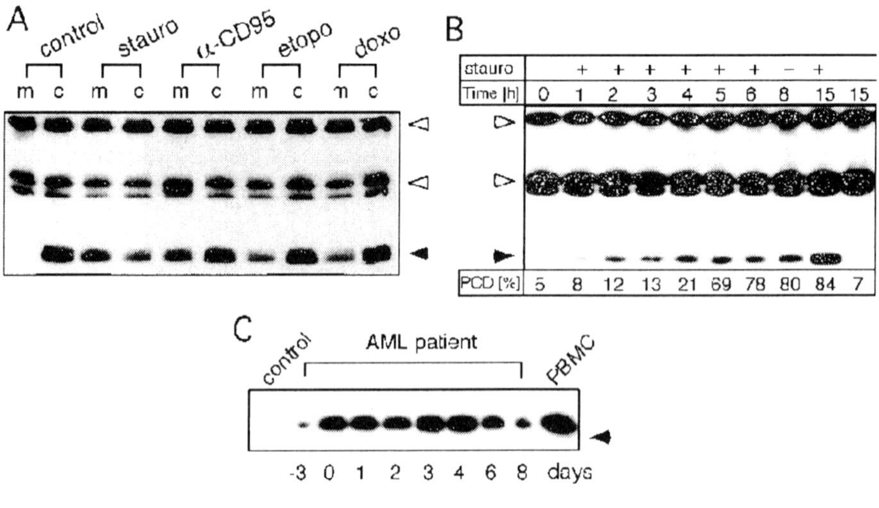

Figure 1. Various apoptotic stimuli lead to rapid Cc release into the extracellular space in vitro and in vivo. (A) Jurkat cells were either left untreated (control) or stimulated with staurosporine (stauro, 2.5 μM), anti-CD95 mAb (α-CD95, 1 μg/ml), etoposide (etopo, 25 μg/ml) or doxorubicin (doxo, 2 μg/ml) for 16 h. Cc was precipitated from the culture medium (m) or cellular extracts (c) with antibody against native Cc. (B) Cc release is a rapid process. Jurkat cells were treated with staurosporine (stauro) for the indicated time. Cc release was determined by immunoprecipitation (IP) of the medium fractions and subsequent immunoblotting. In parallel, PCD was determined by measurement of hypodiploid DNA. (C) Detection of Cc in the serum of a chemotherapy-treated acute myeloid leukemia (AML) patient or of a healthy individual (control). The first day of chemotherapy was considered as day 0. As a positive control, cellular extracts from 10^6 peripheral blood mononuclear cells (PBMC) of control blood were used. Open arrowheads indicate heavy and light chain of anti-Cc mAb, black arrowheads indicate Cc. *METHODS: Serum sample processing.* Sera (4 ml)

from 4 tumor patients (3 males, 1 female, age 20-48) were analyzed. All patients received standard chemotherapy. Sera were collected before and during the therapy. Control samples were obtained from age and sex-matched laboratory personnel. All samples were precleared by centrifugation at 10 000 g, 4 °C for 15 min. The immunoglobulin content was reduced by 2 rounds of extraction with 1 ml of protein G-Sepharose for 1 h. As a positive control PBMC from healthy donors were isolated by Ficoll-Paque gradient, washed twice in PBS and extracted in lysis buffer as described below. *Cell extracts, IP and Western blotting.* To determine the cellular Cc content, cells were washed in PBS and extracted in cold lysis buffer (50 mM Tris, pH 7.4, 150 mM NaCl, 1% Triton-X100, 3 µg/ml aprotinin, 3 µg/ml leupeptin, 3 µg/ml pepstatin A and 2 mM PMSF). Prior to the IPs fractions of the culture medium and lysates were precleared by centrifugation. IPs were performed in a 4 ml volume at 4 °C in a rotator for 4 h using anti-Cc mAb 6H2.B4 (0.5 µg/ml, PharMingen, Hamburg, Germany). The Cc-mAb complexes were then precipitated for 1 h with 40 µl of 50% protein G-Sepharose in PBS, harvested by centrifugation (2000 rpm, 10 sec, 4 °C) and washed four times with cold wash buffer (20 mM HEPES, pH 7.4, 150 mM NaCl, 10% glycerol, 0.1% Triton X-100 containing 1 µg/ml aprotinin and 1 µg/ml leupeptin). The precipitates were separated under reducing conditions on a 12% SDS-polyacrylamide gel and analyzed by Western blotting [8].

Next, we investigated the time course and specificity of Cc liberation. The release of Cc from the cell was a rapid process. Already 1 h after death induction with staurosporine Cc could be detected in the medium of Jurkat (Fig. 2B) or L929 cells (data not shown). The fast kinetic of Cc release corresponded to recent studies demonstrating that Cc release into the cytosol is an all-or-nothing event and completed within a few minutes[9]. Cc release into the medium was observed earlier than other features of apoptosis. Parallel to the release of Cc, the progression of apoptosis was monitored by the detection of hypodiploid DNA. No increase of this classical apoptotic event was detected within the first 5 h, whereas Cc release into the extracellular compartment was already observed 1 h after death induction. Thus, extracellular detection of Cc is an early and sensitive death indicator.

Since the release of Cc was induced by diverse apoptotic stimuli, we postulated that it should be also detectable during cell death *in vivo*, such as in anticancer therapy. Therefore, we screened sera from 4 leukemic patients. Compared to healthy controls, all of them contained elevated Cc levels. The Cc release during chemotherapy of one representative AML patient is shown in Fig. 1C. Already before therapy, elevated Cc was detected. During the first days of treatment with cytarabine, daunoblastine and thioguanine the Cc serum levels increased dramatically. The therapy reduced the white blood cells from 19,800/µl at day 0 to 1,200/µl at day 8 and consequently serum Cc level decreased between day 6 and day 8. Comparable results were obtained with the other patients. The elevated basal level of Cc in the serum of cancer patients may indicate an increased cell turnover and apoptosis in these individuals.

3. CONCLUSIONS

In summary, we show that Cc, a key regulator of the apoptosome, is released not only into cytosol but also leaves the cell. This early event does not only occur in experimental settings but also *in vivo* during chemotherapy of leukemic patients. Our data therefore identify Cc release as a promising marker for monitoring induction of apoptosis and cell turnover *in vivo*.

ACKNOWLEDGMENTS

This work was supported by grants from the Deutsche Forschungsgemeinschaft (LO 823/1-1 and SFB 293).

REFERENCES

1. Golstein, P., Ojcius, D.M., and Young, D., 1991, Cell death mechanisms and the immune system. *Immunological Reviews* 121: 29-65.
2. Los, M., Wesselborg, S., and Schulze-Osthoff K., 1999, The role of caspases in development, immunity, and apoptotic signal transduction: lessons from knockout mice. *Immunity* 10: 629-639.
3. Yang, J., Liu, X., Bhalla, K., Kim, C.N., Ibrado, A.M., Cai, J., Peng, T.I., Jones, D.P., and Wang, X., 1997, Prevention of apoptosis by Bcl-2: release of cytochrome c from mitochondria blocked. *Science* 275: 1129-1132.
4. Kluck, R.M., Bossy-Wetzel, E., Green, D.R., and Newmeyer, D.D., 1997, The release of cytochrome c from mitochondria: a primary site for Bcl2 regulation of apoptosis. *Science* 275: 1132-1136.
5. Desagher, S., Osen-Sand, A., Nichols, A., Eskes, R., Montessuit, S., Lauper, S., Maundrell, K., Antonsson, B., and Martinou, J.C., 1999, Bid-induced conformational change of Bax is responsible for mitochondrial cytochrome c release during apoptosis. *J. Cell. Biol.* 144: 891-901.
6. Jurgensmeier, J.M., Xie, Z., Deveraux, Q.,. Ellerby, L, Bredesen, D., and Reed ,J.C., 1998, Bax directly induces release of cytochrome c from isolated mitochondria. *Proc. Natl. Acad. Sci. U.S.A.* 95: 4997-5002.
7. Li, P., Nijhawan, D., Budihardjo, I., Srinivasula, S.M., Ahmad, M., Alnemri, E.S., and Wang, X., 1997, Cytochrome c and dATP-dependent formation of Apaf-1/Caspase-9 complex initiates an apoptotic protease cascade. *Cell* 91: 479-489.
8. Renz A., and Fackelmayer, F.O., 1996, Purification and molecular cloning of the scaffold attachment factor B (SAF-B), a novel human nuclear protein that specifically binds to S/MAR-DNA. *Nucleic Acids Res.* 24: 843-849.
9. Goldstein, J.C., Waterhouse, N.J., Juin, P., Evan, G.I., and Green, D.R., 2000, The coordinate release of cytochrome c during apoptosis is rapid, complete and kinetically invariant. *Nat. Cell. Biol.* 2: 156-162.

CD 56 (N-CAM) antigen and mRNA expression in human endocrine glands

JAN ŻEROMSKI, RENATA JENEK, ZOFIA NIEMIR, and WLODZIMIERZ LIEBERT

Departments of Immunology, Nephrology and Neurosurgery Karol Marcinkowski University of Medical Sciences, 49 Przybyszewskiego Str. 60 355 Poznan, Poland

1. INTRODUCTION

CD56/N-CAM molecule is well known as a differentiation antigen of NK cells. It is also widely distributed in neural and neuro-muscular tissues, where it is involved in homophilic cell-cell interactions. Several tumors express CD56 [1]. CD56 has been, however, also shown on epithelial cells of both, rat and human endocrine glands.

In particular, some of us have been able to demonstrate CD56 on follicular cells of human thyroid. The molecule had higher expression than that on NK cells and could be shown by various procedures [2]. The aim of this study was to extent the search of CD56 to other human endocrine glands and to confirm its expression by molecular techniques.

Progress in Basic and Clinical Immunology, Edited by Mackiewicz *et al.*
Kluwer Academic/Plenum Publishers, New York, 2001

2. MATERIALS AND METHODS

2.1 Tissues

Fresh surgical samples of various human endocrine glands were studied. Tissues included thyroid operated because of Graves disease (n=4), Hashimoto thyroiditis (n=2), papillary carcinoma (n=2), resected fragments of adrenal glands because of cortical hyperplasia or adenoma (n=3), fragment of pancreas removed because of insulinoma (n=1), portions of adenohypophysis resected due to adenoma (n=5). Portions of tissues were snap frozen and stored in –70°C.

2.2 Immunohistochemistry (IHC)

Cryostat sections of tissue samples were fixed in a cold acetone, incubated with anti CD56 monoclonal antibodies (MoAbs) from various sources and subsequently subjected to alkaline phosphatase-anti alkaline phosphatase (APAAP) IHC. MoAbs used are shown in the Table 1.

Table 1. Monoclonal antibodies used in this study

Name	CD	Specificity	Source
Leu-19	56	140 kD isoform of N-CAM	Becton Dickinson (BD)
ERIC-1	56	As above	Novocastra
VLA-4	49d	$\alpha4\beta1$ integrin	Serotec

2.3 Isolation of RNA and dot blot hybridization assay

The total RNA was isolated from endocrine glands using a Total RNA Isolation System kit (Promega, USA). For preparation of CD56 probe the N-CAM/CDM8 plasmid (generously supplied by Dr Louis Lanier, San Jose, CA) was linearized and 325 bp fragment was amplified by a polymerase chain reaction (PCR) using the following primers: the forward one 5'- GAA TTC ATC CTT GTT-3' and the reverse one 5'- GGA CTG GCT GCG TCT-3'. The purified PCR product serving as a template was used for a synthesis of cDNA probe to N-CAM mRNA by means of asymmetric amplification PCR. The probe was finally digoxygenine labelled. Appropriately prepared samples of RNA were overlayered on Hybond N nylon membranes (Amersham), dried and fixed at 80^{0}C. Denatured probe was added to the hybridization buffer and hybridization was carried on for 18 hrs. at 68^{0}C. The bound probe was detected by means of horseradish peroxidase (HRP) labelled anti digoxygenine antibodies (Boehringer, Manheim). Several control RNAs from various human tissues were tested in parallel.

3. RESULTS

3.1 Immunohistochemistry

Thyroid – in all hyperactive glands there was strong membrane bound staining of follicular cells with both anti CD56 MoAbs in APAAP reaction.The staining was patchy in Hashimoto thyroiditis and almost absent in papillary carcinoma of thyroid (Table 2).

Table 2. APPAP reaction. .Expression of CD56 on endocrine epithelial cells

Tissues	Leu-19 MoAb	ERIC-1 MoAb	VLA-4 MoAb
Thyroid:	Positive	Positive	Negative
Graves disease	+++	+++	---
Adenoma	+++	+++	---
Hashimoto thyroiditis	+ -- (patchy)	+-- (patchy)	---
Papillary carcinoma	--+ (trace)	---	---
Adrenal gland	Positive	Positive	Negative
Cortical hyperplasia	+++	+++	---
Adenoma (Cushing s.)	+++	+++	---
Cortical carcinoma	++ (cytoplasmic)	+ ---	---
Pancreas	Negative	Negative	Negative
Insulinoma	---	---	---
Adenohypophysis	Positive	Positive	Negative
Adenoma	++	+ (focal)	---

Immunostaining: +++ strong, ++ moderate, --- negative

Adrenal cortex – in both adrenal hyperplasia and in adenoma cell membranes of all cortical zones were positive, but with various intensity. In cortical carcinoma of adrenal the reaction was evident but mostly cytoplasmic.

Pancreas (insulinoma) – endocrine cells were uniformly negative in APAAP reaction with CD56 MoAbs.

Hypophyseal adenoma – the reaction was positive in cell membranes but was rather irregular and in some sites focal. Its intensity was weaker than that of thyroid or adrenal cortex (Table 2).

3.2 RNA hybridization assay

RNAs from human and rat kidney were uniformly negative with CD56 probe. In contrast, RNAs from human tonsil and lymph node were reactive and served as a positive control. Interestingly, RNAs from 3 thyroids and 1 adrenal were also positive (Table 3).

Table 3. Dot blot hybridization assay. Reaction of RNA extracted from various human and animal tissues with CD56 DNA probe.

RNA from	Hum. Kidney	Rat kidney	Hum. tonsil	Hum. lymph node	Control buffer
	---	---	++	++	---
RNA	Thyroid 1	Thyroid 2	Thyroid 3	Adrenal cortex	Buffer
	++	++	++	++	---

4. DISCUSSION

Results of this study show, that epithelial cells of at least some human endocrine glands express CD56/N-CAM molecule. Expression of CD56 appears to be mainly confined to cell membranes. Interestingly, CD56 expression seems to be strongest in the conditions of high secretory activity of endocrine glands tested.

Cell genomic machinery for CD56 synthesis appears to be permanent finding as its mRNA could be traced by dot blot hybridization in all thyroids and one adrenal tested. It indicates that expression of this molecule really depends on inherent production by a given cell and is not just an effect of absorption from the neighboring microenvironment.

Jin et al[3] were able to detect N-CAM proteins in various human tumors but not in the follicular carcinoma of the thyroid, by means of polyclonal anti N-CAM antibody. These authors also searched for mRNA of N-CAM by *in situ* hybridization. They found that the cells of adenoma of parathyroid, while negative with anti N-CAM antibody, were positive for mRNA of N-CAM. This finding suggests that also parathyroids may produce this molecule in particular conditions.

N-CAM appears to be widely distributed in rodents. Langley et al.[4] have demonstrated N-CAM in various endocrine cells of rat, using polyclonal anti N-CAM antibody and immunoblotting. The latter technique permitted them to show differences in N-CAM expression between neurohypophysis and adenohypophysis. In the former predominated 180 kDa N-CAM polypeptides, while the latter 140 kDa ones. As 140 kDa polypeptide is considered identical with CD56 antigen, our results concerning human adenohypophysis, demonstrating CD56 on the cell surface, correspond to theirs made in the rat.

REFERENCES

1. Patel, K., Frost, G., Kiely, F., Phimister, E., Coakham, H.B., Kemshead, I.T., 1991, Expression of the cluster 1 antigen (neural cell adhesion molecule) in neuroectodermal tumors. *Br J Cancer, 63:* 20 - 23 (suppl).
2. *Żeromski, J., Bagnasco, M., Paolieri, F., Dworacki, G., 1992, Expression of CD56 (NKH-1) differentiation antigen in human thyroid epithelium.* Clin exp Immunol, 89: *472 - 478.*
3. Jin, L., Hemperly, J.J., Lloid, R.V., 1991, Expression of neural cell adhesion molecule in normal and neoplastic human neuroendocrine tissues. *Am J Pathol, 138*: 961 – 969.
4. Langley, O.K., Aletsee-Ufrecht, M.C., Grant, N.J., Gratzl, M., 1989, Expression of the neural cell adhesion molecule NCAM in endocrine cells. *J Histochem Cytochem, 37*: 781-791.

CANCER IMMUNOTHERAPY

Glycodendrimeric ligands of c-type lectin receptors as therapeutic agents in experimental cancer

MILOSLAV POSPIŠIL, LUCA VANNUCCI*, ANNA FIŠEROVA, KATHERINA KRAUSOVA, ONDREJ HORVATH, VLADIMIR KŘEN, FRANCO MOSCA*, THISBE. K. LINDHORST**, KASHINATH SADALAPURE**, and KAREL BEZOUŠKA.

*Institute of Microbiology, Div. Immunology, Lab. Natural Cell Immunity, Academy of Sciences of the Czech Republic, Prague; *Dpt. Oncology, Transplantation and New Technologies in Medicine, Div. General Surgery, University of Pisa, Italy; ** Institute of Organic Chemistry, Christiana Albertina University of Kiel, Germany*

1. INTRODUCTION

The increased knowledge about the receptor-ligand relationships of the cytotoxic effector cells is suggesting modalities for new systems of immunomodulation. The lectin receptors on natural killer cells (NK) and their recognition of carbohydrate ligands are part of these new perspectives.

1.1 NK cells and C-type lectin-like receptors

Investigating the receptor system on NK and other cytotoxic cells, a large amount of new structures were and are continuously identified, building the picture of a complex network of integrated inhibition – activation pathways. The C-type lectin receptors are either homodimeric or heterodimeric Ca^{++} dependent molecules with the domain (CRD) recognizing carbohydrate moieties. They are expressed not only on the NK cells but also on NKT lymphocytes, dendritic cells and some monocytes, basophils, mast-cells. NKR-P1 (NK1.1 in the mouse, CD 161 in the man) and CD 69 receptors are involved in the carbohydrate mediated NK cell activation. The carbohydrate

Progress in Basic and Clinical Immunology, Edited by Mackiewicz *et al.*
Kluwer Academic/Plenum Publishers, New York, 2001

dependant cytotoxic response could play a pivotal role in the perspective of the anti-tumor immunotherapies. In fact, glycosylated structures undergo important modifications according to the process of malignant transformation.

2. NKR-P1 CARBOHYDRATE LIGANDS AND MULTIVALENT COMPOUNDS.

A large part of the tumor markers used in the clinical approach are glycoproteins.. Their constitution consequent to the variations of the glycosylation enzymatic pathways, on one side can alert the natural cell immunity and on the other may mask possibly useful epitops. In such a situation, the C- type lectin receptors on the NK cells and other cytotoxic lymphocytes may play an important role either to recall the inhibited immune response or to be involved in the tumor escaping, depending on their ligands. It is known that the NKR-P1 activating receptor has a peculiar scale of affinity for oligosaccharide ligands, as it was described after a large series of *in vitro* tests (Bezouska K. et al., Nature 372: 150-157, 1994). The possibility to increase the cancer control by a carbohydrate dependent modulation was confirmed by experiments on *in vivo* colorectal cancer model (1). Following the line of these experiences, we chose the N-acetyl-glucosamine (GlcNAc) and the mannose (Man) as reference carbohydrates. Neoglycoconjugates with a polyamidoamine (PAMAM) core with a different number of branches (bi-, tri-, tetra- penta-, octa- dendrimers), functionalized with GlcNAc moieties, were produced and tested to evaluate the possibility to enhance the anticancer effect. The octadendrimers resulted the only structures able to create aggregates with the recombinant NKR-P1 receptors (2), demonstrating their very high affinity as ligands. They also increased the cytotoxic activity of the NK cells. Man octadendrimers didn't display similar physical properties, also if they produced a positive modulation of the cytotoxicity in the *in vitro* assays. They were used as a control compound.

2.1 Aims

Because of the availability of these glycoconjugates and their peculiar bounding properties to the NK cell activating receptor NKR-P1, the further step was to control if the *in vitro* results could be doubled in the *in vivo* conditions. Therefore, we investigated the possibility to obtain a valuable biological effect and to induce an immune modulation useful for anticancer treatment.

3. *IN VIVO* EXPERIMENTAL MODELS, TREATMENTS AND RESULTS

Two animal models were used for the *in vivo* tests: azoxymethane-bile induced colorectal carcinogenesis in rats (3) and transplanted B16 melanoma in C57BL/6 mice. In both cases, abundant glycosylated structures are presented on the transformed cell surface enabling the immune carbohydrate mediated recognition. The treatment was performed either with GlcNAc or with Man octadendrimers (PAMAM-GlcNAc$_8$ and PAMAM-Man$_8$), at the dosage of 1.5 mg/dose in the rat and 0.15 mg/dose in the mouse (dosages were derived from the *in vitro* tests). To investigate the possibility to enhance the activity of the dendrimers and to deduce their stability according to the biological response, we used both free and liposome-entrapped forms.

In the rats, the treatment started 5 days after the end of the complete initiation-promotion protocol to evaluate the possible reduction of neoplastic events. Instead, mice were treated since 10 days after the syngeneic B16 cell subcutaneous inoculation, in the presence of developed tumors. In both cases, the schedule consisted in one dose administrated intraperitoneally every third day, for a total of three doses. FACS analysis and ^{51}Cr releasing cytotoxicity assay were performed in the scheduled time during and at the end of the experiments, using blood and spleen cells. The incidence of tumors was investigated in the rat, while survival and growth rate of the neoplasms were followed in the mice. Valuable animals at the end of the experiments were 45 rats and 52 mice (plus 45 mice for the immunological evaluations). The results are summarized in the Tables 1 and 2.

TABLE 1

Groups	No.rats with tumors vs no. rats per group	%
1. Untreated	5/7	71.42
2. Simple liposomes	6/8	75.00
3. Liposomes + PAMAM-Man$_8$	4/8	50.00
4. Liposomes + PAMAM-GlcNAc$_8$	2/6	33.33
5. PAMAM-Man$_8$	5/8	62.50
6. PAMAM-GlcNAc$_8$	3/8	37.50

TABLE 2

Groups	Mean survival (days)	(min-max)
1. Untreated	27.33	19-37
2. Simple liposomes	31.87	24-46
3. Liposomes + PAMAM-Man_8	28.60	20-46
4. Liposomes + PAMAM-$GlcNAc_8$	29.88	22-43
5. PAMAM-Man_8	25.90	19-39
6. PAMAM-$GlcNAc_8$	41.66	25-58

In both the models a significant benefit occurred from the PAMAM-$GlcNAc_8$ treatment, especially in the free form. Instead, PAMAM-Man_8 was able to produce some protective effect only in the colorectal carcinogenesis model. Liposomes did not add peculiar advantages. In both models was also possible to observe different dynamics of the various subpopulations of lymphocytes during and after the treatment, with involvement of cytotoxic cells (NKR-$P1^+CD3^-CD8a^+$ and NKR-$P1^+CD3^+CD8a^+\alpha\beta^+$, assumed as NK and NKT lymphocytes). A specific killing activation of the spleen derived NK cells depending on the free glycodendrimers, prevalently after the PAMAM-$GlcNAc_8$ treatment, was demonstrable only in the late period assays (at 7 weeks).

4. CONCLUSIONS

Carbohydrate ligands of the lectin receptors can be a very promising tool in the future of the anticancer immunotherapy, but not only. NKR-P1receptors expressed on rat NK cells stimulates phosphoinositide turnover and human NKR-P1 (CD 161) associates with Src-family protein kinases (4). The modifications of the natural history of the treated tumors are depending on the activities of cytotoxic cells induced by the glycodendrimers (PAMAM-$GlcNAc_8$). However, the mechanism(s) engaged in tumor control needs to be further studied.

ACKNOWLEDGMENTS

This work was supported by grant 312/98/KO34 of the Grant Agency of the Czech Republic, grant A 7020006 of the Academy of Sciences of the Czech Republic and by ARPA Foundation-Pisa, Italy.

REFERENCES

1. Pospíšil M, Vannucci L, Horváth O, Fišerova A, Krausová A, Bezouška K. and Mosca F: Cancer immunomodulation by carbohydrate ligands for the lymphocyte receptor (NKR-P1). Intern J Oncol 16: 267-276, 2000.
2. Bezouška K., Křen V., Kieburg C., Lindhorst T.K.: GlcNAc-terminated glycodendrimers form defined precipitates with the soluble dimeric receptor of rat natural killer cells, sNKR-P1A. FEBS Lett. 426: 243-247,1998.
3. Vannucci L., Huggins C.B. and Mosca .F: A new experimental model for colorectal carcinogenesis in the rat. J Environ Pathol Toxicol Oncol 13:59-61,1994.
4. Černý J., Fišerová A., Horváth O.,Bezouška K., Pospíšil M.,Horejši V.:Association of human NK cell surface receptors NKR-P1 and CD94 with Src-family proteine kinases. Immunogenetics 46(3):231-6, 1997.

Exosomes in cancer immunotherapy: preclinical data

F.ANDRE*, M.ANDERSEN*, J. WOLFERS*, A. LOZIER*, G.RAPOSO+, V.SERRA$, C.RUEGG$, C.FLAMENT*, E.ANGEVIN*, S.AMIGORENA# AND L. ZITVOGEL*

Immunology Unit, Institut Gustave Roussy, Villejuif, France, + : UMR 144 CNRS Institut Curie, Paris and # : Unité INSERM U520, Institut Curie, Paris, France, $: APCells Company, Menlow Park, CA, USA

1. INTRODUCTION

1.1 Dendritic cells in cancer immunotherapy : results of pioneering clinical trials

Tumor cells present tumor antigens, but they are not immunogenic. To circumvent this lack of immunogenicity and induce expansion of specific cytotoxic T lymphocytes (CTL), some investigators have proposed to use dendritic cells in cancer immunotherapy. Dendritic cells (DC) are unique professional antigen presenting cells that are able to uptake and cross-present class I and class II restricted antigens to CD8+ and CD4+ T lymphocytes. Importantly, mature DC are also capable of priming naive T lymphocytes through expression of costimulatories molecules (CD80, CD86). Proof of principle of the role of dendritic cells in clinical trials has been reported in normal volunteers by Dhodapkar (1). Indeed, DC pulsed with antigens, but not DC alone, nor peptides alone, were able to induce primary and to boost secondary antigen specific T cell based immune response. Some clinical trials using this strategy for metastatic cancer treatment have been reported. Using ex-vivo propagated DC, pulsed with either peptides or tumor cell lysates, Nestlé et al (2) reported 5 clinical responses in 16 melanoma

Progress in Basic and Clinical Immunology, Edited by Mackiewicz *et al.*
Kluwer Academic/Plenum Publishers, New York, 2001

patients. Using fusion between DC and tumor cells, Kugler et al (3) reported 4 complete responses in 17 metastatic renal cancer patients.

1.2 Dendritic cells in cancer immunotherapy: prospect and limitations

Monocytes derived and CD34 derived DC pulsed with peptides or lysates or apoptotic bodies are currently tested in several clinical trials. Preliminary data ascertain their lack of toxicity. DC appear to elicit Ag specific antitumor immune response in patients leading to some objective tumor regressions. They are currently tested in phase III clinical trial in patients with prostate cancer and melanoma.

Although it is a promising therapy for cancer patients, some shortcoming need to be mentionned. Two major points are of importance. As any autologous cell therapy, there is a phenotypic variability as a function of patient clinical condition. This represents a hindrance for exploitation and dissemination plans in term of upscale and manufactoring. The option of replacing DC by a component that exhibit immunostimulatory properties of DC but pharmaceutical properties of a drug (stable phenotype, well defined composition, dosage, manufacturing process, allogenic use) is particularly interesting. The second important point to be considered in DC therapy is the method for pulsing. Pulsing must be performed with components that allow a polyepitopic CTL expansion to avoid tumor immunoselection. In addition, the Ag delivery system for optimal DC loading must take into account the optimal pathway of antigen cross-presentation. To date, only apoptotic bodies (4) and immune complexes (5) have been shown to induce antigen cross-presentation. Finally, the method used for DC pulsing must be well characterized for optimal therapeutic use.

1.3 Exosomes: a cell derivative for biotechnology

Exosomes have been described as small membrane vesicles of 60-90 nm released by reticulocytes (6). Later on, Raposo et al (7) found that B-lymphocytes were also able to release exosomes. Molecular characterisation showed that reticulocytes-derived exosomes contain Transferin-receptor, $\alpha 4\beta 1$ integrins, Heat Shock Protein (HSP) and that B Lymphocytes derived exosomes exhibit functional MHC class II/peptides complexes on their surface.

Therefore, exosomes originate from late endosome and are released by a broad array of hematopoietic cells. They contain protein involved in functions of the cells from which they derive. Considering these data and the immunostimulatories properties of DC, we investigated the ability of DC to secrete immunostimulatory exosomes.

2. DENDRITIC CELL-DERIVED EXOSOMES: A POTENTIAL CELL-FREE ALTERNATIVE TO DC THERAPY

2.1 Tumor peptide-pulsed DC secrete exosomes that induce tumor growth suppression in mice (8)

Immunoelectronic microscopy studies have shown that murine dendritic cells secrete exosomes (Dex) that exhibit high amounts of MHC class I and II molecules and tetraspanin (CD63). Therefore, we tested the immunogenicity of such exosomes and their potential antitumor effet in mice. BM-DCs were pulsed with acid-eluted tumor peptides from P815 and DC supernantant were harvested to purify Dex. After a single intradermal injection of these Dex, 40 to 60% of P815 bearing mice were free of tumor at day 60. In addition, these animals rejected lethal injection of the syngeneic P815, while no rejection occured after injection of irrelevant L1210 tumor cells. These findings suggest that Dex were able to induce a long lasting antitumor immune response. No effect of Dex were found in Athymic Nu/Nu mice, indicating that T cells are required for the exosome-induced antitumor immune response *in vivo*.

2.2 Molecular composition of murine Dex: enrichment in proteins involved in the immunological network (8,9)

To unravel the molecular basis of the immune effects of Dex, a molecular characterization has been performed. Dex exhibit large amounts of MHC class I and II molecules and tetraspanins (CD63, CD81, CD82, CD9) on their surface. Analysis of protein profile of the Dex identified eight more dominant proteins. Three are transmembrane (Mac-1α chain, MHC class IIB chain and CD9), one is associated to membranes (MFG-E8), and four are cytosolic (Gi2α, annexin II, gag from MRV provirus, hsc73). Two of these components seem especially relevant for Dex functional activity. The first is hsc73, expressed constitutively and reported to be immunogenic (10). The other interesting component is MFG-E8. This protein has been initially described at the surface of milk fat globule. This is a protein involved in cell-cell contact and interacts through $\alpha V\beta 3$ and $\alpha V\beta 5$ integrins (11).

2.3 Human MD-DC secrete exosomes that bear functional MHC class I/peptide complexes (12)

Electronic microscopy and western-blot analysis showed that human ex-vivo propagated MD-DC secrete exosomes. These exosomes contain MHC class I and II molecules. In vitro data suggest that human Dex are antigenic on CTL clones and therefore bear functional MHC class I and class II/ peptides complexes on their surface.

2.4 Conclusion and perspectives

Exosomes are 60-90 nm membranes vesicles originating from late endosomes and constitutively secreted by DC. They mediate T cell-based immunogenicity *in vitro* and in tumor bearing mice. Dex represents an alternate immunotherapy strategy to DC in *in vivo* preclinical models. Exosomes are stable and well defined and could be manufactured in biotechnology. A clinical grade upscale production of Dex and quality control parameters have been recently established. This translational research allowed implementation of such a cancer vaccine strategy into the clinic. A phase I clinical trial in metastatic melanoma and lung cancer has been recently launched. Research aimed at identifying the critical molecules involved in Dex biogenesis and function is underway and may allow de novo neosynthesis of bioactive exosomes.

3. TUMOR CELL-DERIVED EXOSOMES (TEX): A NEW ANTIGEN DELIVERY SYSTEM FOR DC LOADING (13)

3.1 Results

Tumor cell lines in mouse and human systems release HSP and Class I containing exosomes. Interestingly, western blot analysis revealed that Tex also vehicle tumor antigens such as Mart1, tyrosinase related proteins (TRP). Tex from a HLA-A2$^-$ Mart1+ tumor cell line induce cross-presentation of Mart1 tumor antigen to a CTL clone. In addition, Tex pulsed onto DC protect mice against tumor challenge. Exosomes were immunogenic across histology since MC38 derived exosomes (colon cancer) were efficient to protect mice against TS/A challenge (breast cancer).

3.2 Perspectives

Tex are constitutively released by tumor cells, and are a source of tumor rejection antigens for CTL cross-priming. They are immunogenic across tumor histology and MHC class I barriers. Compared with other methods of polyepitopic DC pulsing (apoptotic bodies, tumor lysates, mRNA...), they exhibit properties that render them attractive. They are stable, their composition can be well defined, and their storage and safety profile might comply with regulatory agencies requirements. Apart for being an attractive method for DC pulsing, Tex are also a novel source of tumor rejection antigens. Cloning of CTL induced by DC pulsed with Tex should allow identification of new tumor epitopes.

REFERENCES

1. Dhodapkar MV, Steinman RM, Sapp M, Desai H, Fossella C, Krasovsky J, Donahoe SM, Dunbar PR, Cerundolo V, Nixon DF, Bhardwaj N, 2000, Rapid generation of broad T-cell immunity in humans after a single injection of mature dendritic cells.*J Clin Invest* 10: 19-14
2. Nestle FO, Alijagic S, Gilliet M, Sun Y, Grabbe S, Dummer R, Burg G, Schadendorf D, 1998, Vaccination of melanoma patients with peptides- or tumor lysate-pulsed dendritic cells. *Nat Med* 4 : 328-32
3. Kugler A, Stuhler G, Walden P, Zoller G, Zobywalski A, Brossart P, Trefzer U, Ullrich S, Muller CA, Becker V, Gross AJ, Hemmerlein B, Kanz L, Muller GA, Ringert RH, 2000, Regression of human metastatic renal cell carcinoma after vaccination with tumor cell-dendritic cell hybrids. *Nat Med* 6 : 332-6
4. Albert, M. L., Sauter, B. and Bhardwaj, N., 1998, Dendritic cells acquire antigen from apoptotic cells and induce class I-restricted CTLs, *Nature* 392. 86-89
5. Regnault, A., Lankar, D., Lacabanne, V., Rodriguez, A., Thery, C., Rescigno, M., Saito, T., Verbeek, S., Bonnerot, C., Ricciardi-Castagnoli, P. and Amigorena, S., 1999, Fc gamma receptor-mediated induction of dendritic cell maturation and major histocompatibility complex class I-restricted antigen presentation after immune complex internalization, *J. Exp. Med.* 189. 371-380
6. Johnstone, R. M., Adam, M., Hammond, J. R., Orr, L. and Turbide, C., 1987, Vesicle formation during reticulocyte maturation, *J. Biol. Chem.* 262. 9412-9420
7. Raposo, G., Nijman, H. W., Stoorvogel, W., Leijendekker, R., Harding, C. V., Melief, C. J. M. and Geuze, H. J., 1996, B lymphocytes secrete antigen-presenting vesicles, *J. Exp. Med.* 183. 1161-1172
8. Zitvogel, L, Regnault A, Lozier A, Wolfers J, Flament C, Tenza D, Ricciardi-Castagnoli P, Raposo G, Amigorena S, 1998, Eradication of established murine tumors using a novel cell-free vaccine: dendritic cell-derived exosomes. *Nat. Med.* 4, 594-600

9. Thery, C., Regnault, A., Garin, J., Wolfers, J., Zitvogel, L., Ricciardi-Castagnoli, P., Raposo, G. and Amigorena, S., 1999, Molecular characterization of dendritic cell-derived exosomes: selective accumulation of the heat shock protein hsc73, *J. Cell. Biol.* 147. 599-610

10. Srivastava, P. K., Menoret, A., Basu, S., Binder, R. J. and McQuade, K. L., 1998, Heat shock proteins come of age: primitive functions acquire new roles in an adaptive world, *Immunity*. 8. 657-665

11. Andersen MH, Graversen H, Fedosov SN, Petersen TE, Rasmussen JT, 2000, Functional analysis of two cellular binding domains of bovine lactadherin. *Biochemistry* 39 : 6200-6

12. Wolfers J, Andre F, Ruegg C, D. Shu, V. Serra, O. Dhellin, G. Raposo, C. Thery, S.Amigorena, J. Crouzet, T.Tursz and L.Zitvogel, 2000, Dendritic cell-derived exosomes are effective cancer vaccine : preclinical data towards a clinical trial. *Proc Am Ass Cancer Res*, A5556

13. Wolfers J, Lozier A, Raposo G, Regnault A, Thery C, Masurier C, Flament C, Pouzieux S, Faure F, Tursz T, Angevin E, Amigorena S, Zitvogel L, 2001, Tumor-derived exosomes are a source of shared tumor rejection antigens for CTL cross-priming. *Nat Med*, in press

Bone marrow dendritic cell-based anticancer vaccines

MARIE INDROVÁ*, LUIS MENDOZA*, MILAN REINIŠ*, VLADIMÍR VONKA#, MICHAL ŠMAHEL#, ŠÁRKA NĚMEČKOVÁ#, TÁŇA JANDLOVÁ*, and JAN BUBENÍK*

**Institute of Molecular Genetics, Academy of Sciences of the Czech Republic, 16637 Prague 6, Czech Republic, #Institute of Haematology and Blood Transfusion, 12820 Prague 2, Czech Republic*

1. INTRODUCTION

Dendritic cells (DC), capable of activating naïve T cell population and of inducing primary immune responses, play an important role as the most potent antigen-presenting cells. Recently, it has been possible to generate large quantities of mature DC *in vitro* and to pulse them with a variety of antigens. This study is focused on investigation the priming ability of murine bone marrow dendritic cells (BMDC) loaded either with tumour lysates of the HPV 16-induced carcinoma MK 16[1,2] stably producing E7 and activated *ras* oncoproteins or with the HPV 16 E7 peptide RAHYNIVTF. Moreover, the priming capacity BMDC and two established lines of dendritic cells, DC2.4 and JAWS II, were compared

2. RESULTS

To examine the in vitro priming effect of DC on syngeneic, nonadherent murine C57BL/6 (B6) spleen cells, BMDC cultivated *in vitro*, JAWS II (ZymoGenetics, Seattle, WA) and DC2.4[3] cells were pulsed with tumour lysates or with the synthetic HPV 16 $E7_{(49\text{-}57)}$ peptide RAHYNIVTF (for Materal and Methods, see ref. 4, 5). The *in vitro* priming activity of MK 16 tumour lysate exibited significant diference ($P < 0.05$) in comparison with unpulsed DC; the priming activity of the HPV 16 $E7_{(49-57)}$ peptide was substantially weaker than the priming activity of tumour lysate. Comparative experiments utilizing a lysate from an unrelated, chemically induced sarcoma Mc12[5] as a standard, moderately immunogenic tumour preparation demonstrated a similar activity of both lysates (Fig. 1). In Fig. 2, the in vitro priming activity of BMDC pulsed with MK 16 tumour lysate or RAHYNIVTF petide was compared with that of established syngeneic DC lines JAWS II and DC2.4 pulsed with the same lysates. It has been found that both of these DC lines are able to prime the mitogenic activity of syngeneic nonadherent spleenocytes, but the priming activity of pulsed BMDC is substantially stronger than that of the established DC lines JAWS II and DC2.4 pulsed with the same antigens.

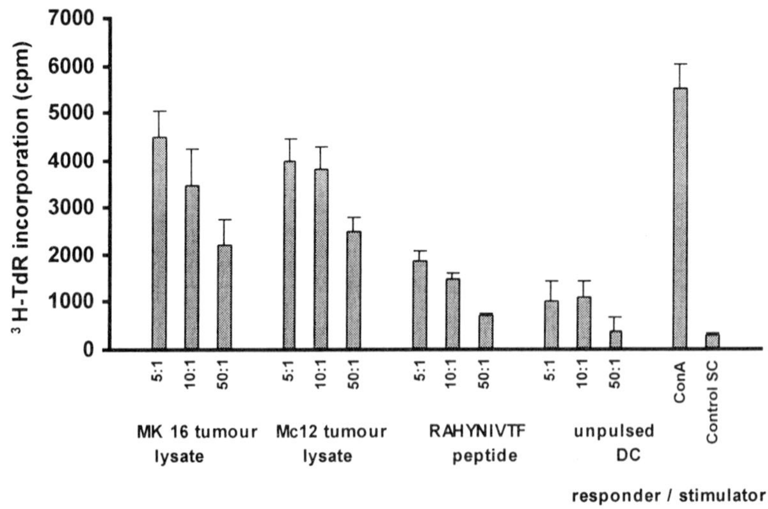

Figure 1. In vitro priming of proliferative spleen cell responses by BMDC pulsed with tumour lysates or HPV 16 $E7_{49-57}$ RAHYNIVTF peptide. Con A - spleen cells were incubated in the presence of 1μg/ml Concanavalin A/ml; control SC - spleen cells only. For Material and Methods, see Ref. 4, 5.

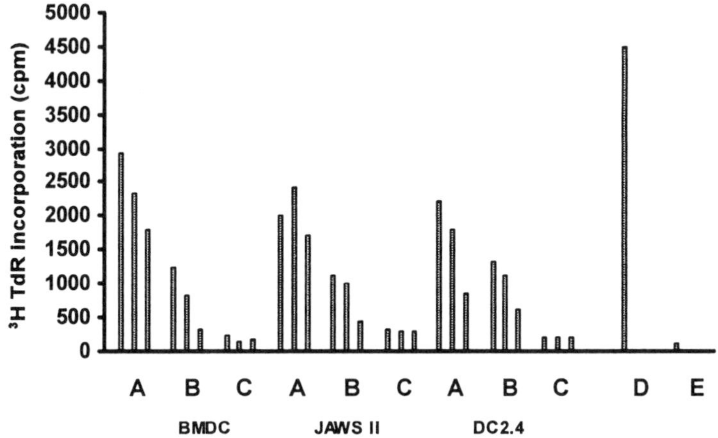

Figure 2. In vitro priming of proliferative spleen cell response by BMDC, JAWS II and DC2.4 cells. A - pulsed with MK 16 tumour lysate; B - pulsed with HPV 16 $E7_{49\text{-}57}$ RAHYNIVTF peptide; C – unpulsed. D - spleen cells incubated in the presence of 1μg/ml Concanavalin A/ml; E - spleen cells only. Columns represent responder: stimulator cells ratio 5:1, 10:1 and 50:1, respectively. For Material and Methods, see Ref. 4, 5.

3. CONCLUSIONS

We have utilized murine carcinoma MK 16 to compare the efficacy of loading the DC with tumour lysates and the synthetic peptide RAHYNIVTF (HPV 16 $E7_{49\text{-}57}$). It has been found that (1) loading the DC with tumour lysate is more efficient for *in vitro* priming of syngeneic spleen cells than loading with the imunodominant RAHYNIVTF peptide; (2) both established dendritic cell lines, JAWS II and DC2.4, are also able to prime the mitogenic activity of syngeneic spleen cells after loading with antigen.

Taken together, the priming ability of loaded DC supports a rationale for the construction of dendritic cell-based vaccines for the therapy of HPV 16-induced tumours[5,7].

ACKNOWLEDGEMENTS

This work was supported by grant No. NC/5526-3 from the Grant Agency of the Ministry of Health of the Czech Republic; No. 312/98/0826, 312/99/0542, 301/00/0114 and 301/01/0985 from the Grant Agency of the Czech Republic; No. A7052002 from the Grant Agency of the Academy of Sciences of the Czech Republic; and by Czech Terry Fox Foundation.

REFERENCES

1 Šmahel, M., Sobotková, E., Bubeník, J., Šímová, J., Žák, R., Ludvíková, V., Hájková, R., Kovařík, J., Jelínek, F., Povýšil, C., Marinov, J., and Vonka, V., in press, Metastatic MHC class I negative mouse cells derived by transformation with human papillomaviruses type 16: A model for studies on vaccination against papillomavirus-associated tumours.. *Brit. J.Cancer.*

2 Bubeník, J,, Šímová, J., Hájková, R., Sobota, V., Jandlová T, Šmahel, M., Sobotková, E., Vonka, V., 1999, Interleukin 2 gene therapy of residual disease in mice carrying tumours induced by HPV 16. *Int J Oncol* 14: 593-597.

3 Shen, Z., Reznikoff, G., Dranoff, G., Rock, K.L., 1997, Cloned dendritic cells can present exogenous antigens on both MHC class I and class II molecules. *J. Immunol.* 158: 2723-2730.

4 Mendoza, L., Indrová, M., Hájková, R., Reiniš, M., Šmahel, M., Vonka, V., Bubeník, J., Jandlová, T., 2000, Peritumoral administration of antigen-unstimulated bone marrow-derived dendritic cells inhibits tumour growth. *Folia Biol (Praha)* 46: 91-97.

5 Indrová, M.., Bubeník, J., Šímová, J., Vonka, V., Němečková, Š., Mendoza, L., Reiniš, M., 2001, Therapy of HPV 16-associated carcinoma with dendritic cell-based vaccines: *In vitro* priming of the effector cell responses by DC pulsed with tumour lysates and synthetic RAHYNIVTF peptide. *Int. J.Molec. Med.* 7: 97-100.

6 Bubeník, J., Indrová, M., Němečková, Š,, Malkovský, M., von Broen, B., Pálek, V., Anderlíková, J., 1978, Solubilized tumour-associated antigens of methylcholanthrene-induced mouse sarcomas. Comparative studies by in vitro sensitization of lymph node cells, macrophage electrophoretic mobility assay and transplantation tests. *Int J Cancer* 21: 348-355.

7 Bubeník, J., Šímová, J., Vonka, V., Šmahel, M., Mikyšková, R., Mendoza, L., in press, Dendritic cell-based vaccines for therapy of HPV 16-induced tumours. *Adv. Exp, Med. Biol.,* this issue.

Dendritic cell-based vaccines for therapy of HPV16-induced tumours

JAN BUBENÍK*, JANA ŠÍMOVÁ*, VLADIMÍR VONKA[#], MICHAL ŠMAHEL[#], ROMANA MIKYŠKOVÁ*, AND LUIS MENDOZA*
**Institute of Molecular Genetics, Academy of Sciences of the Czech Republic, Flemingovo nám. 2, 166 37 Prague, Czech Republic; [#] Institute of Haematology and Blood Transfusion, U Nemocnice 1, 128 20 Prague, Czech Republic*

1. INTRODUCTION

Dendritic cells (DCs) are the most potent professional antigen-presenting cells with exquisite capacity to interact with T cells and initiate their responses; the antigen-presenting capabilities of DCs make them attractive vehicles for the delivery of therapeutic cancer vaccines. The working hypothesis for utilization of DC-based cancer vaccines is that lack of efficient tumour antigen presentation on mature DCs, which is frequently observed in tumour-bearing individuals, can be bypassed by direct loading of DCs with oncoproteins *in vitro*, thus ensuring the transfer of immunostimulatory peptides on the respective antigen-presenting molecules.

Progress in Basic and Clinical Immunology, Edited by Mackiewicz *et al.*
Kluwer Academic/Plenum Publishers, New York, 2001

2. RESULTS

To examine the in vivo effects of DC-based tumour vaccines in a mouse model system mimicking human HPV16-associated carcinomas, murine kidney cells were malignantly converted by in vitro co-transfection with a mixture of activated ras, HPV16 E6/E7, and neomycin resistance gene DNA. Immunization with HPV16 E6/E7 plasmid DNA could specifically inhibit growth of the HPV16-induced tumour, designated as MK16, in the immunized mice and the stable expression of E7 and activated ras oncoproteins was proved by immunoblotting. After subcutaneous transplantation, the MK16 tumours grew locally. However, in the majority of inoculated animals metastases were regularly observed in lungs and lymph nodes[1,2]. Priming of the proliferative anti-MK16 responses was efficient when the bone marrow-derived DC (BMDC) were pulsed with lysates of MK16 cells and co-cultivated in vitro with syngeneic spleen cells[3]. In an attempt to evaluate the role of increased local DC concentration in defence against the MK16 carcinoma, C57 BL/6 mice were pretreated twice on days 0 and 21 with $2{,}5x10^6$ antigen-unstimulated bone marrow-derived DC (for detail Materials and Methods, see ref. 4) and challenged on day 35 with a dose of $1x10^5$ syngeneic MK16 carcinoma cells. As can be seen from Fig. 1 and Table 1, local pretreatment with DC substantially inhibits growth of a subsequent inoculum of the MK16 cells ($P<0.05$) and reduces the number of lung metastases.

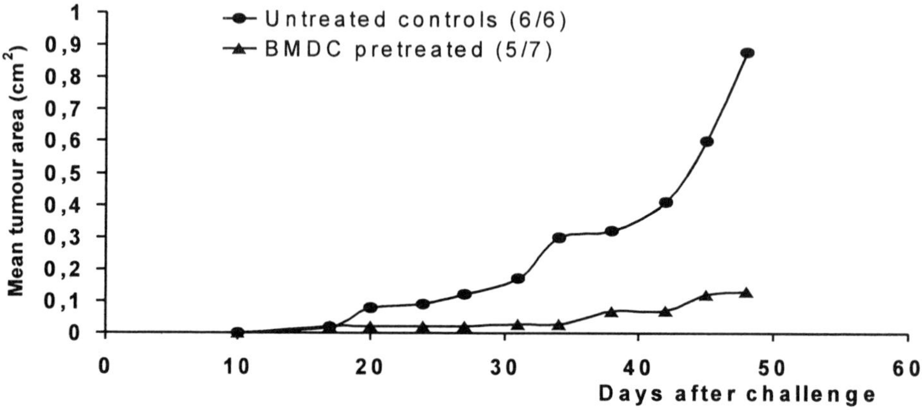

Figure 1. The effect of local DC pretreatment on s.c. growth of MK16 carcinoma transplants in syngeneic mice

Table 1. The effect of local pretreatment with DC or DC plus MK16 cells on s.c. growth of a subsequent challenge inoculum of the MK16 cellsa

Mice pretreated with	No. of mice with tumour/total No. of mice	No. of lung metastases/mouse
MK16 (2.5x10^6 cells/mouse)	6/6	4
DC (2.5x10^6 cells/mouse)	10/12	3
MK16+DC	6/6	0.5
Untreated controls	18/18	7

[a] Mice were pretreated with irradiated (MK16) or non-irradiated (DC) cells on day 0 and 21 and challenged with 1x10^5 MK16 cells on day 35

In subsequent experiments, peritumoral treatment of 5-day MK16 tumours was performed with 3x10^6 antigen-unstimulated DC (for detail Materials and Methods, see ref.4) or 3x10^6 MK16 lysate-pulsed DC (for detail Materials and Methods, see ref. 3). As shown in Fig. 2, both the unpulsed and MK16 lysate-pulsed DC inhibited tumour growth, the MK16 lysate-pulsed DC being more efficient.

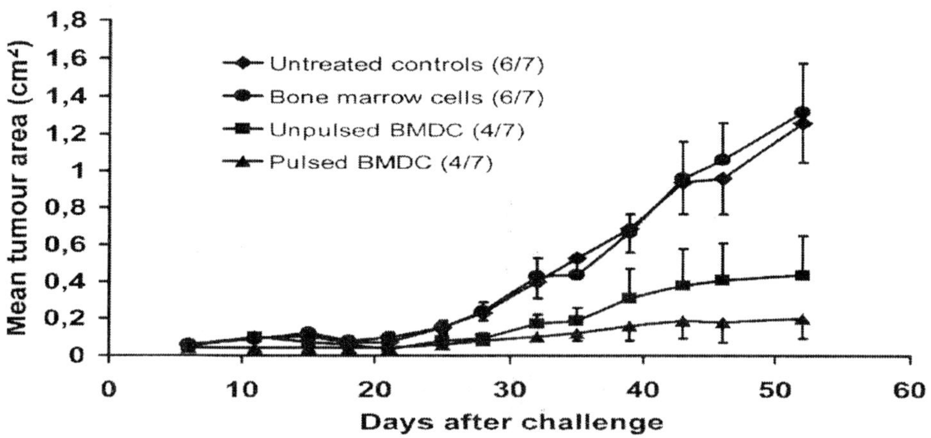

Figure 2. Peritumoral treatment of 5-day MK16 tumours with MK16 lysate--pulsed DC

Similarly, local treatment of surgically induced minimal residual MK16 tumour disease (for detail Materials and Methods, see ref. 1) with MK16 lysate-pulsed DC was performed (Fig. 3). Briefly, C57 BL/6 mice were inoculated s.c. with 1x10^6 MK 16 cells. In 25-30 days, 100% of mice developed s.c. carcinoma of approximately 8-12 mm in diameter. The tumours were surgically removed and the recurrence rate of the completely extirpated tumours was 77%.

Vaccination performed 3 days after the operation decreased the tumour recurrence rate to 53% (p = 0.0382, log-rank and Cox-Mantel tests).

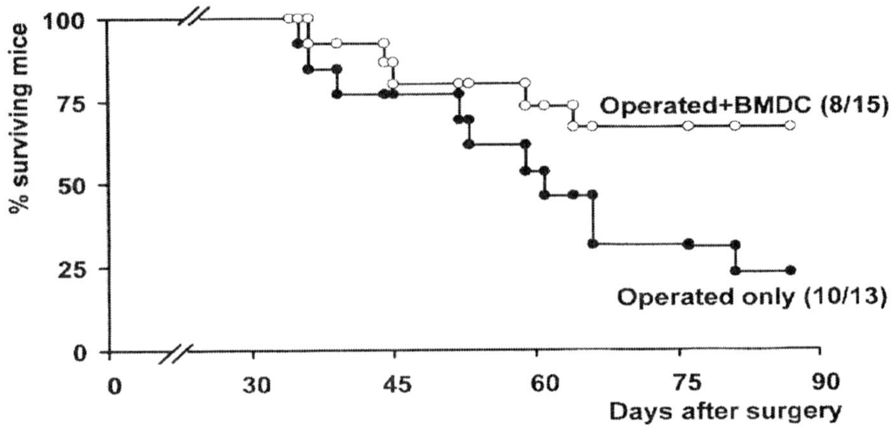

Figure 3. Local treatment of surgically induced minimal residual MK16 disease with MK16 lysate-pulsed DC

3. CONCLUSIONS

These results suggest that the activating and co-stimulatory signals delivered by oncoprotein-pulsed antigen presenting cells should be considered in the construction of vaccines for treatment of human HPV16-associated carcinomas.

ACKNOWLEDGEMENTS

This work was supported by grants No. NC/5526-3 and NC/4501-3 from the Grant Agency of the Ministry of Health of the Czech Republic; No. 312/98/0826, 312/99/0542, and 301/00/0114 from the Grant Agency of the Czech Republic: No. A7052002 from the Grant Agency of the Academy of Sciences of the Czech Republic; and by Czech Terry Fox Foundation.

REFERENCES

1. Bubeník, J., Šímová, J., Hájková, R., Sobota, V., Jandlová, T., Šmahel, M., Sobotková, E., and Vonka, V., 1999, Interleukin 2 gene therapy of residual disease in mice carrying tumours induced by HPV16. Int. J. Oncol. 14: 593-597.
2. Šmahel, M., Sobotková, E., Bubeník, J., Šímová, J., Žák, R., Ludvíková, V., Hájková, R., Kovařík, J., Jelínek, F., Povýšil, C., Marinov, J., and Vonka, V., in press, Metastatic MHC class I negative mouse cells derived by transformation with human papillomavirus type 16: A model for studies on vaccination against papillomavirus-associated tumours. Brit. J. Cancer.
3. Indrová, M., Mendoza, L., Reiniš, M., Vonka, V., Šmahel, M., Němečková, Š., Jandlová, T., and Bubeník, J., in press, Bone marrow dendritic cell-based anticancer vaccines. Adv. Exp. Med. Biol., this issue.
4. Mendoza, L., Indrová, M., Hájková, R., Reiniš, M., Šmahel, M., Vonka, V., Bubeník, J., and Jandlová, T., 2000, Peritumoral administration of antigen-unstimulated bone marrow-derived dendritic cells inhibits tumour growth. Folia biol. (Praha) 46: 91-97.
5. Vlk, V., Rössner, P., Indrová, M., Bubeník, J., and Sobota, V., 1998, Interleukin-2 gene therapy of surgical minimal residual tumour disease. Int. J. Cancer 76: 115-119.

Cytokine gene transfection for autologous and allogeneic melanoma vaccines

S TODRYK*, L BIRCHALL, R ERLICH, N HALANEK, JK ORLEANS-LINDSAY AND A DALGLEISH
**Tumour Immunology Group, Institute for Immunology, Department of Biology, National University of Ireland Maynooth, Ireland; and Division of Oncology, St George's Hospital Medical School, London.*

1. INTRODUCTION

Whole tumour cells are a logical basis for generating immunity against the cancers they comprise or represent[1]. Allogeneic (MHC-disparate) tumour cells offer a useful avenue as vaccines because tumours of the same histological type often share antigens, and immune priming will occur via host antigen-presenting cells. A number of human trials have been initiated using cytokine-transfected whole tumour cells of autologous or allogeneic origin as vaccines. Although precedent exists for the efficacy of autologous-transfected vaccines in animal models, little preclinical evidence confirms that these findings will extrapolate to allogeneic-transfected vaccines[2].

2. RESULTS

In order to directly address this issue, a murine melanoma cell line (K1735) was retrovirally transfected to secrete interleukin (IL)-2, IL-4, IL-7 or GM-CSF; cytokines currently in use in clinical trials. Cytokine secretion levels by cell clones were similar to those published previously. The efficacy of these cells as vaccines was tested head-to-head in syngeneic (C3H; H-2^k) mice and in MHC-disparate (C57BL/6; H-2^b) mice, the former being subsequently challenged with K1735 cells and the latter with naturally-cross-reactive B16-F10 melanoma cells. Vaccine cells were irradiated (100Gy) and administered subcutaneously. Whilst the GM-CSF-secreting vaccine was the most effective at generating protection (80%) in C3H mice, little enhancement in protection above the wild-type vaccine (30%) was seen with any of the transfections for the allogeneic vaccines (Fig.1).

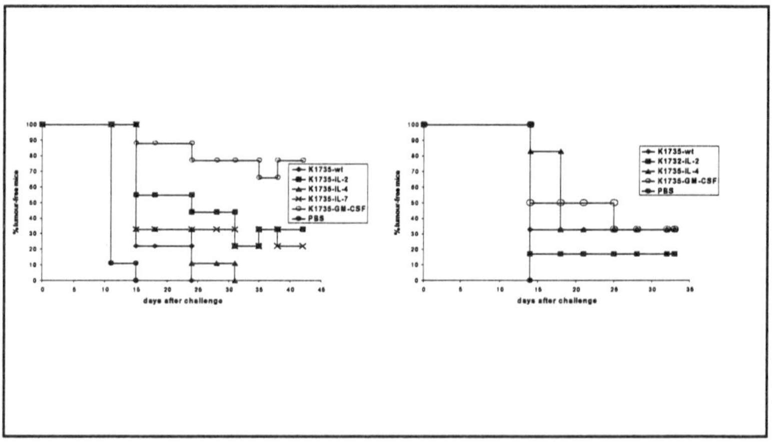

Figure 1. Protection from autologous tumour challenge following autologous (C3H; left) or allogeneic (C57BL/6; right) vaccination.

Following vaccination, anti-tumour CTL activity was investigated in spleen cells *in vitro* against autologous tumour cells, and was detected in both models, but did not appear to correlate well with protection (Fig.2).

In vitro anti-tumour IFNγ secretion tended to be higher following the GM-CSF-secreting vaccine for both autologous and allogeneic vaccines (Fig.3) although the differences between vaccines were small.

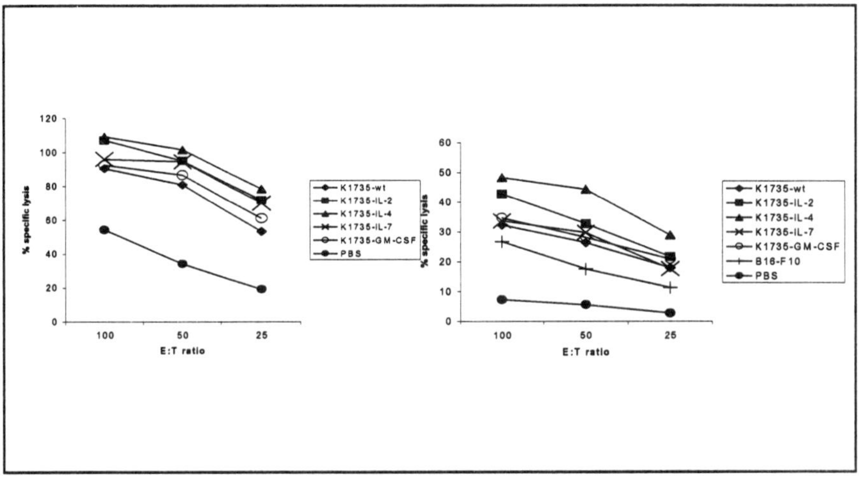

Figure 2. CTL activity *in vitro* following autologous (C3H; left) or allogeneic (C57BL/6; right) vaccination.

Cytokine transfection of vaccines generally, increased anti-tumour CTL activity and IFNγ secretion. Further studies in other model systems are required to confirm this apparent lack of benefit of cytokine transduction in allogeneic vaccines, and to determine which *in vitro* assays will correlate best with protection *in vivo*. Preliminary data suggest that an immune response to allogeneic MHC molecules at the vaccine priming site may be contributing to the adjuvant effect.

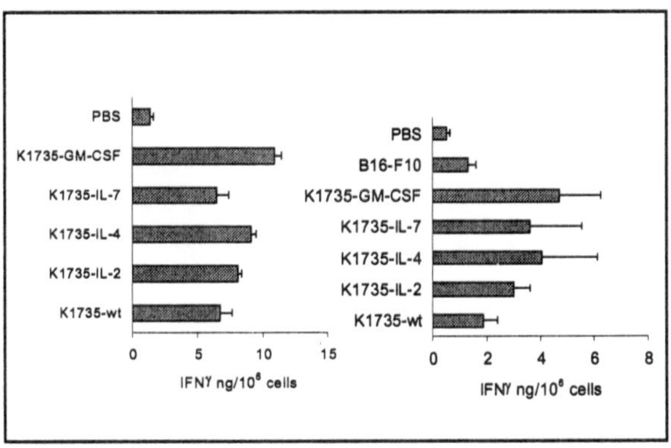

Figure 3. IFNγ secretion *in vitro* following autologous (C3H; left) or allogeneic (C57BL/6; right) vaccination.

3. CONCLUDING REMARKS

Transfection of allogeneic tumour vaccines to secrete cytokines does not necessarily improve upon the adjuvant effect provided by the allogeneic molecules in a prophylactic vaccine setting.

ACKNOWLEDGEMENTS

This data is reproduced with permission from Blackwell Scientific, from a manuscript[3] which is in press in Immunology. This work was funded by Onyvax Ltd.

REFERENCES

1. Pardoll DM . 1998. Cancer vaccines. Nat Med 4(5 Suppl):525-31
2. Kayaga, J., Souberbielle, B., Sheikh, N., Morrow, W., Scott-Taylor, T., Vile, R., Chong, H., Dalgleish, A. 1999. Anti-tumour activity against B16-F10 melanoma with a GM-CSF secreting allogeneic tumour cell vaccine. Gene Ther. 6, 1475.
3. Todryk SM, L Ashworth, R Erlich, N Halanek, J Kayaga and AG Dalgleish. 2001. Efficacy of cytokine gene transfection differs for autologous and allogeneic tumour cell vaccines. Immunology in press

Brain Tumor Treatment with IL-2 and IL-12 Producing Autologous Cancer Cell Vaccines

SZILVIA DESAKNAI[1], KATALIN LUMNICZKY[1], EGON J. HIDVEGI[1], HIROFUMI HAMADA[2] and GEZA SAFRANY[1*]

[1]Department of Molecular and Tumor Radiobiology, National Research Institute for Radiobiology and Radiohygiene, Budapest, Hungary; [2]Department of Molecular Medicine, Biomedical Research Center, Sapporo Medical University, Sapporo, Japan; [*]corresponding author

1. INTRODUCTION

In humans, gliomas constitute about 30-45% of all intracranial tumours. Conventional therapy for high-grade gliomas consists of surgery that is followed by radiation therapy and/or by chemotherapy. The life expectancy of patients with glioblastoma is less than one year from the time of diagnosis[1], therefore development of new therapeutic approaches is necessary. Animal models have demonstrated the efficacy of cytokine gene therapy of melanomas using autologous cancer cèlls producing various cytokines[2,3]. We decided to study the therapeutic effect of cytokine expressing cancer cell vaccines for the treatment of high-grade gliomas.

2. METHODS

To isolate cytokine-producing vaccines mouse glioma (Gl261)[4] cells were transduced at different multiplicity of infection (moi) with adenoviral vectors[5,6] encoding either mouse IL-2 (AdexCAmIL-2) or the 35S (AdexCAmIL-12p35) and 40S (AdexCAmIL-12p40) subunits of IL-12 (the two subunits were cloned into two different constructs). The cytokine production was measured in the culture supernatant of infected cells by

Progress in Basic and Clinical Immunology, Edited by Mackiewicz *et al.*
Kluwer Academic/Plenum Publishers, New York, 2001

conventional ELISA kits (Endogen and BIOSOURCE) two days after transduction. Cytokine-producing cells were irradiated with 20 Gy ^{60}Co-γ radiation to stop cell division and 1×10^6 cells were injected subcutaneously to vaccinate tumour-bearing mice. Brain tumours were induced by intracranial injection of $1\text{-}2 \times 10^4$ Gl261 cells. Mice were vaccinated 3 days after tumour induction with cytokine producing cells and survival rates followed. Statistical analysis was performed by Mantel-Cox test. A P value of <0.02 was considered as significant.

3. RESULTS AND CONCLUSION

First, we investigated the transduction efficiency of adenoviral vectors in Gl261 cells. A construct (Adex1CAlacZ) encoding the bacterial lacZ gene was introduced into Gl261 cells at different multiplicity of infection (moi) and the presence of lacZ activity measured[5]. At ten moi about 50-70% of the cells was transduced. The transduction efficiency increased linearly up to 100 moi when all of the cells were infected (not shown). This proved that Gl261 cells could be transduced with high efficiency by adenoviral vectors.

The IL-2 expressing vaccine was prepared by introducing mouse IL-2 encoding adenoviral vector into Gl261 cells at different moi. The IL-2 level increased linearly in the culture medium even beyond 100 moi (Figure 1) showing that the cells could be overloaded by the virus. IL-12 expressing cells were produced by co-transduction of the cells with vectors encoding the 35S and the 40S subunits of mouse IL-12. The IL-12 level was much lower in the culture medium than the IL-2 level (Figure 1). The ELISA kit used for the analysis of IL-12 expression detected the mature mouse IL-12 protein. The formation of the mature IL-12 protein requires both the expressions of the 35S and 40S subunits within the same cell and an efficient maturation process. This might explain the lower IL-12 levels.

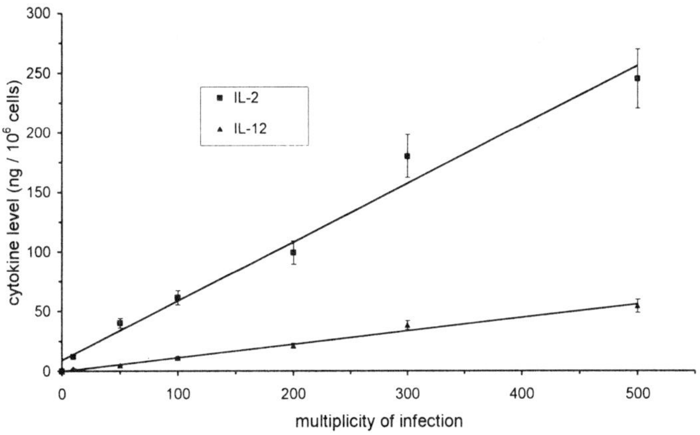

Figure 1. Expression of cytokines in Gl261 cells. Gl261 cells were transduced at different moi with adenoviral vectors encoding mouse IL-2 and IL-12. Cytokine production was measured in the culture medium 48 h after transduction.

The therapeutic effect of cytokine expressing autologous cancer cell vaccines was studied on a mouse brain tumour model using glioma 261 (Gl261) cells. Brain tumours were induced by intracranial transplantation of Gl261 cells. Three days after tumour induction tumour-bearing mice were treated with cytokine producing vaccines. To isolate the vaccines, Gl261 cells were transduced at different moi (10, 50, 100 and 200 for IL-2; 50, 100, 200 and 300 for IL-12) with the vectors. This ensured that the cells expressed different levels of cytokines (Figure 1). The *therapeutic* effect of the vaccines strongly depended on the cytokine production. Only the vaccines produced at 200 moi cured any of the mice (Figure 2). Vaccines made by infecting the cells at other than 200 moi proved to be ineffective (data not shown).

In conclusion, glioma cells can be infected with adenoviral vectors with high efficiency. Glioma-bearing mice might be cured with IL-2 and IL-12 expressing autologous cancer cell vaccines, however the therapeutic effect strongly depends on the cytokine level produced by the vaccine.

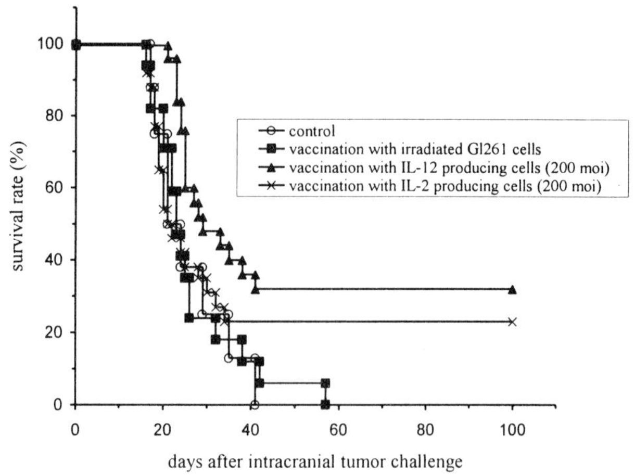

Figure 2. Therapeutic effect of cytokine producing cancer cell vaccines. Brain tumour bearing mice were vaccinated with IL-2 and IL-12 expressing Gl261 cells and survival followed. P values were <0.002 for the IL-12 and <0.02 for IL-2 vaccine.

ACKNOWLEDGEMENTS

This work was supported by the following grants to G.S.: ICGEB CRP/HUN98-02(t2), OMFB 96-97-65-1201, ETT T01/053/2000 and 247/1996. The authors thank Maria Frigyesi and Erzsebet Fekete for technical assistance.

REFERENCES

1. Shoenberg, BS. (1983) In MD Walker (ed). Oncology of the Nervous System. Martinus Nijhoff: Boston, pp. 1-30.
2. Dranoff G., Jaffee E, Lazenby A., Golumbek P., Levitsky H., Brose K., Jackson V., Hamada H., Pardoll D. and Mulligan RC. (1993) Proc. Natl. Acad. Sci USA 90. 3539-3543.
3. Forni, G., Foa R., Santoni A., Frati L. (eds) (1994) Cytokine-induced tumor immunogenicity. Academic Press, San Diego, CA
4. Shapiro, WR., Ausman, JI. and Rall, DP. (1970) Cancer Res. 30. 2401-2413.
5. Yamaguchi, S., Wakimoto, H., Yoshida, Y., Kanegae, Y., Saito, I., Aoyagi, M., Hirakawa, K., Amagasa, T. and Hamada, H. (1995) Nucleic Acids Res. 23. 2080-2081.
6. Nakamura, Y., Wakimoto, H., Abe, J., Kanegae, Y., Saito, I., Aoyagi, M., Hirakawa, K. and Hamada, H. (1994) Cancer Res. 54. 5757-5760.

IL-11 is a potent anti-melanoma factor

HANNA DAMS-KOZLOWSKA, DARIUSZ IZYCKI, ANDRZEJ MACKIEWICZ
Department of Cancer Immunology, Academy of Medicine, GreatPoland Cancer Center, Poznan, Poland.

1. INTRODUCTION

Interleukin 11 (IL-11) is a pleiotropic cytokine initially identified as a factor stimulating proliferation of IL-6-dependet murine plasmacytoma cell line T1165[1]. Today IL-11 is known to interact with variety of haematopoietic and nonhematopoietic cell types (for review see ref. 2). Many of the biological effects of IL-11 are shared with IL-6 since both cytokines share a common receptor subunit β (gp130).

IL-6, displays anti-tumour activity in various animal models[4-6]. However, anti-tumour properties of IL-11 have not been demonstrated so far. In this report we demonstrate anti-melanoma activity of IL-11 in tumour rejection model. The IL-11 cDNA was introduced into murine melanoma cell line B78H1, and the tumour growth as well as tumour protection were analysed. Moreover, the cellular mechanisms responsible for IL-11 activity were studied.

2. MATERIAL AND METHODS

B78H1 cell line was kindly provided by dr LH Graf, Chicago, USA. The retroviral vector carrying human IL-11 was a gift from Dr. RG Hawley, Toronto, Canada. The stable modified B78H1 cells were generated via transduction by using recombinant retroviruses produced by packaging cell

Progress in Basic and Clinical Immunology, Edited by Mackiewicz *et al.*
Kluwer Academic/Plenum Publishers, New York, 2001

line (PA 317/IL-11). Expression of IL-11 was measured by ELISA (R&D) and was found to be (30ng/ml/10^6 cells/24h).

The mock transduced and IL-11 modified B78H1 cells ($5x10^5$) were injected into C57BL/6xC3H and SCID mice subcutaneously (s.c.). The tumour growth and survival were monitored. The ability of B78H1/IL-11 cells to stimulate long lasting anti-tumour immunity was studied by injecting s.c. B78H1/IL-11 or control cells (left flank) and re-challenging s.c. with parental B78H1 cells (right flank) after 2 weeks. The tumour size and survival were observed.

Infiltration of tumour cells by immune cells was studied by excision of B78H1 cells injection site at days 2, 5, 9, 11 and immunohistochemistry. For assessment of infiltrating cells the following scale was used: "-"- no stained cells, "-/+"- bellow 5% of stained cells, "+"- 5-20%, "++"- 20-50% and "+++"- above 50% of stained cells.

3. RESULTS AND DISCUSSION

Transduction of IL-11 into B78H1 cells inhibited tumour growth when compared with mock transduced cells. 100% of animals injected with control cells developed tumours at 3rd week, while at the same time only 30% of mice vaccinated with B78H1/IL-11 had tumours (Fig. 1.a). At 7th week half of animals injected with B78H1/IL-11 group developed tumours and to the

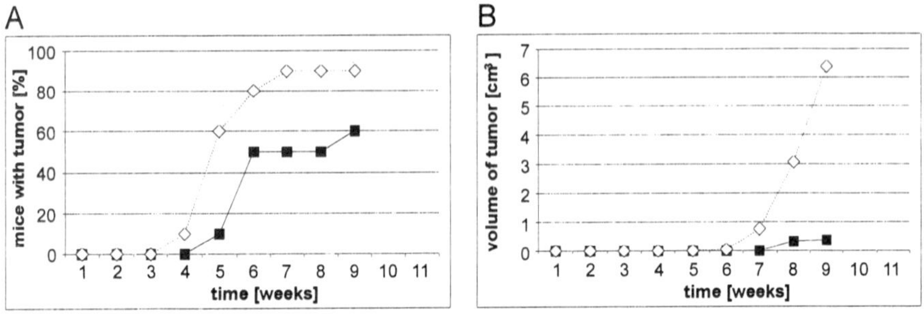

Figure1. Tumour formation (A) and kinetic of tumour growth (B) in C57BL/6xC3H mice after injection the "mock" (◊) and IL-11 (■) transduced B78H1 cells.

end of experiment the number of mice with tumours did not increase. There were also significant differences in tumour volume (Fig. 1.b) and in survival rate.

The ability of B78H1/IL-11 cells to stimulate long lasting anti-tumour immunity was studied by injecting s.c. B78H1/IL-11 or control cells (left leg) and rechallenging s.c. after 2 weeks with parental B78H1 cells (right leg). Control mice started to develop tumours 4 weeks after injection, while IL-11 group one week later (Fig.2.a). At 7th week 90% of mice vaccinated with B78H1 cells had tumours, while in B78H1/IL-11 immunised group 50% of animals. There was a significant difference in tumour volume between both groups (Fig. 2.b).

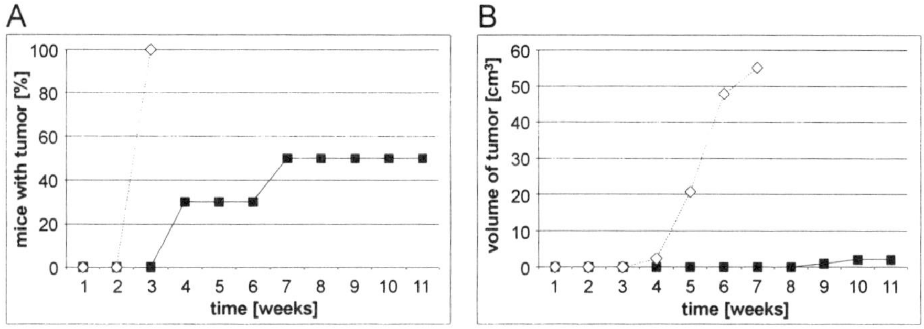

Figure 2. Tumor formation (A) and kinetic of tumor growth (B) in C57BL/6xC3H mice vaccinated with B78H1 (◇) and B78H1/IL-11 (■) cells after rechallenging with parental B78H1 cells.

In another set of experiments, SCID mice were used. They lack T and B cells, but possess NK cells, what allows evaluation of the role of these cells in primary tumour rejection mediated by IL-11. We observed that in mice which received B78H1/IL-11 cells tumours appeared a week later than in control mice (5 animals in each group). The survival of SCID mice injected with B78H1/IL-11 cells was one week longer when compared to the B78H1 group. The tumour volume was not significantly different in both analysed groups (data not shown). These results indicate, that anti-tumour activity of IL-11 is rather not depend on NK cells. This subpopulation of immune cells does not play the major role in IL-11-induced inhibition of primary tumour growth.

Table 1. Immunological cells infiltrating control and gene modified murine melanoma B78H1 cells

day after injection	B78H1			B78H1/IL-11		
	CD4	CD8	NK	CD4	CD8	NK
2	-	-	+	-	-	-
5	-	-	-	+++	+++	-
9	++	+	+	-	-	+
11	-	-	-	-	-	-

Table 2. Immunological cells infiltrating B78H1 cells after immunization with control and gene modified B78H1 cells

day after rechallenging	B78H1			B78H1/IL-11		
	CD4	CD8	NK	CD4	CD8	NK
2	-	-	+	+++	+++	+
5	+	-	+	+	-	-/+
9	-/+	-	-/+	+++	-	+
11	-	-	+	+++	-	+

In order to understand the cellular mechanisms responsible for IL-11 anti-melanoma activity we analysed the tumour infiltrates in the induction and effector phases of immune response. The induction phase was studied by injecting control and IL-11-modified melanoma cells into unprimed mice and analysing immune cell infiltration (Table 1). Control B78H1 cells were infiltrated by a single CD4+ and CD8+ T lymphocytes, while B78H1/IL-11 cells were densely infiltrated by CD4+ and CD8+ cells. B78H1 and B78H1/IL-11 cells were infiltrated by NK cells at the low level. These observations indicate that in induction phase of anti-melanoma response elicited by IL-11 CD4+ and CD8+ cells might be involved. Results obtained in SCID mice, that NK cells are not important in suppression of primary tumour growth were confirmed in these experiments as well. In the effector phase, in which the pre-immunised mice were rechallenged with parental B78H1 cells, infiltrates of single CD4+ cells were observed in control mice (Table. 2), while in mice immunised with B78H1/IL-11 cells tumours were densely infiltrated by CD4+ cells. In addition at the second day a severely infiltration of CD8+ cells was observed. Single NK cells infiltrated tumours in both groups. Presented results demonstrate that a major effector cells attracted by IL-11 are CD4+ lymphocytes and in the early phase CD8+ cells as well. Phenotyping of the tumour infiltrating cells does not reflect the activity of these cells thus, the immunological mechanisms induced by IL-11 in anti-melanoma activity require further studies.

ACKNOWLEDGMENTS

Supported by Collaborative Research Project CRP/POL98-03(t1) from the International Centre for Genetic Engineering and Biotechnology

REFERENCES

1. Paul SR, Bennett F, Calvetti JA, Kelleher K, Wood CR, O'Hara RM Jr, Leary AC, Sibley B, Clark SC, Williams DA, YangYC, 1990, Molecular cloning of a cDNA encoding interleukin 11, a stromal cell-derived lymphopoietic and hematopoietic cytokine. *Proc Natl Acad Sci U S A.* 87:7512-6.
2. Du X, Williams DA, 1997, Interleukin-11: review of molecular, cell biology, and clinical use. *Blood.* 89:3897-908.
3. Mackiewicz A, Koj A, Sehgal PB, 1995, Interleukin-6-type cytokines. *Ann NY Acad Sci.* 762.
4. Katz A, Shulman LM, Porgador A, Revel M, Feldman M, Eisenbach L, 1993, Abrogation of B16 melanoma metastases by long-term low-dose interleukin-6 therapy. *J Immunother.* 13:98-109.
5. Porgador A, Tzehoval E, Katz A, Vadai E, Revel M, Feldman M, Eisenbach L, 1992, Interleukin 6 gene transfection into Lewis lung carcinoma tumor cells suppresses the malignant phenotype and confers immunotherapeutic competence against parental metastatic cells. *Cancer Res.* 52:3679-86.

6. Mackiewicz A, Wiznerowicz M, Roeb E, Karczewska A, Nowak J, Heinrich PC, Rose-John S, 1995, Soluble interleukin 6 receptor is biologically active in vivo. *Cytokine.* 7:142-9.

IL-6 and GM-CSF in tumor rejection model of renal cell cancer

PIOTR J. WYSOCKI*, DARIUSZ W. KOWALCZYK*, DARIUSZ IZYCKI*, PIOTR GRABARCZYK*, ZBIGNIEW KWIAS[#] and ANDRZEJ MACKIEWICZ

[*]Department of Cancer Immunology, University School of Medical Sciences, at GreatPoland Cancer Center, Poznań, Poland. [#]Department of Urology, University School of Medical Sciences, Poznań, Poland

1. INTRODUCTION

Tumors developing within a host induce a state of immune tolerance to tumor antigens. Number of concepts are tested in order to activate the antitumoral immune response to recognize and destroy tumor cells. Tumor vaccines genetically modified with cytokine genes (GMTV) are one of strategies currently examined. Different cytokines display different patterns of antitumoral immune response activation but the perfect cytokine or a combination of cytokine are still to be found. Here we present two GMTVs one consisting of cells producing IL-6 and the second producing GM-CSF in a murine tumor rejection model of Renal Cell Carcinoma (RenCa).

2. MATERIALS AND METHODS

2.1 Tumor cells and transduction

The RenCa cells expressing IL-6 or GM-CSF were generated by transduction using bicistronic, doublecopy retroviral vector – DCCMV IRES

Neo. The murine GM-CSF cDNA was excised from pT-easy-mGM-CSF plasmid by NotI restriction enzyme and cloned into NotI site of the vector. The IL-6 cDNA was excised from pEXIL-6 plasmid as SalI fragment and cloned into SalI site of DCCMV IRES Neo. Production of corresponding cytokines was measured by ELISA (R&D, Mineapolis, MN). As control mock transduced RenCa cells were used.

2.2 Analysis of growth kinetic of modified tumor cells in naive mice

6-10 weeks old Balb/c mice were inoculated s.c. with $5x10^5$ genetically modified RenCa cells into a right leg flank. The kinetic of tumor growth was evaluated in 7 days intervals.

2.3 Analysis of growth kinetics of RenCa cells in preimmunized mice

Balb/c mice were inoculated s.c. with $5x10^5$ irradiated (8 Gy) RenCa cells modified with IL-6, GM-CSF or mock control cells in a right leg flank. 2 week later mice were rechallenged s.c. into an opposite leg flank with $5x10^5$ wild type RenCa cells. The tumor take and growth kinetic were subjects of evaluation every week.

2.4 Analysis of immune cells infiltrating the administered genetically modified RenCa cells.

Balb/c mice were injected sc. with $2x10^6$ cells, incorporated into a Matrigel®. 7 days later 'matrigel tumors' were excised and the infiltrating cells were isolated and analysed by flow cytometry, using following antibodies: CD4, CD8, CD25, CD69, CD11c, CD40, CD80.

3. RESULTS

3.1 RenCa cells modified with the IL-6 gene showed the slowest growth in vivo

Within 3 weeks after administration of RenCa cells all groups animals begun to develop tumors. All Balb/c mice that received 'mock' transduced cells were bearing palpable tumors at this time. Within 5 weeks all animals in each group developed tumors. There was a visible difference between the GM-CSF and IL-6 group. During the first 4 weeks of experiment mice that received the IL-6 RenCa cells were developing tumors slower than the GM-CSF group (Fig. 1) Moreover the mean tumor volume was significantly ($p<0,05$) smaller as assessed 5 weeks after inoculation (data not shown).

3.2 The slowest formation of tumors in mice immunized with RenCa cells expressing GM-CSF

Mice immunized with irradiated control cells begun to develop tumors within 3 weeks after rechallenge with wild type cells (Fig. 2). The mice immunized with IL-6 GMTV started to form tumors one week later than the control group. Mice immunized with irradiated cells expressing GM-CSF displayed the slowest dynamic of tumor formation. Tumors developed in this group in 100% of animals 7 weeks after rechallenge with wild type cells. The mean tumor volume in the GM-CSF immunized group was significantly smaller ($p<0,05$) then in other groups studied (data not shown).

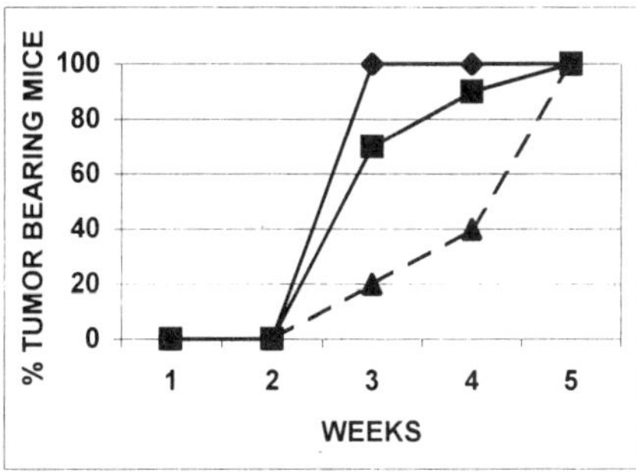

Figure 1. Tumor take in mice, that received genetically modified cells. ◆ - control cells; ■ - GM-CSF; ▲ - IL-6

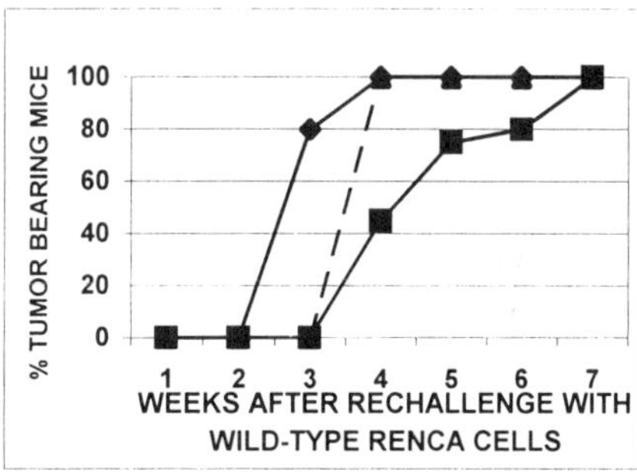

Figure 2. Tumor take in mice preimmunized ith following GMTVs: ◆ - control cells, ■ - GM-CSF, ▲ - IL-6

3.3 IL-6 or GM-CSF induce antitumoral immune response by different patterns.

Seven days after administration of genetically modified cells the tumors were excised and the infiltrating immune cells were analyzed by flow cytometry. RenCa-IL-6 cells were heavily infiltrated by activated CD4+ and CD8+ cells. The number of activated T cells infiltrating tumors formed by control cells was much lower, however it was still higher than in the case of

GM-CSF-transduced cells, which were infiltrated mainly by inactivated CD4+ and CD8+ cells (Table 1)

GM-CSF-transduced cells were attracting high number of acitated dendritic cells (DCs) as assessed by expression of CD40 and CD80 (B-7.1) costimulatory molecules on the CD11c+ cells. Tumors formed by control cells were infiltrated by a lower number of activated dendritic cells than the GM-CSF secreting tumors. In case of animals that received RenCa cells modified with IL-6 the number of tumor infiltrating DCs was even lower.

Table 1. Immunophenotype of cells infiltrating particular tumors.

	% of double-positive tumor infiltrating cells		
	RenCa	RenCa IL-6	RenCa GM-CSF
CD4 CD25	21,7	55	20,3
CD4 CD69	37,2	59,3	28
CD8 CD25	19,2	39,9	2,6
CD8 CD69	14,5	60,5	16,7
CD11c CD40	20,8	3,2	31,8
CD11c CD80	63	57	75

4. CONCLUSIONS

GM-CSF expressing GMTVs has been demonstrated to be effective in inducing immune response towards renal cell cancer in preclinical models[1,2]. However, we are not aware of any studies on renal cell cancer gene therapy with IL-6 gene, although it was widely studied in other types of cancers[3,4]. We have demonstrated that IL-6 displays an antitumoral activity, which is not as effective as in the case of GM-CSF. By using the Matrigel, for the first time we were able to analyse the immunological phenomena at the site of GMTV administration. The GM-CSF secreting cells attract mainly DCs, which are required for induction of specific antitumoral immune response. The tumors expressing IL-6 are mainly infiltrated by activated lymphocytes, which are the effectory arm of antitumoral immune response. In our studies the GM-CSF GMTV turned out to be more efficient than the IL-6 and to act in different way. However, the different antitumoral mechanisms mediated by these cytokines may act synergistically in order elucidate an immune mediated rejection of established tumors.

ACKNOWLEDGMENTS

This work was supported by grant from Polish State Committee For Scientific Research (Grant No. KBN P05/97 and PBZ-K002/PO4/99).

REFERENCES

1. Ali SA, McLean CS, Boursnell ME, Martin C, Holmes CL, Reeder S et al. Preclinical evaluation of "whole" cell vaccines for prophylaxis and therapy using disabled infectious single cycle-herpes simplex virus vector to transduce cytokine genes. 2001 *Cancer Res.*; 60: 1663-70
2. Wang LG, Ju DW, Sun Y, Tao Q, Qian S, Mi J, Hamada H, Cao X. The potential antitumor effects of combined p16 gene and GM-CSF gene therapy through efficient induction of antitumor immunity. 2001 *J Cancer Res Clin Oncol.*; 127: 101-108
3. Porgador A, Tzehoval E, Katz A, Vadau E, Revel M, Feldman M, Eisenbach L. Interleukin 6 gene transfection into Lewis lung carcinoma tumor cells suppresses the malignant phenotype and confers immunotherapeutic competence against parental metastatic cells. 1992 *Cancer. Res; 52: 3679-86*
4. Mackiewicz A, Wiznerowicz M, Roeb E, Karczewska A, Nowak J, Heinrich PC, Rose-John S. Soluble interleukin 6 receptor is biologically active in vivo. 1995 *Cytokine*; 7: 142-49
5. Drakesmith H, O'Neil D, Schneider SC, Binks M, Medd P et al. In vivo priming of T cells against cryptic determinants by dendritic cells exposed to interleukin 6 and naïve angigen. 1998 *Proc. Natl. Acad. Sci; 95: 14903-08.*

The effects of peritumoral therapeutic vaccination with IL-2-secreting cells on growth of MC38 colon tumours in mice, local NO production and sentinel lymph node cells activation

ELŻBIETA PAJTASZ–PIASECKA[#], HALINA KUŚNIERCZYK[#], KRZYSZTOF P. KRAWCZYK[*], EGBERT PIASECKI[#], MARTYNA ELAS[*], and CZESŁAW RADZIKOWSKI[#]
[#]*Institute of Immunology and Experimental Therapy, P.A.S, R. Weigl St 12, Wrocław, Poland*
[*]*Institute of Molecular Biology, Jagiellonian University, A. Mickiewicz Av. 3, Kraków, Poland*

1. INTRODUCTION

The antitumor effects of cytokines used in cancer immunotherapy depend on the actual balance between the host immune system and a growing tumor. One of the most potent regulatory molecules that play a critical role in generating a successful immune response is interleukin-2 (IL-2), which like other cytokines, acts in a paracrine and autocrine manner. The cytokine induces a broad spectrum of biological events, which in some cases lead to tumor regression. Among others IL-2 stimulates the proliferation of $CD8^+$ T cells and their IFN-γ production. By initiation of cascade of secondary cytokines, especially IFN and TNF-α, IL-2 is also involved in activation of macrophages. Activated macrophages produce nitric oxide (NO), defined as an effector molecule that can kill or inactivate target cells.

Systemic application of IL-2 is greatly limited by toxic side effects as well as rapid degradation and elimination of the cytokine from the circulation. When applied locally, IL-2 acts at the site of immune reaction (the tumor and draining lymph nodes); therefore local delivery of IL-2 seems to be a more rational approach.

Repeated administrations of recombinant IL-2 directly into a tumor or in the proximity of a draining lymph nodes (LN) may result in tumor rejection[1]. To secure prolonged secretion of the cytokine at the tumor site other approaches than multiple injections of the protein, for instance immuno-gene therapy seem more rational.

In our model of IL-2 immunotherapy murine plasmocytoma cells transfected with the cytokine gene were repeatedly administered in the vicinity of unrelated tumours growing subcutaneously (s.c.) in syngeneic, semi-syngeneic or semi-allogeneic mice[2, 3].

In the presented study the immunomodulating effect of the cellular vaccine was evaluated by estimation *in vitro* of the production of IL-2 and IFN by primed *in vivo* LN cells (LNc) and by NO production in the tumour tissue.

2. RESULTS

Mice bearing advanced s.c. colon tumours were injected peritumorally with IL-2-transfected cells (X63mIL-2). Usually about 10^7 cells/mouse/inj. were given once a week in 4-7 injections altogether. Therapeutic effect of the treatment was evaluated by tumour growth delay, increase in life-span, and complete tumour regressions: altogether 15% of treated mice (18 out of 120, data cumulated from 11 independent experiments) were cured. Tumour-free survival was a life span long and mice were found to be resistant to the tumour rechallenge. Figure 1 illustrates changes in MC38 tumour growth during X63mIL-2 therapy in one of these experiments.

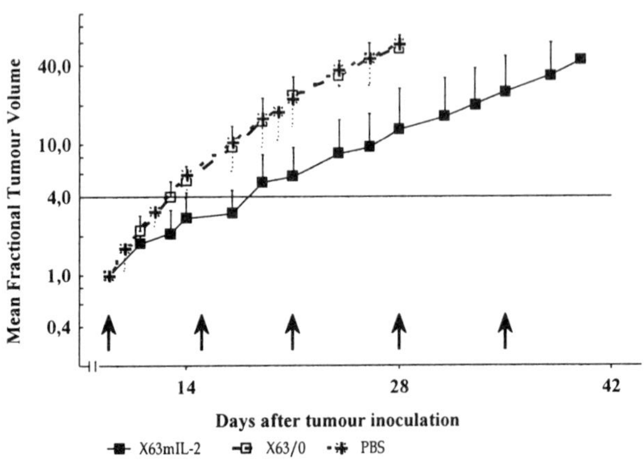

Figure 1. MC38 tumour growth in mice treated with IL-2-secreting cells.
Mice with s.c. tumours (10 in each group) were given peritumoural injections of X63mIL-2 cells or PBS once a week (arrows).

Lymph nodes were harvested 7 days after each injection of IL-2-secreting cells and LNc were maintained in culture for 24h, with or without Con A.

IL-2 and IFN activities in supernatants were estimated in the appropriate bioassays. The level of IL-2 decreased gradually with consecutive injections of X63mIL-2 cells, both in Con A$^-$ and in ConA$^+$ supernatants. The stepwise increase in IFN level was observed only in Con A stimulated cultures; in Con A$^-$ supernatants IFN activity did not exceed 6 LU/ml. These results are shown in figure 2.

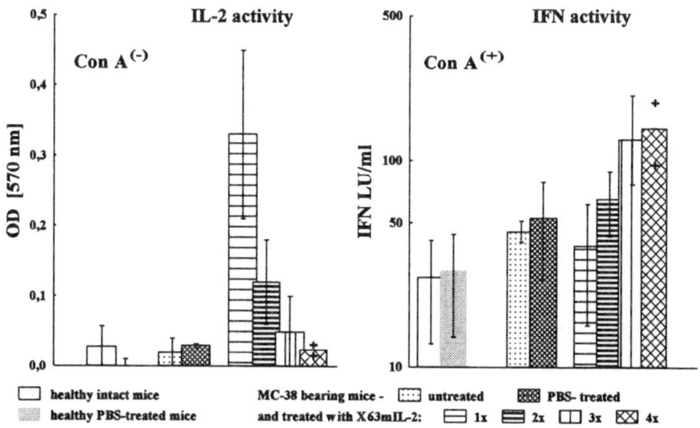

Figure 2. IL-2 and IFN activity in culture supernatants of LNc harvested from mice inoculated with X63mIL-2 cells.

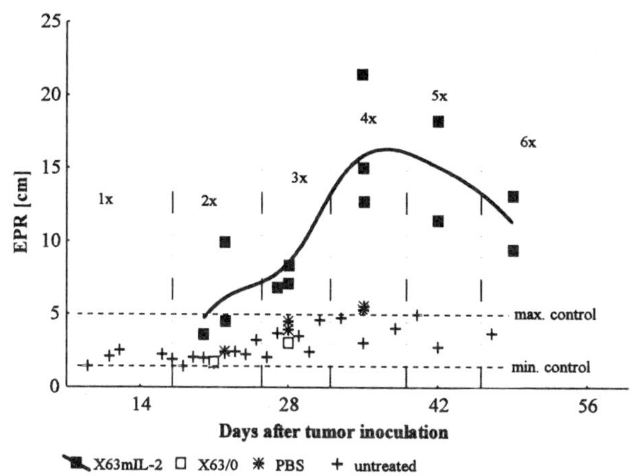

Figure 3. Nitric oxide levels in MC38 tumors. In treated mice tumors were excised 4 days after each injection.

Nitric oxide production at the tumour site was measured by estimation of the amplitude of the 2nd hyperfine line of a nitrosohemoglobin triplet (EPR) in MC38 tumors excised from treated mice 2, 4 or 7 days after each injection. Nitric oxide level before treatment (day 11) was low and did not increase significantly in untreated mice during observation period of 47 days.

Multiple peritumoural injections of PBS or wild type plasmocytoma cells did not cause marked elevation of NO production. However, gradual increase in NO level in tumour tissue was observed after consecutive injections of IL-2-secreting cells. The significant, up to five-fold increase was detected after 3 or more injections of tranfectants. Figure 3 shows changes in NO level in MC38 tumours taken 4 days after administration of PBS, X63/0 or X63mIL-2 cells.

3. CONCLUSION

Local administrations of IL-2-secreting cells has therapeutic effect expressed by tumour growth retardation, increase in life-span and 15% complete response rate. Cured mice were protected against tumour rechallenge. Gradual decrease in IL-2 production and increase of IFN secretion by draining LN cells *in vitro* was observed. At the tumour site marked elevation of nitric oxide production was detected after three or more injections of IL-2-producing cells.

ACKNOWLEDGMENTS

The work from our laboratory was supported by grant 4 P05A 123 14 from the Committee for Scientific Research (KBN) of the Republic of Poland.

REFERENCES

1. Kaplan B., and Moy R.L., 2000, Effect of Perilesional Injections of PEG-Interleukin-2 on Basal Cell Carcinoma. *Dermatol. Surg.* 26: 1037-1040.
2. Pajtasz-Piasecka E., Glazman-Kuśnierczyk H., Salwa J., Konarski L., and Radzikowski C., 1995, Growth inhibition of transplantable tumors in mice by mIL-2-secreting murine plasmocytoma cells used alone or in combination with a cytostatic agent. *Arch. Immunol. Ther. Exp.* 43: 281-292.
3. Kuśnierczyk H., Pajtasz-Piasecka E., and Radzikowski C.: 1999, Synergistic antitumour effects of chemo-immunotherapy with an oxazaphosphorine drug and interleukin-2-secreting cells in a mouse colon cancer model. *Medical Oncology* 16: 267-278.

Improving the retroviral vector (RV) systems for immunotherapy of cancer

PIOTR GRABARCZYK[*,#], KATARZYNA GRYSKA[*], PIOTR J. WYSOCKI[*], DARIUSZ IŻYCKI* and ANDRZEJ MACKIEWICZ*
[*]*Department of Cancer Immunology, University School of Medical Sciences at GreatPoland Cancer Center, Poznań, Poland;* [#]*Postgraduate School of Molecular Medicine, Warsaw, Poland*

1. INTRODUCTION

Most protocols of gene therapy clinical trials are based on immunotherapy strategies with genetically modified tumor vaccines (GMTV). The major issue when designing GMTV is gene delivery system; RV proven to be very useful for ex vivo transduction of therapeutic genes. The advantages of RV include: easy manipulation of small viral genome, stable integration of transduced gene and safety. Most frequently, Gibbon Ape Leukemia Virus (GaLV) and Amphotropic Murine Leukemia Virus (A-MuLV) envelope proteins are used to pseudotype RV-based vectors. Such vector pseudotypes infect target cells by their specific receptors: PiT1 and PiT2, respectively. Both receptors belong to the same family[1], and despite high degree homology, no cross interference is observed.

Since human cells differ in the transducilbility and the correlation between PiT1 and PiT2 mRNA levels and GaLV and A-MuLV mediated infectibility was reported[2,3], it was of our interest if such relation could be established for tumor cell lines, derived from human melanoma and renal cell carcinoma. Another goal was to determine which vector pseudotype is more efficient for the transduction of appropriate cells.

Progress in Basic and Clinical Immunology, Edited by Mackiewicz *et al.*
Kluwer Academic/Plenum Publishers, New York, 2001

2. MATERIALS AND METHODS

2.1 Cells and vector pseudotypes

PA317, TE-FLY-A, TE-FLY-GA, renal cell carcinoma (P54, P58, P66, P138) and human melanoma cell lines (A375, WM9, WM35, WM339, WM902b) were cultured in standard conditions.

The bicistronic retroviral vector, encoding enhanced green fluorescent protein (EGFP) was constucted basing of MSCV2.1 RV. The construct pMINV-EGFP was introduced into PA317 cells by electroporation, followed by selection in G418 (800μg/ml). The infection medium was used to transduce TE-FLY-A and TE-FLY-GA packaging cells. GaLV and A-MuLV pseudotypes carrying pMINV-EGFP vectors were harvested, filtered (0.45μm pore size), titrated and used for infection assays. Relative virus concentration was measured by whole virion dot-blott hybrydization, with radiolabeled EGFP-specific probe. Media of equal virus concentration were used for all transduction assays. Cells were infected by 24h exposure to the virus containing medium with Polybrene (4μg/ml). The transduction efficiency was evaluated by FACS analysis of EGFP expressing cells.

2.2 Quantitative, competitive RT-PCR

Competitive templates were generated by amplification of PiT1, PiT2 and GAPDH fragments, ligation into T-easy vector and introduction of 86 bp random stuffer sequence. Total RNA isolated from target cells were reverse transcribed and amlpified with various amounts of competitive templates, using pairs of primers: GA: ATGAGCCCCAGGCTTCTCCAT, GS: GGTCGGAGTTCAACGGGATTT, P1A: CAGCAACGGTGCTCCAG, P1S: GTGTGGCAACTCGTGGCTTC, P2A: GCTGGTCATGAGAGAGCCGTG, P2S: CGGAACATCTTCGTGGCCTG. PCR products were analyzed by agarose gel electrophoresis and Vilber Lourmat gel documentation system.

3. RESULTS AND CONCLUSIONS

Quantitative RT-PCR analysis revealed PiT1 and PiT2 expression in all lines studied. The amounts of receptor mRNAs was different not only between melanoma and renal cell carcinoma cell lines, but also between cells derived from the same tumor. Generally, PiT1 was present at higher levels than PiT2. Both receptors were more abundant in melanoma cells than renal cell carcinoma cells (Table 1.). The highest level of PiT1 and PiT2 receptors was observed in WM902b cells, 24,7% and 4,5%, respectively, compared to GAPDH, as an external standard. Among renal cell carcinoma, P54 showed the highest amounts of both receptors, but the expression was markedly lower, compared to melanoma.

Table 1. PiT1 and PiT2 mRNAs in renal cell carcinoma and human melanoma cells (% of GAPDH) compared to transduction efficiency.

	PiT1 mRNA and GaLV transduction		PiT2 mRNA and A-MoMLV transduction	
Melanoma cells	PiT1 mRNA	EGFP posit. cells	PiT2 mRNA	EGFP posit. cells
A375	12,6 ± 1,34	10,3 ± 1,3	2,8 ± 0,4	14,95 ± 1,12
WM9	0,99 ± 0,23	18,9 ± 2,1	0,25 ± 0,1	6,07 ± 0,7
WM35	5,38 ± 0,63	2,84 ± 0,26	2,16 ± 0,24	6,77 ± 0,42
WM239	12,8 ± 1,44	27,5 ± 2,51	1,48 ± 0,2	18,2 ± 2,1
WM902B	24,7 ± 0,9	10,44 ± 0,15	4,5 ± 0,041	15,21 ± 2,3
Renal cancer cells				
P54	2,25 ± 0,51	7,8 ± 0,7	1,44 ± 0,23	2,7 ± 0,28
P58	0,74 ± 0,21	8,52 ± 0,6	0,52 ± 0,11	2,71 ± 0,4
P66	0,64 ± 0,12	0,36 ± 0,12	0,006± 0,003	3,87 ± 0,5
P138	0,13 ± 0,05	7,04 ± 1,2	0,007± 0,002	0,81 ± 0,12

To investigate, whether receptor mRNA levels correlate with infectibility, 4 renal cell carcinoma and 5 human melanoma lines were exposed to GaLV and A-MuLv pseudotyped vectors carrying EGFP. Genarally, human melanoma lines were susceptible to infection by both GaLV and A-MuLV pseudotyped vectors, while renal cell carcinoma were only poorly transducible (Table 1.). The transduction efficiency varied for both pseudotypes, but the differences in EGFP positive cells did not reflect the various expression of PiT1 and PiT2 mRNAs. Higher receptor mRNA did not provide the better transduction efficiency. Cells with over 12- fold lower PiT1 mRNA level (WM9 and A375) could be infected 2-times better (Fig.1). The same could be demonstrated, when both receptors in one cell line were considered. All cell lines analyzed, expressed less PiT2 than PiT1 mRNA, but some of them could be transduced with higher efficiency by A-MuLV than GaLV pseudotypes (P66 and A375). The data presented here revealed that the expression of RV receptors, on the mRNA level, did not correlate with the susceptibility to infection by appropriate vector pseudotype. The lack of correlation was observed both between two types of tumor-derived cell lines and even between cells derived from the same kind of tumor.

The results suggest, that retroviral receptor mRNA is not predictive of transducibility by A-MLV and GaLV pseudotyped vectors. Although both receptors can be detected on both types of cell lines and in some cases the levels of expression seem to correlate with transduction efficiency, the extended analysis does not confirm that. This is in agreement with other observations[4], however there was no data comparing cells derived from the same tumor type. We showed, that the different susceptibility to transduction is not restricted to different tissue or tumor.

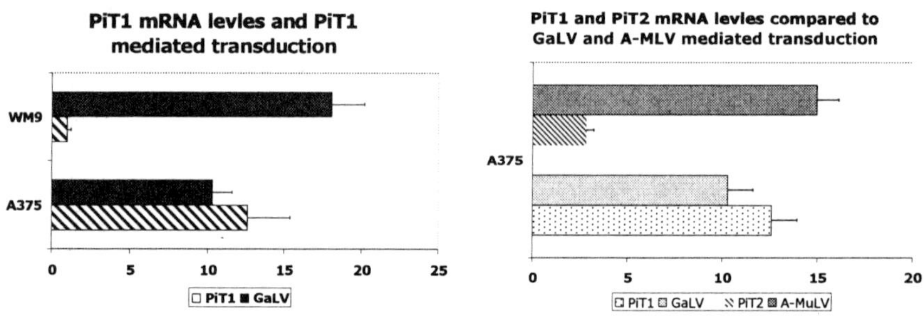

Figure 1. Lack of correlation between expression of PiT1 and PiT2 mRNAs and transduction efficiency with PiT1 and PiT2 targeted retroviral vectors.

ACKNOWLEDGMENTS

This work was supported by grant from Polish State Committee For Scientific Research (PBZ-K002/PO4/99).

REFERENCES

1. O`Hara B., Johann S.V., Klinger H.P., Blair D.G., Rubinson H., Dunn K.J., Sass P., Vitek S.M. and Robins T. (1990) Characterization of human gene confering sensitivity to infection by gibbon ape leukemia virus. Cell Growth Differ. 1, 119-127.
2. Bauer T.R. Jr., Miller A.D. and Hickstein D.D. (1995) Improved transfer of the leukocyte integrin CD18 subunit into hematopoietic cell lines by using retroviral vectors having gibbon ape leukemia virus envelope. Blood 86, 2379-2387.
3. Orlic D., Girard L.J., Jordan C.T., Anderson S.M., Cline A.P., and Bodin D.M. (1996) The level of mRNA encoding the amphotropic retrovirus receptor in mouse and human hematopoietic stem cells is low and correlates with the efficiency of retrovirus transduction. Proc. Natl. Acad. Sci. U.S.A., 93, 11097-11102.
4. Uckert W., Willimsky G., Pedresen F.S., Blankenstein T., and Pedersen L. (1998) RNA levels of human Retrovirus Receptors PiT1 and PiT2 do not correlate with infectibility by three retroviral vector pseudotypes. Human Gene Ther. 9:2619-2627.

Tumor immunity in mice immunized with fibroblasts transfected with tumor DNA

EDWIN F. de ZOETEN, DONGHUA LI and EDWARD P. COHEN*
*Department of Microbiology and Immunology, *University of Illinois, Chicago, Illinois 60612*

1. INTRODUCTION

Accumulating evidence from multiple sources[1] indicates that cancer cells form unique tumor associated antigens (TAAs). Under appropriate circumstances, they can become the targets of immune-mediated attack. Immunization of tumor-bearing animals, and patients, with tumor vaccines can stimulate anti tumor immune responses[2,3] leading to tumor rejection.

Several approaches have been used to prepare tumor vaccines for use in cancer therapy. Vaccines were prepared by the introduction of expression-competent genes for various immune-augmenting cytokines into malignant cells[4-6]. Immunization of experimental animals with the cytokine-secreting cells led to the rejection of both the modified as well as unmodified tumor cells. Genes for foreign (to the host) MHC-determinants or genes specifying co stimulatory molecules such as B7.1[7] have also been introduced into tumor cells to augment their immunogenic properties. Since, in most instances, normal, nonmalignant cells of the immunized, tumor-bearing host were not affected, the anti tumor immune responses were directed toward unique TAAs expressed by the malignant cells.

Other approaches have involved pulsing dendritic cells (DCs) with tumor antigens in the form of whole cell lysates[8], peptides[9], protein[10], or RNA[11]. Primary class I or class II restricted T-cell responses that resulted in anti tumor effects developed in immunized experimental animals and patients.

We investigated an alternative approach that has important practical benefits[12]. We found that undefined, weakly antigenic TAAs were expressed in a highly immunogenic form by a fibroblast cell line that was transfected with genomic DNA from cancer cells[12-13]. Immunization of mice with the DNA-transfected cells resulted in potent anti tumor cellular immune responses that were specific for the type of tumor from which the DNA was obtained. The advantages were that an effective vaccine can be prepared with only small quantities of DNA from primary neoplasms, the vaccine encompasses an array of TAAs that characterize the neoplasm, and the cells used as DNA-recipients can be selected for special characteristics such as the expression of allogeneic MHC-determinants to enhance their immunogenic properties.

In prior studies, the cells used as DNA-recipients were modified before DNA-transfer to secrete IL-2. Here, to further simplify this approach, we tested the immunogenic properties of IL-2-nonsecreting allogeneic fibroblasts transfected with DNA from either of two different mouse neoplasms, melanoma and squamous cell carcinoma. The rejection of cells expressing allogeneic MHC-determinants by the tumor-bearing host might be a sufficient stimulus to the secretion of various immune-augmenting cytokines into the site of injection of the vaccine. The results indicated that mice immunized with (IL-2 non-secreting) transfected fibroblasts developed robust anti tumor responses that were capable of prolonging the survival of tumor-bearing mice.

2. MATERIALS AND METHODS

2.1 Cell lines and experimental animals

Pathogen-free C57BL/6J ($H\text{-}2^b$) or DBA/2 ($H\text{-}2^d$) mice were obtained from the Jackson Laboratory (Bar Harbor, ME). They were maintained in the animal care facilities of the University of Illinois according to NIH Guidelines for the Care and Use of Laboratory Animals. The mice were 8 to 12 weeks old when used in the experiments.

B16 cells, a highly malignant melanoma cell line derived from a spontaneous neoplasm occurring in a C57BL/6 mouse, were obtained from I. Fidler, (M.D. Anderson Cancer Center, Houston, TX). KLN/205 cells, a squamous cell carcinoma cell line derived from a tumor arising in the lung of a DBA/2 mouse, were from the American Type Culture Collection (Rockville, MD). Both tumor cell lines were maintained by serial passage in histocompatible C57BL/6J or DBA/2J mice respectively, or at 37^0C in a humidified 7% CO_2/air atmosphere in standard growth medium (Dulbecco's modified Eagle's medium supplemented with 10 % fetal bovine serum and antibiotics). LM cells were obtained from the American Type Culture Collection. The cells were maintained at 37^0C in a humidified 7% CO_2/air atmosphere in growth medium.

2.2 Modification of LM cells for the secretion of IL-2 and for the expression of H-2K^b class I-determinants

LM cells were modified for IL-2-secretion by transduction with a retroviral vector, pZipNeoSVIL-2 (from M.K.L. Collins, University College, London, England) (LM-IL-2 cells) as described previously[18]. Every third passage, the transduced cells were maintained in growth medium containing 400 ug/ml G418. A plasmid, pBR327H-2K^b (Biogen Research Corp., Cambridge, MA), specifying H-2K^b-determinants was used to modify LM-IL-2 cells for the expression of H-2K^b-determinants (LM-IL-2K^b cells), as described previously [14].

2.3 Immunofluorescent staining and cytofluorometric measurements

Quantitative immunofluorescence measurements were used to detect the expression of B7.1 and H-2K^b-determinants by LM-IL-2 cells as described previously[14]. The measurements were performed in an Epic V flow cytofluorograph (Coulter Electronics, Hialeah, FL) equipped with a multiparameter data-acquisition and display system (MDADS). At least 10^4 cells were analyzed to generate one-parameter fluorescence histograms.

2.4 Transfection of LM mouse fibroblasts with genomic DNA from B16 melanoma or KLN205 squamous cell carcinoma cells

High molecular weight DNA from B16 or KLN205 cells was used to transfect LM, LM-IL-2 and LM-IL-2K^b fibroblasts as described previously[12]. Briefly, genomic DNA from the tumor cells was sheared by passage through a number 25 gauge needle. Afterward, 100 ug of sheared DNA was mixed with 10 ug pHyg, a plasmid that encodes the *E. Coli* enzyme hygromycin B phosphotransferase gene, conferring resistance to hygromycin B. The sheared DNA and pHyg were mixed with Lipofectin according to the manufacturer's instructions and added to a population of 1 X 10^7 LM fibroblasts that had been divided into ten 100 mm plastic cell culture plates 24 hrs. previously. Eighteen hrs. after adding the DNA/Lipofectin mixture to the cells, the medium was replaced with fresh growth medium containing

500 ug/ml hygromycin B (Boehringer Mannheim, Indianapolis, IN). In some instances, DNA from tumor cells was omitted and 10 ug of pHyg alone was mixed with Lipofectin and added to an equivalent number of the fibroblasts. One hundred percent of non-transfected fibroblasts maintained in the hygromycin-growth medium died within 14 days in growth medium. The surviving colonies (more than 2 X 10^4 in each instance) of hygromycin-resistant fibroblasts transfected with pHyg and DNA from the tumor cells, or with pHyg alone (LM-IL-2K^b) were pooled and used in the experiments.

2.5 Statistical analyses

The Student *t* test was used to determine the statistical differences between the survival and cytotoxic activities in mice in various experimental and control groups. A *p* value equal to or less than 0.01 was considered significant.

3. RESULTS

3.1 Modification of LM cells, a fibroblast cell line for the expression of H-2K^b class I determinants

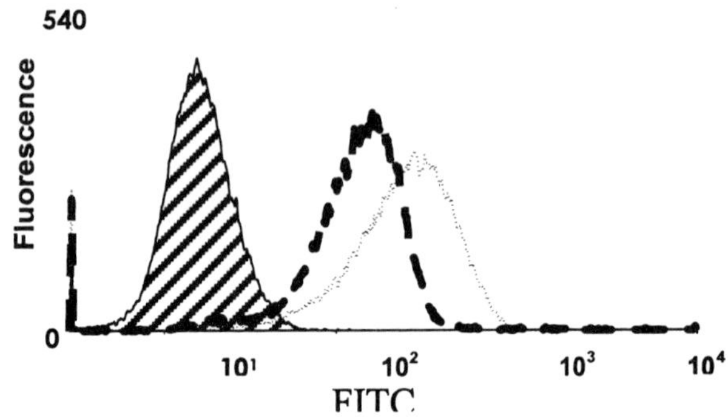

Figure 1. Immunofluorescent staining of LM-IL-2 cells transfected with pBR327H-2K^b with mAbs for H-2K^b-determinants. LM-IL-2 cells transduced with the plasmid pBR327H-2K^b (LM-IL-2K^b cells) were dissociated from 100 mm^2 tissue culture petri dishes with EDTA (0.1mM), and then incubated for 1 hr. at 4° with FITC-conjugated anti-H-2K^b (thick line), or FITC-conjugated anti-H-2K^k (thin line). As a control, aliquots of the cell suspensions were treated in the same way except that FITC-conjugated-IgG_{2a} isotype serum (shaded curve) was substituted for the mAbs.

LM fibroblasts were modified to express H-2K^b class I determinants by transfection with the plasmid pBR327H-2K^b. A second plasmid, pBabePuro (conferring resistance to puromycin) was included to increase the likelihood that the puromycin-resistant cells had taken up the vector specifying H-2K^b – determinants as well (10 ug of pBR327H-2K^b to 1 ug pBabePuro). The cells were grown in puromycin containing media to select for transfected cells. As determined by quantitative immunofluorescence measurements (Figure 1), the transfected cells (LMK^b) stained positively with H-2K^b monoclonal antibodies (mAb). The cells, of C3H mouse origin, also stained with H-2K^k mAbs, the natural MHC determinant. The expression of H-2K^b-determinants by the transfected cells was stable. The cells stained with equivalent intensity with H-2K^b mAbs after three months of continuous culture.

3.2 Comparison of the survival of C57BL/6J mice with B16 melanoma treated by immunization with IL-2-secreting or non secreting LMKb fibroblasts transfected with genomic DNA from B16 cells

A melanoma vaccine was prepared by transfecting (IL-2-nonsecreting) LMK^b fibroblasts with genomic DNA from B16 cells (LMK^b/B16 cells). The immunotherapeutic properties of the vaccine were determined by injecting C57BL/6J mice s.c. with B16 cells and LMK^b/B16 cells, followed by two subsequent injections at weekly intervals of LMK^b/B16 cells alone. The results (Figure 2) indicated that mice injected with B16 cells and the vaccine survived significantly ($P < .01$) longer than mice injected with an equivalent number of B16 cells alone. The survival of mice injected with B16 cells and (non DNA-transfected) LMK^b cells was not significantly different than that of mice injected with B16 cells alone. It was significantly less than that of mice with melanoma treated with fibroblasts transfected with DNA from the melanoma cells.

The survival of C57BL/6J mice injected with B16 cells and IL-2-secreting or non-secreting transfected fibroblasts was compared to determine if IL-2-secretion contributed significantly to the cells' immunogenic properties. As indicated (Figure 2), the survival of mice with melanoma treated by immunization with the cytokine-secreting or non secreting transfected cells was not significantly different ($P > .01$). Mice in both groups survived significantly longer than mice in various control groups including naive C57BL/6J mice injected with B16 cells and (non DNA-transfected) LM-IL-2 cells. The difference in the survival of mice injected with B16 cells alone, and with B16 cells and LM-IL-2 cells was not significant ($P > 0.1$) consistent with the expression of melanoma associated antigens by the DNA-transfected cells.

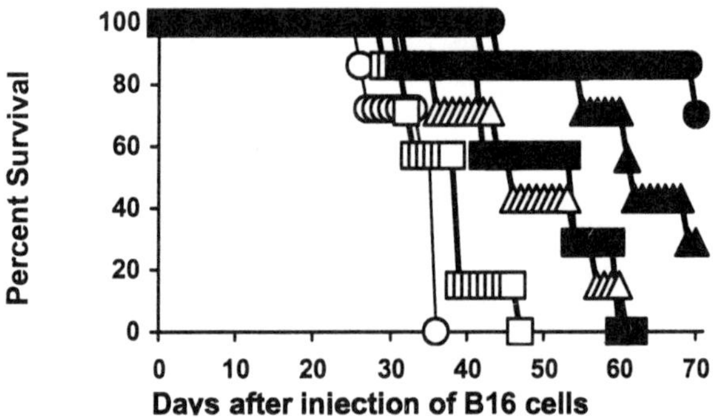

Figure 2. C57BL/6 mice (7 per group) were injected s.c. with a mixture of 5 x 10^3 B16 cells and 2 x 10^6 LM-K^b/B16 cells (closed triangles). At the same time, the mice received a second injection i.p. of 2 x 10^6 LM-K^b/B16 cells alone. As controls, other naive C57BL/6J mice were injected according to the same protocol with equivalent numbers B16 cells and LM-IL-2K^b/B16 cells (closed circles), with B16 cells and LM-IL-2 cells (closed squares), with B16 cells and LM-IL-2K^b cells (open triangles), with B16 cells and LM-K^b cells (open squares), or with B16 cells alone (open circles). The mice in each treatment group were injected twice more, at weekly intervals, with the same number of the relevant cell type or with media, but without additional B16 cells.

H-2K^b class I-determinants, syngeneic in C57BL/6J mice, augmented the cells' immunogenic properties. The survival of mice injected with B16 cells and fibroblasts that expressed both syngeneic and allogeneic MHC-determinants (LM-IL-2K^b/B16 cells) was significantly longer than the survival of mice injected with B16 cells and (K^b non expressing) LM-IL-2/B16 cells ($P < .001$, these data are not presented).

Thus, the greatest therapeutic benefit was in the group of mice treated with transfected cells that expressed both syngeneic and allogeneic MHC-determinants. IL-2-secretion by the transfected cells had no significant effect on the immunotherapeutic properties of the vaccine.

3.3 Survival of mice with squamous cell carcinoma (SCC) treated by immunization with (non cytokine-secreting) LM fibroblasts transfected with genomic DNA from SCC

The vaccine was prepared by transfection of (non cytokine-secreting) LM fibroblasts with DNA from KLN205 cells, a squamous carcinoma cell line. Three protocols were used to test the cells' immunotherapeutic properties in DBA/2 mice, syngeneic with the SCC. In the first, the mice were injected with the vaccine before they were injected with the malignant cells. In the second, mice injected with small numbers of SCC were treated by immunization with the vaccine, and in the third, mice with larger, established tumors received treatment with the vaccine. The results (Figure 3) indicate the efficacy of the non cytokine-secreting transfected cells. None of the mice immunized with the DNA-based vaccine before injection of the carcinoma cells developed tumors. They survived indefinitely (more than 70 days after tumor injection). Mice with small tumor burdens (injected with 2 X 10^5 SCC at the same time as the first injection of the vaccine) and mice with larger established tumors (injected with 5 X 10^5 cells two weeks before the first therapeutic injection of the vaccine) survived significantly (P = .01) longer than mice injected with an equivalent number of SCC cells alone (Figure 3). An analogous protocol was followed to determine if IL-2-secretion by the transfected fibroblasts augmented the immunogenic properties of the vaccine. The results indicated that the survival of mice with larger tumor burdens treated with cytokine-secreting cells or non secreting tansfected cells were not significantly different (these data are not presented).

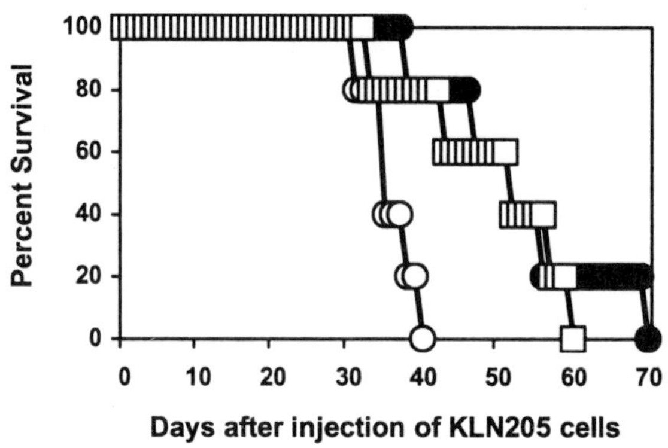

Figure 3. DBA/2mice (5 per group) were injected s.c. with 5 x 10^5 KLN205 cells. 2 weeks later, the mice were injected with 2 x 10^6 LM/KLN205 cells (closed circles). At the same time, the mice received a second injection i.p. of 2 x 10^6 LM/KLN205 cells alone. As controls, other naive C57BL/6J mice were injected according to the same protocol with equivalent numbers KLN205 cells and LM/KLN205 cells simultaneously (open squares), or with KLN205 cells alone (open circles). The mice in each treatment group were injected twice more, at weekly intervals, with the same number of LM/KLN205 cells, or media, but without additional KLN205 cells.

4. DISCUSSION

In prior studies, we found that tumor immunity was generated in mice immunized with IL-2-secreting fibroblasts transfected with genomic DNA from different mouse neoplasms. The immunity, mediated predominantly by

NK/LAK and $CD8^+$ cells, was directed toward the type of tumor from which the DNA was obtained. This was the case for mice with melanoma, lymphoma, and breast cancer. The immunizations were non-toxic, and did not lead to autoimmune disease.

Here, we asked if the cells' immunogenic properties were dependent on the secretion of IL-2. We found that the survival of mice with melanoma treated solely by immunization with IL-2-secreting or IL-2 non-secreting transfected fibroblasts were not significantly different from each other. For mice with SCC, animals with small tumor burdens, or with established tumors, treated with IL-2-nonsecreting transfected cells survived significantly longer than untreated mice. Mice immunized with the DNA-based vaccine before injection of the SCC failed to develop tumors.

Genetic modification of a highly immunogenic cell line expressing allogeneic MHC determinants, rather than modification of the tumor itself was chosen for two non exclusive reasons. The first is that the vaccine can be prepared inexpensively under standard laboratory conditions. Thus, large numbers of cancer patients might receive treatment. The second is that only microscopic amounts of tumor tissue are required to prepare the vaccine. A needle biopsy of the patient's tumor might provide sufficient quantities of DNA to prepare an effective vaccine. In addition, the vaccine has been found to be non-toxic. Autoimmune disease has not been observed in mice immunized with the DNA-based vaccines.

REFERENCES

1. Boon, T., Cerottini, J-C, Van den Eynde, B., van der Bruggen, P. And Van Pel, A. Tumor antigens recognized by T lymphocytes. Annul Rev Immunol 12: 337-360, 1994
2. Boon T. Tumor antigens recognized by cytolytic T lymphocytes: present perspectives for specific immunotherapy. Int. J. Cancer, *54:* 177-180, 1993.
3. Storkus, W.J., Zeh, H.J. III, Maeurer, MJ., Salter, R.D. and Lotze, M.T. Identification of human melanoma peptides recognized by class I restricted tumors infiltrating T lymphocytes. J. Immunol. 151: 3719-3727, 1993
4. Cavallo, F., Pierro, F.D., Giovarelli, M., Gulino, A., Vacca, A., Stoppacciaro, A., Forni, M., Modesti, A., and Forni, G. Protective and curative potential of vaccination with interleukin-2-gene-transfected cells from a spontaneous mouse mammary adenocarcinoma. Cancer Res. 53: 5067-5070, 1993.
5. Golumbek, P.T., Lazenby, A.J., Levitsky, H.I., Jaffee, L.M., Karasuyama, H., Baker, M., and Pardoll, D.M. Treatment of established renal cancer by tumor cells engineered to secrete interleukin-4. Science 254: 713-716, 1991.
6. Mullen, C.A., Coale, M.M., Levy, A.T., Stetler-Stevenson, W.G., Liotta, L.A., Brandt, S., and Blaese, R.M. Fibrosarcoma cells transduced with the IL-6 gene exhibit reduced tumorigenicity, increased immunogenicity, and decreased metastatic potential. Cancer Res. 52: 6020-6024, 1992.

7. Townsend S. E. and Allison, J.P. 1993. Tumor rejection after direct costimulation of CD8$^+$ T cells by B7 transfected melanoma cells Science 259:368.

8.Geraghty PJ, Fields RC, Mule JJ. Vaccination with tumor-pulsed splenic dendritic cells mediates immunity to poorly-immunogenic tumor. Surg. Forum 47: 459-461, 1996.

9.Mayordomo JI, Zorina Y, Storkus WJ, Zitvogel L, Celluzzi C, et al Bone marrow derived dendritic cells pulsed with synthetic tumor peptides elicit protective and therapeutic anti tumo rimmunity. Nat Med 1: 1297-1302, 1995

10.Palgia P, Chiodoni C, Rodolfo M and Colombo MP. Murine dendritic cells loaded in vitro with soluble protein prime cytotoxic T lymphocytes against tumor antigen in vivo. J Exp Med 183: 317-322, 1996

11.Boczkowski D, Nair SK, Nam JH, Lyerly HK, Gilboa E. Induction of tumor immunity and cytotoxic T lymphocyte responses using dendritic cells transfected with messenger RNA amplified from tumor cells. Cancer Res . 2000 Feb 15;60(4):1028-34.

12.Kim, T.S., Russell, S.J., Collins, M.K.L., and Cohen, E.P. Immunity to B16 melanoma in mice immunized with IL-2-secreting allogeneic mouse fibroblasts expressing melanoma associated antigens. Int. J. Cancer 51: 283-289, 1992

13.Kim, T. S. and E. P. Cohen. 1994. Interleukin-2-secreting mouse fibroblasts transfected with genomic DNA from murine melanoma cells prolong the survival of mice with melanoma. *Cancer Research* 54 (May):2531-2535.

14.deZoeten, E.F., Carr-Brendel, V., Cohen, E.P. Resistance to melanoma in mice immunized with semiallogeneic fibroblasts transfected with DNA from mouse melanoma cells. *J. Immuno* 160: 2915-2922, 1998.

T cell response to tumor antigens and its therapeutic use in cancer patients

GIORGIO PARMIANI, CHIARA CASTELLI, PIERO DALERBA and LICIA RIVOLTINI
Unit of Immunotherapy of Human Cancer, Istituto Nazionale Tumori, Via G. Venezian 1, 20133, Milano, Italy

1. INTRODUCTION

The molecular characterization of human tumor antigens has allowed a rapid translation of information gained in basic research into clinical protocols. Melanoma is the tumor that was more frequently studied thanks to several clinical reports suggesting its antigenicity and to the availability of tumor cell lines and autologous T lymphocyte lines or clones that can be obtained from the majority of patients and used for *in vitro* studies[1]. However, several other tumor histotypes have been also analyzed though with less clear-cut results.

Molecular techniques were used to clone genes encoding protein antigens through the screening of cDNA tumor library by cytotoxic T lymphocytes (CTL) clones[2]. An alternative approach to the identification of tumor antigens was adopted which is also dependent on the availability of patients' T cell clones but is based on extraction/elution of antigenic peptides from MHC/peptide complexes expressed on the cell surface of tumor cells, their fractionation by reverse phase HPLC, screening by anti-tumor specific T cells and use of mass spectrometry to sequence the peptide of interest[3].

By using either of these approaches many new tumor antigens (mostly in melanoma) and their epitopes recognized by T cells in the context of class I HLA have been described (see Renkvist *et al.*[4]). More recently, techniques became available that permit molecular characterization of class II HLA-

Progress in Basic and Clinical Immunology, Edited by Mackiewicz *et al.*
Kluwer Academic/Plenum Publishers, New York, 2001

restricted epitopes recognized by CD4 T helper lymphocytes, a finding which paves the way to more effective vaccines for the immunotherapy of cancer patients (for a full list of these antigens see Renkvist *et al.*[4]).

2. CLASSIFICATION OF TUMOR ANTIGENS RECOGNIZED BY T CELLS

According to their molecular nature and tissue distribution, tumor antigens can be classified as follows.

2.1 Antigens Predominantly Expressed by Tumor Cells (or Cancer/Testis Antigens)

These antigens include normal proteins expressed in different tumors but not by normal tissues with the exception of testis. The prototype is MAGE-1 (melanoma antigen-1), the first human tumor antigen recognized by HLA class I-restricted T cells that has been molecularly characterized[2]. In addition to the well known MAGE, BAGE and GAGE families of antigens, recently a new cancer/testis antigen has been described and called NY-ESO-1 which was isolated from esophageal cancer by using patient's serum antibodies and the SEREX technique[5]. NY-ESO-1 mRNA expression is found in 20-30% of melanomas, lung, breast, ovarian and bladder cancers but not in colon or renal cancers[5]. Antibodies to NY-ESO-1 were detected in 40-50% of patients with antigen-expressing tumors.

The *in vitro* and *in vivo* immunogenicity of these antigens is rather weak and no tumor-infiltrating lymphocytes (TIL) could ever be found in cancer patients directed against these families of antigens. Generation of anti-MAGE-3 immunity, however, was recently obtained by using dendritic cells (DC) for its presentation to the immune system[6].

2.2 Differentiation Antigens Recognized by Class I HLA-Restricted T Cells

These antigens are shared between tumor and normal cells from which tumor derives, and have been found mostly in melanomas where these lineage-related normal proteins are involved in the biosynthesis of melanin[7]. These antigens are recognized by peripheral blood lymphocytes that can be stimulated *in vitro* to develop antigen-specific CTL[8]. Therefore, melanocyte differentiation antigens appear to be immunogenic at least in a fraction of patients with a hierarchy that indicates Melan-A/MART-1 as the most immunogenic one.

2.3 Widely Expressed Antigens

Other class I-restricted antigens consist of normal proteins widely expressed both on neoplastic and normal tissues (e.g. p15, Her2/neu, p53). It is possible that many normal protein epitopes expressed by normal tissues are below the threshold level of T-cell recognition, while their overexpression in tumor cells can trigger an anti-cancer response even by breaking a previously established tolerance.

2.4 Tumor-Specific, Class I HLA-Restricted Unique and Shared Antigens

Tumor-specific antigens include two subgroups. Antigens generated by point mutation of normal proteins and expressed by one single tumor only (unique antigens), like CDK4 and β-catenin in melanoma or caspase-8 in head and neck tumors (see Renkvist *et al.*[4]), which, up to now, are of impossible use in vaccination trials owing to the difficulty to prepare peptide-based vaccines from unique antigens at the single patient level. The other subgroup encompasses antigens that are shared among tumors without being found in normal tissues. This kind of antigens, if enough immunogenic, will represent the ideal vaccine that may allow immunization of many patients without generating toxic effects being the normal tissues spared from any harmful immunological reaction. At least two members of this subgroup of tumor antigens (NA17-A and TRP-2/INT2) have been molecularly characterized; in both cases the immunogenic epitopes were created by the translation of retained intronic sequences[9, 10].

In particular, our TRP-2/INT2 antigen was found to be expressed in 70% of melanomas thus lending itself to prospective vaccination studies which, up to now, appear to be limited by the low frequency of the HLA-A68 allele that is necessary to present the antigen[10] though TRP-2/INT2 peptides recognized in the context of HLA-A2 have been recently identified (Sensi *et al.*, manuscript in preparation).

2.5 Class II HLA-Restricted Cancer Antigens

Immunogenicity of class I HLA-restricted tumor antigens is usually weak and only occasionally patients do develop a strong CTL reactivity after immunization with molecularly defined vaccines. Among the many possible reasons of such a phenomenon, the lack of activation of T helper cells may be crucial inasmuch as CD4 T cells appear to be instrumental in eliciting a strong and sustained immune response against tumor antigens. It is a relevant step forward that several class II HLA-restricted epitopes have been recently described. They fall into the group of differentiation antigens of melanoma (e.g. tyrosinase[11]) and cancer/testis antigens (e.g. NY-ESO-1)[12] but several additional epitopes were found to result from point mutations or chromosomal rearrangements of a variety of normal genes (for a complete list of such antigens and their features see Renkvist *et al.*[4]).

Though the molecular identification of many tumor antigens represents a crucial progress in tumor immunology, only peptides generated from cross-reacting, shared normal antigens have been used in clinical trials. In fact, unique antigens that are truly tumor-specific and immunogenic cannot be characterized in a time compatible with their use in metastatic cancer patients in whom tumor is rapidly progressing. However, the use of heat-shock proteins (HSP) which, at least in the mouse system, are known to bind the full repertoire of immunogenic tumor peptides, including the unique ones, and serve as chaperons for the presentation of such peptides by antigen presenting cell (APC), may allow to bypass the need of antigen identification[13]. In fact, we have recently shown that HSP-70 purified from human melanoma efficiently present known melanoma antigens to patients' T cells[14]. This approach appears feasible at single patient's level provided enough tumor tissue is available.

3. RECOGNITION OF TUMOR ANTIGENS BY T CELLS

Most of the antigens discussed above are recognized by patients' T lymphocytes *in vitro* after repeated stimulations and with a variable frequency in a population of cancer patients. Results obtained by this approach, however, do not allow to distinguish between patients whose immune system was already primed *in vivo* against tumor antigens owing to "natural" growth of the neoplasm, from patients whose T cells were primed *in vitro* by the repeated antigenic stimulations. Such a distinction, however, could be made by studies of *ex vivo* enumeration of melanoma antigen-specific T lymphocytes with tetramers[15]. The availability of such a technology has allowed to conclude that 40% of untreated metastatic melanoma patients possess Melan-A/MART1-specific CD45R0+ memory T cells which display tumor cytotoxicity after *in vitro* culture with IL-2 while being ineffective within metastatic lesions despite the presence of the HLA-A2 restricting molecule and of the cognate antigen as shown by immunohistochemistry[15]. These studies thus suggest that tumor growth *in vivo* may activate a specific T-cell response, this response being then unable to effectively counteract tumor growth.

4. THERAPEUTIC USE OF TUMOR ANTIGENS

Thanks to the above findings the development of therapeutic vaccines to treat cancer patients has become a reality. Of the many new, molecularly defined T cell epitopes, several have been used in clinical trials of vaccination in advanced patients with histologically different tumors. The below Table 1 summarizes this situation.

Table 1. Tumor antigens recognized by T cells and their use in clinical studies

Antigen	Tumor	Phase of clinical study
MUC-1	Breast, pancreas	I
CEA	Colon	II
RAS	Colon, pancreas	I-II
MART-1,gp100, tyrosinase	Melanoma	II
PSA, PSMA	Prostate	II, III
MAGE-1,-3	Melanoma, bladder, H/N	I, II
Idiotype	Non-Hodgkin's lymphoma	I, II

The major problem in this first generation of vaccination trials based on the use of well characterized tumor antigens, was the vaccine formulation. In fact, these antigens or their epitopes have been administered by a variety of schedules and routes of injection. Moreover, thanks to the striking progress in the biology and in technical handling of dendritic cells (DC) that can now be easily obtained from cancer patients[16], it became possible to inject autologous DC pulsed with different antigens. This resulted in a significant increase of immunogenicity thus allowing immunization with apparently weakly immunogenic antigens like MAGE-3[17].

We have participated in a multicenter trial of vaccination of metastatic (stage IV) melanoma patients given a MAGE-3.A1 peptide after assessing the expression of such antigen in their tumor cells by PCR. Though the peptide was given without adjuvants, clinical responses were obtained in 7 out of 25 eligible patients (3 CR and 4 PR, 28% RR), most of which durable despite a lack of detectable CTL reaction in the peripheral blood[18].

Tumor antigens have also been injected along with traditional adjuvants like IFA but the only successful trial using such an antigen formulation is that of Rosenberg and co-workers[19]. These authors vaccinated metastatic melanoma patients with the modified gp100-2M peptide in IFA followed by systemic administration of high dose IL-2 and achieved a 38% clinical response rate but again without association with a vaccine-specific CTL response that was detected in the blood of a minority of such patients.

4.1 Unique *vs.* Shared Antigens in Vaccination

As discussed in the previous sections, unique antigens appear to be the most immunogenic ones, at least in the mouse system[13]. In an attempt to use similar antigens to immunize cancer patients, HSP, which should bind a full repertoire of antigenic peptides, including those deriving from unique antigens were purified from autologous tumors. Such an approach has been applied in phase I-II studies of gastro-intestinal tumors and renal cancers with some encouraging results both at clinical and immunological levels[20].

Thus the use of HSP appears to open the possibility of immunizing patients with unique antigens without the need of their previous chracterization. However, it is crucial to demonstrate that such antigens do have a better T cell stimulatory activity *in vitro* as compared to shared antigens obtained from the same human tumor. This evidence is still unavailable and further studies are thus necessary to better characterize human unique antigens before their systematic use in clinical protocols.

ACKNOWLEDGMENTS

The authors' work was supported by the Italian Association for Cancer Research (Milano), by Italian Ministry of Health (Rome) and by the European Commission (EC Grant QLK3-1999-00064).

REFERENCES

1. Parmiani, G., Anichini, A., and Fossati, G., 1990, Cellular immune response against autologous human malignant melanoma: are in vitro studies providing a framework for a more effective immunotherapy? J. Natl. Cancer Inst. USA 82: 361-370.
2. Van der Bruggen, P., Traversari, C., Chomez, P., Lurquin, C., De Plaen, E., Van den Eynde, B., Knuth, A., and Boon, T., 1991, A gene encoding an antigen recognized by cytolytic T lymphocytes on a human melanoma. Science 254: 1643-1647.
3. Cox , A.L., Skipper, J., Chen, Y., Henderson, R.A., Darrow, T.L., Shabanowitz, J., Engelhard, V.H., Hunt, D.F., and Slingluff, C.L. Jr., 1994, Identification of a peptide recognized by five melanoma-specific human cytotoxic T cell lines. Science 264: 716-719.

4. Renkvist, N., Castelli, C. Robbins, P., and Parmiani, G., 2001, A listing of tumor antigens recognized by T cells. Cancer Immunol. Immunother., in press.
5. Chen, Y.T., Scanlan, M.J., Sahin, U., Tureci, O., Gure, A.O., Tsang, S., Williamson, B., Stockert, E., Pfreundschuh, M., and Old, L.J., 1997, A testicular antigen aberrantly expressed in human cancers detected by autologous antibody screening. Proc. Natl. Acad. Sci. USA 94: 1914-1918.
6. Schuler-Thurner, B., Dieckmann, D., Keikavoussi, P., Bender, A., Maczek, C., Jonuleit, H., Roder, C., Haendle, I., Leisgang, W., Dunbar, R., Cerundolo, V., von den Driesch, P., Knop, J., Brocker, E.B., Enk, A., Kampgen, E., and Schuler, G., 2000, Mage-3 and influenza-matrix peptide-specific cytotoxic T cells are inducible in terminal stage HLA-A2.1+ melanoma patients by mature monocyte-derived dendritic cells. J. Immunol. 165: 3492-3496.
7. Anichini, A., Maccalli, C., Mortarini, R., Salvi, S., Mazzocchi, A., Squarcina, P., Herlyn, M., and Parmiani, G., 1993, Melanoma cells and normal melanocytes shared antigens recognized by HLA-A2 restricted cytotoxic T cell clones from melanoma patients. J. Exp. Med. 177: 989-998.
8. Rivoltini, L., Kawakami, Y., Sakaguchi, K., Southwood, S., Sette, A., Robbins, P.F., Marincola, F., Salgaller, M., Yannelli, J.R., Appella, E., and Rosenberg, S.A., 1995, Induction of tumor-reactive CTL from peripheral blood and tumor-infiltrating lymphocytes of melanoma patients by in vitro stimulation with an immunodominant peptide of the human melanoma antigen MART-1. J. Immunol. 154: 2257-2265.
9. Guilloux, Y., Lucas, S., Brichard, V.G., Van Pel, A., Viret, C., De Plaen, E., Brasseur, F., Lethé, B., Jotereau, F., and Boon, T., 1996, A peptide recognized by human cytolytic T lymphocytes on HLA-A2 melanomas is encoded by an intron sequence of the N-acetylglucosaminyltransferase V gene. J. Exp. Med. 183: 1173-1183.
10. Lupetti, R., Pisarra, P., Verrecchia, A., Farina, C., Nicolini, C., Anichini, A., Bordignon, C., Sensi, M., Parmiani, G., and Traversari, C., 1998, Translation of a retained intron in tyrosinase-related protein (TRP) 2 mRNA generates a new cytotoxic T lymphocyte (CTL)-defined and shared human melanoma antigen not expressed in normal cells of the melanocytic lineage. J. Exp. Med. 188: 1005-1016.
11. Topalian, S.L., Rivoltini, L., Mancini, M., Markus, N.R., Robbins, P.F., Kawakami, Y., and Rosenberg, S.A., 1994, Human CD4+ T cells specifically recognize a shared melanoma-associated antigen encoded by the tyrosinase gene. Proc. Natl. Acad. Sci. USA 91: 9461-9465.
12. Zeng, G., Touloukian, C.E., Wang, X., Restifo, N.P., Rosenberg, S.A., and Wang, R-F-, 2000, Identification of CD4+ T cell epitopes from NY-ESO-1 presented by HLA-DR molecules. J. Immunol. 165: 1153-1159.
13. Srivastava, P.K., Menoret, A., Basu, S., Binder, R.J., and McQuade, K.L., 1998, Heat shock proteins come of age: Primitive functions acquire new roles in an adaptive world. Immunity 8: 657-665.
14. Castelli, C., Ciupitu, A.-M.T., Rini, F., Rivoltini, L., Mazzocchi, A., Kiessling, R, and Parmiani, G., 2001, Human HSP70-peptide complexes specifically activate anti-melanoma T-cells. Cancer Res. in press.
15. Anichini, A., Molla, A., Mortarini, R., Tragni, G., Bersani, I., Di Nicola, M., Gianni, A.M., Pilotti, S., Dunbar, R., Cerundolo, V., and Parmiani, G., 1999, An expanded peripheral T cell population to a cytotoxic T lymphocyte (CTL)-defined melanocyte-specific antigen in metastatic melanoma patients impacts on generation of peptide-specific CTLs but does not overcome tumor escape from immune surveillance in metastatic lesions. J. Exp. Med. 190: 651-667.

16. Di Nicola, M., Anichini, A., Mortarini, R., Bregni, M., Parmiani, G., and Gianni, M., 1998, Human dendritic cells: natural adjuvants in antitumor immunotherapy. Cytok. Cell. Mol. Ther. 4: 265-273.
17. Thurner, B., Haendle, I., Roder, C., Dieckman, D., Keikavoussi, P., Jonuleit, H., Bender, A., Maczek, C., Schreiner, D., von den Driesch, P., Brocker, E.B., Steinman, R.M., Enk, A., Kampgen, E., and Schuler, G., 1999, Vaccination with Mage-3A1 peptide-pulsed mature, monocyte-derived dendritic cells expands specific cytotoxic T cells and induces regression of some metastases in advanced stage IV melanoma. J. Exp. Med. 190: 1669-1678.
18. Marchand, M., van Baren, N., Weynants, P., Brichard, V., Dréno, B., Tessier, M.H., Rankin, E., Parmiani, G., Arienti, F., Humbler, Y., Bourlond, A., Vanwijck, R., Liénard, D., Beauduin, M., Dietrich, P.Y., Russo, V., Kerger, J., Masucci, G., Jäger, E., De Greve, J., Atzpodien, J., Brasseur, F., Coulie, P.G., van der Bruggen, P., and Boon, T., 1999, Tumor regressions observed in patients with metastatic melanoma treated with an antigenic peptide encoded by gene MAGE-3 and presented by HLA-A1. Int. J.Cancer 32: 717-721.
19. Rosenberg, S.A., Yang, J.C., Schwartzentruber, D.J., Hwu, P., Marincola, F.M., Topalian, S.L., Restifo, N.P., Dudley, M.E., Schwarz, S.L., Spiess, P.J., Wunderlich, J.R., Parkhurst, M.R., Kawakami, Y., Seipp, C.A., Einhor, J.H., and White, D.E., 1998, Immunologic and therapeutic evaluation of a synthetic peptide vaccine for the treatment of patients with metastatic melanoma. Nature Med. 4: 321-327.
20. Janetzki, S., Palla, D., Rosenhauer, V., Lochs, H., Lewis, J.J., and Srivastava, P.K., 2000, Immunization of cancer patients with autologous cancer-derived heat shock protein gp96 preparations: a pilot study. Int. J. Cancer 88: 232-238.

Humoral responses to melanoma vaccine, genetically modified with interleukin 6 and soluble interleukin 6 receptor

SERGIUSZ NAWROCKI[1], MARIA ŁACIAK[1], DARIUSZ IŻYCKI[2], KATARZYNA GRYSKA[2], PIOTR J. WYSOCKI[1], PIOTR GRABARCZYK[1] ALDONA KARCZEWSKA[1], ALDONA KACZMAREK[1], PAWEŁ MURAWA[1], JULIAN MALICKI[1], STEFAN ROSE-JOHN[3], ANDRZEJ MACKIEWICZ[1,2]

[1]GreatPoland Cancer Centre, Garbary 15, Poznań, Poland; [2]University School of Medical Sciences, Poznań, Poland; [3] Christian-Albrechts University, Kiel, Germany

1. INTRODUCTION

Production of antibodies directed against the tumour antigens is well recognised in cancer patients. However, role of antibodies in antitumour immune responses and their clinical significance is not clear, especially when specific immune therapies aim boosting of cellular responses to tumour cells[1-3]. Moreover, antagonisms between cellular and humoral responses were observed mainly in animal models[4-5]. Recently, so called immune enhancement, in human colon cancer patients was also demonstrated[6] in which depletion of B lymphocytes correlated with tumour regression. On the other hand, several reports suggested that humoral responses are associated with positive clinical outcomes.[7-10]

Molecularly defined melanoma antigens, which are recognised by autologous cytotoxic T lymphocytes, such as MAGE-1, tyrosinase and NY-ESO-1 were reported to induce production of specific antibodies.[11-13] Allogenic melanoma vaccine *Cancervax*, developed by Morton et al., was able to induce anti-MAGE-1 antibodies in about half of immunised patients,

Progress in Basic and Clinical Immunology, Edited by Mackiewicz *et al.*
Kluwer Academic/Plenum Publishers, New York, 2001

which correlated with a favourable clinical course. In the study of Fuji et al. intratumoral treatment with IFN-gamma induced anti-MAGE-1 humoral responses.[14-15] Autologous vaccine, modified with IFN-gamma, induced anti-MAGE-1 humoral responses in 8 out of 13 immunised patients.[16] The most extensive studies of humoral responses against tumour specific antigens recognised by T cells, in metastatic melanoma patients, were carried out by Stockert et al.[17] She was able to detect anti-MAGE-1 and anti-tyrosinase antibodies only in 3 out of 127 patients.

Since Jan. 1996 we have been treating stage IV (AJCC) melanoma patients with genetically modified cellular vaccine (GMTV), according to the published protocol.[18] The objective was to actively immunise HLA-A1 and/or HLA-A2-positive melanoma patients with an admixture of irradiated autologous tumour cells and allogeneic melanoma cells (Mich-1 and Mich-2) genetically engineered to secrete IL-6 and sIL-6R.[19-20] The allogeneic melanoma cell lines Mich-1 and Mich-2 were transduced with the dicistronic double copy retroviral vector, caring the IL-6 and sIL-6R genes. The Mich-1 and Mich-2 cells express the MAGE-1 and MAGE-3 melanoma antigens and are HLA-A1 and A2 positive. 105 melanoma patients received vaccine between January 96 and November 99.

Clinical responses were evaluable in 45 patients with measurable metastatic disease. Median age of patients was 49 years (range: 23-71). There were 25 women and 20 men. 30 patients were in good general condition (grade 0-1, WHO), 15 patients in moderate condition (grade 2, WHO). 19 patients had metastases confined only to soft tissues, 26 had internal organ metastases at the study entry. 6 patients were treated before with IFN-alfa or/and IL-2; 8 patients were treated with tamoxifen; and 7 patients were treated with chemotherapy. In 16 (35%) patients objective clinical responses were seen after immunisation with GMTV. CR (complete regression of metastases) was seen in 4 patients, PR (a decrease of the sum of longest diameters by min. 30%) in 4 patients, and minor responses (a decrease of the sum of the longest diameters by less than 30%) were seen in 8 patients. Progressive disease was noted in 29 (65%) patients.

The aim of the study was to assess humoral immune responses to the vaccine, using an assay based on flow cytometry. Humoral responses to allogeneic melanoma cells, to autologous cells isolated from metastases and to some melanoma associated antigens: MAGE-1, MAGE-3, MART-1 and tyrosinase were analysed. In order to detect antibodies directed against the melanoma antigens we constructed a panel of rat prostate carcinoma cells, genetically modified with the human cDNAs encoding these antigens. Humoral responses were analysed in 48 patients. Clinical significance of humoral responses was evaluated in 26 out of 45 patients, characterised above. The remaining 22 patients, in whom antibody responses were studied, were immunised following surgical removal of all macroscopic metastases. Thus the clinical responses were not evaluable.

2. MATERIALS AND METHODS

2.1 Preparation of melanoma cells for an analysis of surface and intracellular antigens

Allogeneic melanoma cells used to prepare genetically modified vaccine – Mich-1 and Mich-2 after trypsynizaton, or autologous melanoma cells isolated from resected patients' metastases were centrifuged at 1000 rpm for 5 min in 4^0 C and suspended in buffer (Dulbecco's PBS without Mg^{2+} or Ca^{2+}, 1% heat inactivated FCS, 0,09% sodium azide). 1 μL of heat inactivated (30 min, 56^0 C) patients' sera (in different dilutions) were added to cells and such a mixture was incubated for 30 min on ice. Cells were washed with staining buffer, then 2 μL of FTIC-conjugated mouse monoclonal antibodies (Immunotech, USA) directed against human IgG, IgG1, IgG2, and IgM were added and incubated for 30 min on ice. Cells were spined, washed and resuspended in 50 μL of PBS for flow cytometry. In order to analyse humoral responses to intracellular antigens cells were permeabilized according to manufacturer's instructions (Pharmingen, USA) using Cytofix™ and Perm/Wash Solution™. Flow cytometry was performed using Coulter Epics XL (Coulter, USA).

2.2 Preparation of cells genetically modified with MAGE-1, MAGE-3, MART-1 and tyrosinase cDNAs

cDNAs (Invitrogen Corporation, Belgium) encoding the above melanoma antigens were inserted into retroviral vector – DCCMV-IRES-Neo. Amfotropic packaging cells PA-317 (ATCC, CRL 9078) were transfected with DCCMV IRES Neo – MAGE-1, DCCMV IRES Neo – MAGE-3, DCCMV IRES Neo – MART-1, DCCMV IRES Neo – tyrosinase, using electroporation. Recombinant retroviruses carrying corresponding genes were then used to transduce rat prostate carcinoma MAT-LyLu cells.

The expression of genes was verified at the mRNA level. Total RNA was isolated from transduced MAT-LyLu cells according to the Chomczyński's method. Northern blot with specific probes derived from appropriate cDNAs were performed in standard conditions.

Transduced cells were then incubated with patients sera, FITC-conjugated mouse anti-human Ig antibodies, and analysed by flow cytometry for surface and intracellular antibodies as described above.

2.3 Statistical analysis

Correlations between presence of antibodies against allogenic and autologous cells as well as between antibodies against surface and intracellular antigens were evaluated using the Chi^2 test. Correlation between immune or clinical parameters and objective clinical responses was analysed using the Chi^2 test. Differences between means of CD4+/CD8+ ratio between clinical responders and nonresponders were assessed with the t-Student's test. Overall survival of patients was calculated according to the Kaplan-Meier method. Survival rates were compared with the log-rank test.

3. RESULTS

3.1 Humoral responses to allogenic melanoma cells

Sera from 48 immunised patients were analysed. Preimmune sera (collected before first immunization) were compared with postimmune sera, collected after 2-3 months of immunization with melanoma vaccine. Seroconversion against surface and intracellular antigens (with permeabilized cells) was studied. Seroconversion was seen in 22 out of 48 patients (46%). In that patients antibodies against surface antigens were detected in 18 sera (82%), whereas against intracellular antigens in 13 patients (59%). In 9 out of 22 patients both surface and intracellular antigens were found to be correlated ($p=0.06$). In first 7 patients, in whom IgG antibodies were detected, IgG1, IgG2 and IgM antibodies were also studied, but only IgG1 antibodies were present. Kinetics of antibody production during at least one year of immunisation were analysed in selected patients and correlated with clinical course of the disease. There was no detectable difference in sera reactivity while progression or clinical remissions were observed.

3.2 Humoral responses to autologous melanoma cells

In 17 out of 48 patients, analysed as above, humoral responses to autologous cells were studied. In this subgroup seroconversion to allogenic cells was detected in 11 patients, whereas induction of antibody production to autologous cells in 7 patients. In 5 patients antibodies against allogenic and against autologous cells coexisted. However, the small number of patients does not allow performing any reliable statistical analysis, but it is possible that production of antibodies to allogenic cells may correlate with production of antibodies against autologous melanoma cells.

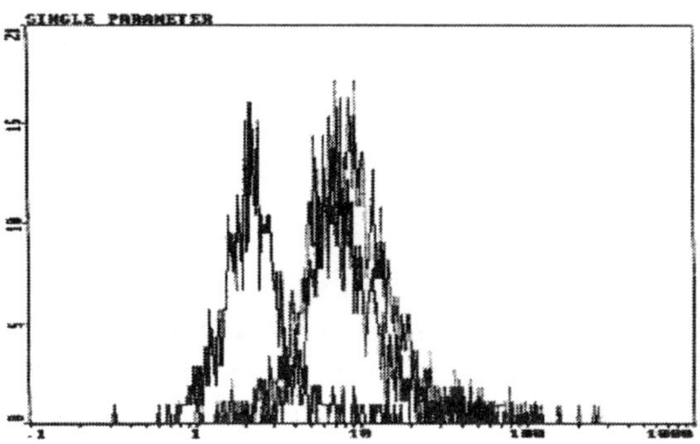

Figure 1. Seroconversion against autologous melanoma cells seen after 3 months of immunisation. Cytofluorometric analysis of the preimmune and postimmune patient's sera.

3.3 Humoral responses against MAGE-1, MAGE-3, MART-3 and tyrosinase

Sera from patients with antibodies against allogenic or autologous melanoma cells, were incubated with a panel of cells genetically modified with melanoma antigens. In no instance, specific antibodies directed against these four antigens were detected.

3.4 Prognostic significance of humoral responses

An induction of humoral responses to allogenic or/and autologous melanoma cells correlated with objective clinical responses (table 1). Clinical remissions (CR+PR+minor responses) were also associated with better performance status of patients, soft tissue metastases and higher CD4+/CD8+ ratio determined mostly by greater absolute CD4+ counts in responders.

Table 1. Correlation between clinical responses to vaccine and patients' characteristics, humoral responses, and CD4+/CD8+ ratio.

	Responders (n=16)	Nonresponders (n=29)	Correlation (p value)
Age	50,7 +/- 13,6 (mean +/- SD) range: 23-72	47 +/- 12,3 (mean +/- SD) range: 29-71	N/S
Sex: f/m	7/9	18/11	N/S
Performance status	Very good and good: 14 moderate: 2	very good and good: 16 moderate: 13	Significant p=0,03*
Soft tissue/internal organ metastases	10/6	9/20	Significant p=0,04*
Humoral response to vaccination	8/12	3/14	Significant p=0,02*
CD4+/CD8+ ratio	1,97 +/- 0,48 (mean +/- SD)	1,22 +/- 0,48 (mean +/- SD)	Significant p=0,0004**

* Chi-square test, ** t-Student test, N/S not significant

In the univariate analysis of prognostic factors, humoral responses were associated with better overall survival of vaccinated melanoma patients (Fig 2). Median survival of patients with humoral responses was 22 months, whereas median survival of patients without detectable seroconversion was only 9 months. 2-year overall survival was about 30% and 7%, respectively. The difference was significant (p=0.01).

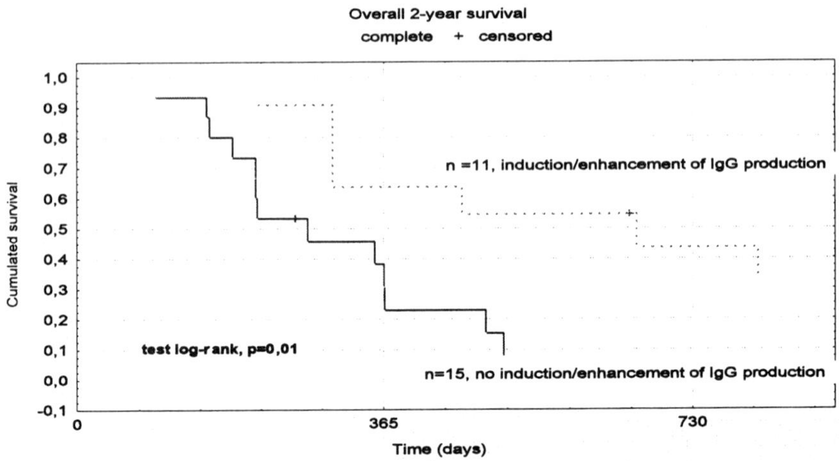

Figure 2. Overall 2-year survival of immunised melanoma patients in relation to humoral responses

4. CONCLUSIONS

Immunisation with allogenic/autologous melanoma vaccine, modified with IL-6/sIL6-R, induces humoral responses of IgG class to allogenic melanoma cells in about 50% of patients. Humoral responses to autologous cells were observed in 40% of patients. We have not detected antibodies against MAGE-1, MAGE-3, MART-1 or tyrosinase. Induction of humoral responses to allogenic or autologous melanoma cells was associated with objective clinical responses, and was a significant prognostic factor predicting longer overall survival. The question is still open if detected antibodies are involved in eliminating metastatic melanoma cells or the observed induction of humoral responses is rather associated with immunocompetence and immunoresponsivness of treated patients.

ACKNOWLEDGEMENTS

Supported by the State Committee for Scientific Research, grant No KBN 0705, KBN 0704

REFERENCES

1. Hellstrom I, Hellstrom KE, Pierce GE i wsp.: Cellular and humoral immunity to different types of human neoplasms. Nature 1969, 220: 1352-1354.
2. Bystryn JC, Oratz R, Roses D, Harris M, Henn M, Lew R: Relationship between immune response to melanoma vaccine immunization and clinical outcome in stage II malignant melanoma. Cancer 1992, 69:1157-1164.
3. Hellstrom I, Hellstrom KE: Immunology: an overview. Ann NY Acad Sci 1993, 690: 204-213.
4. Manson LA: Anti-tumor immune responses of the tumor bearing host: the case for antibody-mediated immunologic enhancement. Clin Immunol Immunopathol 1994, 72: 1
5. Qin Z, Riechter G, Shuler T i wsp.: B cells inhibit induction of T cell –dependent tumor immunity. Nat Med 1998, 4: 627-630.
6. Barbera-Guillem E, Bud-Nelson M, Barr B i wsp.: B lymphocyte pathology in human colorectal cancer. Experimental and clinical therapeutic effects of partial B cell depletion. Cancer Immunol Immunother 2000, 48: 541-549.
7. Hsueh EC, Gupta RK, Morton DL: Correlation of specific immune responses with survival in melanoma patients with distant metastases receiving polyvalent melanoma cell vaccine. J Clin Oncol 1998, 16: 2913-2920.
8. Livingston PO, Kaelin K, Pinsky CM i wsp.: The serologic response of patients with stage II melanoma to allogeneic melanoma cell vaccines. Cancer 1985, 56:2194-2200.
9. Livingston PO, Ritter G, Srivastava P, i wsp.: Characterization of IgG and IgM antibodies induced in melanoma patients by immunization with purified GM2 ganglioside. Cancer Res 1989, 49:7045-7050.

10. Livingston PO: Approaches to augmenting the IgG antibody response to melanoma gangliozyde vaccines. Ann NY Acad Sci 1993, 690:204-213.
11. Jager E, Gnjatic S, Nagata Y i wsp.: Induction of primary NY-ESO-1 immunity: CD8+ T lymphocyte and antibody responses in peptide-vaccinated patients with NY-ESO-1 cancers. Proc Natl Acad Sci 2000, 97: 12198-12203.
12. Jager E, Nagata Y, Gnjatic S i wsp.: Monitoring CD8 T cell responses to NY-ESO-1: correlation of humoral and cellular immune responses. Proc Natl Acad Sci 2000, 97: 4760-4765.
13. Chen YT, Scanlan MJ, Sahin U i wsp.: A testicular antigen aberrantly expressed in human cancers detected by autologous antibody screening. Proc Natl Acad Sci 1997, 94: 1914-1918.
14. Hoon DSB, Yuzuki D, Hayashida M i wsp.: Melanoma patients immunized with melanoma cell vaccine induce antibody responses to recombinant MAGE-1 antigen. J Immunol 1995, 154: 730-737.
15. Fujii S, Huang S, Fong TC i wsp.: Induction of melanoma-associated antigen systemic immunity upon intratumoral delivery of interferon-gamma retroviral vector in melanoma patients. Cancer Gene Ther 2000, 7: 1220-1230.
16. Abdel-Wahab Z, Weltz C, Hester D i wsp.: A phase I clinical trial of immunotherapy with interferon-gamma gene-modified autologous melanoma cells. Cancer 1997, 80: 401-412.
17. Stockert E, Jager E, Chen YT i wsp.: A survey of the humoral immune responses of cancer patients to a panel of human tumor antigens. J Exp Med 1998, 187: 1349-1354.
18. Mackiewicz A, Górny A, Łaciak M i wsp.: Gene Therapy of human melanoma. Immunization of patients with autologous tumor cells admixed with alogenic melanoma cells secreting interleukin 6 and soluble interleukin 6 receptor. Hum Gene Ther 1995, 6:805-811.
19. Mackiewicz A, Wiznerowicz M, Roeb E i wsp. Interleukin 6-type cytokines and their receptors for gene therapy of melanoma. Ann NY Acad Sci 1995; 762: 361-374.
20. Mackiewicz A, Wiznerowicz M, Roeb E i wsp.: Soluble interleukin-6 receptor is biologicaly active in vivo. Cytokine 1995, 7: 142-14.

Clinical studies of human papilloma vaccines in cervical cancer

MALCOLM ADAMS*, LEZEK BORYSIEWICZ+, ALISON FIANDER+, STEPHEN MAN,+ BHARAT JASANI,+ HOSSEIN NAVABI*, ALAN S EVANS+ and MALCOLM MASON+.
*+ University of Wales College of Medicine and * Velindre Hospital*

1. INTRODUCTION

Cervical cancer is the second most common cause of cancer death world wide[1] and is a particular problem in developing countries. Even with optimum treatment approximately 40% continue to die from this disease.[2] There is therefore a need for new strategies to reduce global mortality, including immunotherapeutic intervention.

Human papilloma virus (HPV) infection is now recognised as the cause of this disease.[3] HPV DNA has been identified in 99.8% of invasive cervical tumours world wide.[4] In high grade pre invasive and invasive cervical cancer the open reading frames encoding E6 and E7 early proteins are integrated into the host genome [5] interfering with p53 and Rb functions. Continued expression of E6 and E7 oncoproteins is necessary for the continued growth of the malignant phenotype [6] and these oncoproteins therefore provide a potential immunotherapeutic target for T cell based vaccines.

The rationale for HPV specific immunotherapy is supported by the demonstration of the capacity of peptide or recombinant vaccinia vaccines to induce HPV specific CTL and produce effective prophylaxis and therapy in animal models.[7-10] We have examined two distinct strategies in clinical studies (a) one utilising a recombinant virus encoding HPV 16 and 18 E6 and E7 oncoproteins and the other (b) using autologous dendritic cells

Progress in Basic and Clinical Immunology, Edited by Mackiewicz *et al.*
Kluwer Academic/Plenum Publishers, New York, 2001

loaded with autologous or allogenic cervical tumour lysate as the source of HPV 16 and 18 antigens. The key aims of these studies was to induce an HPV-specific, class 1 restricted CD8+ CTL immune responses in humans and test the safety profile of the vaccines.

1.1 Recombinant vaccinia virus HPV 16 & 18 E6/E7 expressing vaccine (TA-HPV)

1.1.1 Rationale, biological and structural features

A recombinant vaccinia virus engineered to encode modified forms of HPV 16 and 18 E6 and E7 sequences has been developed by Cantab Pharmaceuticals,Cambridge,UK.[11] HPV 16 and 18 oncogenic strains account for between 70-85% of cervical tumours.[12] The backbone of the recombinant is the Wyeth strain of vaccinia which has a long safety record having been employed for smallpox vaccination in 14.2 million individuals in North America.[13] Major complications of vaccinia are rare and largely confined to children and the immunosuppressed. [13] The use of a recombinant vaccinia vector ensures that the target antigens are processed and presented by an antigen presenting cell to induce an MHC class 1 restricted CTL response,[14] which in murine models has been found to be capable of lysing target cells infected with TA-HPV. Further safety features of the construct include (a) the lytic life cycle of vaccinia minimising the risk of the potentially oncogenic inserts[11] (b) reduced neurotoxicity of the construct compared to the parent Wyeth virus in mice[11] and (c) modification of the E7 ORF thereby reducing Rb binding and oncogenicity.[11]

1.1.2 Clinical trial, methods and end points

Three clinical studies[15-17] have been completed in Europe in 49 patients with pre-invasive and invasive cervical cancer (see table1). The key end points of the studies were peripheral cytolytic T cell and antibody responses to the HPV 16 and 18 E6 and E7 inserts of TAHPV and the safety and toxicity of the vaccine. The first study was a phase 1 study in advanced cervical cancer. A second study involved CIN3 volunteers and the third study was a EORTC multi centre phase 2 study in 29 patients with stage 1 and 2 invasive cervical cancer prior to surgery. Anti tumour effect could not be assessed in these studies as TAHPV was given as adjuvant therapy. In the phase 1 study immunosuppresion,[19] low CD4 count associated with recurrent bulky cancer and previous therapies was common. Patients with CD4 counts < 350 –400 /mm were considered to be at potential risk of generalised vaccinia and were therefore excluded. Vaccination was administered by dermal scarification according to the schedules outlined in table 1. In the phase 1 study for regulatory reasons vaccinees remained in an isolation facility and the presence of vaccinia, at various environmental sites monitored. These included swabs from the throat, genitals, vaccination site, dressings and surrounding environment. Vaccinia was found to be confined to the vaccination site and scab. Isolation was consequently not necessary for subsequent studies. An occlusive dressing was maintained until scab dehiscence. Patients in household contact with immunosuppressed individuals and children under 5 years were excluded from the study as these latter individuals were deemed at risk of generalised vaccinia.[13]

Vaccinia -specific IgG was detected by ELISA using Wyeth strain cell lysates as antigen and mock infected cell lysates were used as the control antigen. HPV 16 and 18 E6 and E7 specific antibodies were assayed using a radio immunoprecipitation assay.

In order to assay HPV specific cytotoxic T cells, EBV transformed B-lymphoblastoid cell line (B-LCL) were prepared from each patient for in vitro CTL targets. Peripheral blood mononuclear cells (PBMC) were collected before and after vaccination, cryopreserved and stored in liquid nitrogen. Recombinant adenovirus vectors containing HPV 16 E6/7 sequences (Rad:101) and HPV 18 E6/E7 sequences (Rad:102) were constructed under the control of human cytomegalovirus mIE promoter.[20] To restimulate the HPV- specific CTL in vitro, PHA induced autologous lymphoblasts were infected with Rad:101 and Rad 102, irradiated and then cultured with PMBC in the presence of interleukin 7 for 7 days, before being restimulated and exposed to IL2 on day 10 for CTL assays performed on day 14. CTL cultures were assayed against autologous and allogenic B-LCL targets [37] in a chromium release assay. Target cells were B cell lines infected with TA-HPV or Wyeth strain vaccinia virus.

1.1.3 Clinical Trial Results (see table 1)

No serious toxicities were seen with TA-HPV in these studies. Local erythema with a vaccination lesion appearing at 3-5 days and scab formation after 10-14 days was the norm and mild systemic toxicity unusual. No medium to long term toxicities have been noted with a maximum follow up of 7 years.

An IgG serological response to the vaccinia vector was seen in all the patients in the phase 1 and CIN3 study and 18/29 in the EORTC study. Serological responses to the E6 and E 7 inserts of TAHPV were seen in cancer patients but not CIN3 subjects (see table 1).

One MHC restricted CTL response to HPV 18 was seen in 1/8 patients with advanced cervical cancer in the phase 1 study who had an HPV 16 positive tumour. The response to HPV 16 in the same patient was difficult to assess as a result of non specific back ground lysis of targets expressing the control Wyeth vaccinia virus. This may be due to natural killer activity which may have obscured MHC restricted specific lysis in the assay. The CTL response was detected 9 weeks after vaccination and was not evident at 14 and 20 weeks. This patient is alive and clinically disease free 7 years after vaccination. However it is not possible to attribute her favourable outcome to the vaccination alone as she also received palliative chemotherapy and radiotherapy. Due to the immunosuppression in these patients HPV-specific CTL responses were evaluable in only 3 of the 8 patients.

In the CIN 3 study 3/10 TA-HPV vaccinees exhibited a response to HPV18. However this result may underestimate the HPV specific CTL response since for technical reasons it was not possible to assay HPV 16 specific responses.[16] In the EORTC study one patient with early cervical cancer responded to HPV 18 at 4 weeks and 3 patients with early cervical cancer had a specific CTL response to HPV 16 and 18 at 8 weeks. [17]

Table 1. Results of clinical studies of TAHPV [15-17] (table after Adams et al [18])

Patients Studied	No of Pts.	Dose/schedule of TAHPV	Serological Response Vaccinia vector	Response to E6/E7 vaccine inserts	CTL response
Advanced Cervical Cancer [15] 5/8 recurrent	8+	1 vaccination 10^6 pfu/ml	8/8	3/8)	1/3 evaluable HPV 18 E6/E7
CIN3 [16] volunteers	12+	2 vaccinations 2.5 x 10^5 pfu/ml 4 weeks apart	9/11	0/11	3 /12 evaluable HPV 18 E6/E7
Stage 1-2A[17] cervical cancer	29 +	2 vaccinations 2.5 x 10^5 pfu/ml 4 weeks apart	18/29	8/29	4/29 1 HPV 18/E6/E7 2 HPV 16/E6/E7

1.1.4 Observations and related observations

In all studies the TAHPV vaccine was shown to be safe. The HPV specific CTL responses were only observed at one time point in pre invasive and invasive cancer usually occurring at 8 weeks. There was no evidence to support a boosting effect for two doses of the vaccine which is consistent with animal models. [22-23]

Using a similar protocol HPV specific CTL to HPV 16 and 18 E6 and E7 have been detected in the peripheral blood 6/10 CIN3 non vaccinated subjects. [24] Such HPV specific CTLs are able to lyse autologous targets when presented by multiple alleles including A *0201,A24 and B7. Similar HPV specific CTL have been demonstrated in the cervical tumour, regional lymph nodes and peripheral blood of subjects with early invasive cancer. [25] Unlike invasive cancer CIN3 is known to spontaneously regress in 25-30% of individuals suggesting immunological tumour or virus induced tolerance mechanisms may be reversible. Consequently a further trial is underway to HPV specific CTL responses in the periphery and at sites of disease using more sensitive techniques such as HLA/HPV tetamers.[26]

1.2 Autologous Dendric cells primed with tumour lysate

1.2.1 Rationale and clinical methods

Dendritic cells , professional antigen presenting cells ,are capable of capturing and processing antigens and migrating to lymph nodes to elicit a primary immune response [27] . In contrast tumour cells are weakly immunogenic and are unable to elicit primary CTL response. Immature DC s pulsed with HPV16 tumour antigen peptide are capable of inducing CTL response powerful enough to eradicate established murine tumour expressing HPV 16 [28]. In humans with metastatic melanoma and monocyte derived DC primed with specific tumour peptide antigens or tumour lysate have successfully induced powerful anti tumour responses in humans.[29] In vitro it has proved possible to induce an MHC class 1 restricted CTL response against autologous targets HPV following priming of autologous immature DC in vitro with HPV positive sonicated tumour lysate supporting, the rationale for DC therapy in cervical cancer.[30] Consequently this approach is being tested in a phase 1b trial in patients with advanced recurrent cervical cancer. At present it is unclear what constitutes an optimum DC vaccine since DC populations are heterogeneous in phenotype ,ontogeny and function. It is also unclear whether the immune response depends on the antigen presentation of a specific DC, the nature of the activating signal or the stage of maturation.[31]

Maturation of DC may offer the advantage of a phenotype with optimum migratory capacity to lymph nodes to prime T cells in lymph nodes , optimum Th1 lymphokine[32] production capacity and a stable state which is not susceptible to the cancer- associated tolerogenic influences such as interleukin 10.[33.] Consequently the study is being performed initially with a cohort of HPV tumour lysate primed immature DC followed by a cohort of matured lysate pulsed DC.

2. PATIENTS AND METHODS

To date 9 patients of the first cohort with advanced cervical cancer (7/9with recurrent gross tumour) have been vaccinated. They have received up to 6 subcutaneous vaccinations of $10^6 - 10^7$ immature DC antigen loaded with allogeneic or autologous sonicated HPV positive tumour lysate sonicated. Despite the fact all patients had a CD4 count >400, only 2/9 exhibited a significant DTH response to 1 Pasteur Merieux recall antigen. The study is ongoing and the primary aims are to (1) assess toxicity (2) monitor specific CTL response to HPV antigen and (3) note any anti tumour activity.

No significant DTH response has been seen to HPV antigen following vaccination

A specific HPV class 1 response has been seen in 1 patient with advanced metastatic disease. In this patient the frequency of HPV 16 $E7_{11\text{-}20}$ CTL rose to 2.2% 1 week after the first of 6 vaccinations. Subsequent vaccinations produced no increase in specific CTL. Within 2 weeks of completing 6 vaccinations the tumour was found to progress.

3. OBSERVATIONS

To date the emphasis has been on induction of a MHC class 1 specific CTL response with no objective anti-tumour effect to date. It remains to be seen whether the vaccine can be rendered more effective with the use of mature DC for the vaccine for reasons described above.

4. CONCLUSION

E6 and E7 offer scientifically attractive targets for specific immunotherapies of HPV associated malignancies. Our studies have shown that it is feasible to induce HPV specific CTL responses in patients with cervical cancer and pre invasive disease with a variety of vaccines including TA-HPV and HPV antigen loaded dendritic cells. Future trials will attempt to relate the power and kinetics of HPV specific CTL response to clinical effectiveness.

REFERENCES

1.Pisani, P., Parkin ,D.M., and Ferlay J., 1995 ,Estimates of the world wide mortality from eighteen major cancers in 1985. Implications for prevention and projection of future burden. Int. J. Cancer. 55:891-903.

2.Gatta , G., Lasota ,MB.,Verdecchia , A , and the Eurocare Working Group.,1998 , Survival of European Women with Gynaecological tumours during the period. 1978-1989.Eur.J.Cancer 34(14) :2218-2225.

3.Zur Hausen , H., 1999, Papilloma viruses in human cancer . Proceedings of the Association of American Physicians. 111(6) :581- 587.

4.Walboomers, J.M.M., Jacobs , MV , van Oostveen , JW.,van den Brule , A J C.,. Snijders , PJF., & Meijer ,CJLM.,1997 , Detection of human papilloma virus infections and possible clinical implications. In :Human Papillomavirus Infections in Dermatovenereology.Eds:G.Gross and G.von Krogh,CRC press, London, Tokyo,New York pp. 341-64.

5.Jeon ,S. , and Lambert ,PF.,1995. Integration of human papillomavirus type 16 DNA into the human genome leads to increased stability of E6 and E7 mRNAs: implications for cervical carcinogenesis. Proc Natl Acad Sci USA..,92:1654-8.

6.Crook ,T. , and Vousden KH 1996. HPV oncoprotein function. In: Papilloma virus Reviews: Current research on Papilloma viruses. Ed: Lacey C. Leeds, University Press, Leeds pp.55-60.

7.Feltkamp , MCW., Smits , H. , Vierboom , MPM.,.1993, Vaccination with cytoxic T lymphocyte epitope containing peptide protects against a tumour induced by human papilloma virus type 16 E7 Virology 1,181:62-69.

8.Meneguzzi, G., Cerni , C., Kiery, MP., Lathe, R.,. 1991 ,Immunisation against papilloma virus type 16 tumour cells with recombinant vaccinia viruses expressing the HPV E6 and E7 oncoproteins. Virology 181:62-9.

9.Campo ,MS., Grindley ,GJ., O'Neil , BW., Chandrachud ,LM., McGarvie, GM., Jarret ,WF.1993 , Prophylactic and therapeutic vaccination against mucosal papilloma virus. J Gen Virol 74: 945-53.

10.Lin, K-Y.,Guarnieri , FG., Staveley, O.,Carroll, KF., Levitsky, HI. , August, JT., Pardoll DM. ,Wu , TC . , 1996. Treatment of established tumours with a novel vaccine enhances major histocompatibility class 2 presentation antigen. Cancer Research 56: 21-26.

11.Boursnell, MEG., Rutherford ,E., Hickling ,JK., Rollinson , EA. ,Munro , Rolley , N., Mclean , CS., Borysiewicz,LK., Vousden ,K., and Inglis , SC., 1995 Construction and cells. Eur J Immunol. 23:2242-49.

12.van den Brule ,AJC.,Snijders, PJF.,Meijer, CJLM., and Walboomers., JMM., 1993 , PCR based detection of genital HPV genotypes. An update and future perspectives. Papilloma virus Reports 4: 95-99.

13. Lane, JM., Ruben , FL., Neff , JM., and Millar, JD., 1968, Complications of smallpox vaccination.National surveillance in the United States. New Engl J Med 281:1201-1208.

14.Yewdell, J. , Bennink , Smith ,G. , Moss , B., 1988,Use of recombinant vaccinia viruses to examine cytotoxic T lymphocyte recognition of individual viral proteins.1 Advances in experimental Medicine and Biology 239(151):151-161.

15.Borysiewicz , LK., Fiander, A., Nimako ,M., Man ,S., Westmoreland , D.,Evans ,AS., Adams, M., Stacey SN., Boursnell ,MEG., Rutherford ,E., Hickling ,JK. ,Inglis ,SC., 1996. A recombinant vaccinia virus encoding human papilloma virus types 16 and 18,E6 and E7 proteins as immunotherapy for cervical cancer. Lancet 347 :1523 –27.

16.Fiander ,AS. ,Man ,S., Borysiewicz, L. , 2001 submitted for publication.

17.Rankin ,E., Sommer , H., Schneider, A., Adams ,M., Kitchener , H., Bauknecht , ,T.,Wagner , U., Kroon ,K., Hickling , J.,Stacey , S., Kaufmann , A. , and Zwierzina Heinz , H., EORTC Biology Therapeutics Development Group (BTDG). 2000. TA-HPV ^{TM},A Modified Vaccinia virus carrying HPV 16 and 18 E6 and E7 Proteins induces potent immunity in women with early cervical cancer. (Abstract) Proceedings of AACR 91 st annual meeting 41, abstract 2992. p 469.

18.Adams , M., Borysiewicz ,L.,Fiander , A., Man ,S. , Jasani , B. , Navabi, H., Lippetz, C, Evans, AS, Mason , M. ,2001.Vaccine in press.

19. Fiander , AN., Adams , M. , Evans , AS., Bennett , AJ and Borysiewicz ,LK., 1995. Immunocompetent for imunotherapy? A study of the immunocompetence of cervical cancer patients. Int J Gynecol Cancer. 5: 438-442.

20.Wilkinson, GWG., Akrigg ,A.,1992, Constitutive and enhanced expression from CMV major IE promoter in a defective adenovirus vector. Nucleic Acids Res. 20: 233-39.

21.Borysiewicz ,LK., Hickling ,JK., Graham ,S. ,Sinclair, J., Cranage , MP.,Smith , GL. , Sissons , JG. , 1988 , Human cytomegalovirus specific cytotoxic T cells recognise the 72Kd immediate early proteins and glycoprotein B in recombinant vaccinia viruses. J Exp Med 168, 20 :2233-39.

22.Hodge , JW., Mc Laughlin , JP., Kantor ,JA., Schlom , J. , 1997 , Diversified prime and boost protocols using recombinant vaccinia virus and recombinant non-replicating avian pox virus to enhance T-cell immunity and anti-tumour responses Vaccine115 : 6-7.

23.Irvine , KR. ,Chamberain , RS., 1997 ,Enhancing efficacy of recombinant anti-cancer vaccines with prime/boost regimens that use two different vectors. J Natl Cancer Inst 89(21) : 1595-601.

24. Nimako, M. , Fiander, A. , Wilkinson , GWG., Borysiewicz , LK. , and Man , S., 1997 , Human Papillomavirus-specific Cytotoxic T Lymphocytes in Patients with Cervical Intra epithelial Neoplasia Grade 3. Cancer Research 57:4855-4861.

25. Evans ,E M. ,Man , S. ,Evans , AS. ,and Borysiewicz , LK., 1997. Infiltration of Cervical Cancer Tissue with Human Papillomavirus-specific Cytotoxic T-Lymphocytes Cancer Research 57: 2943 –2950.

26.Youde, S J. , Dunbar ,PR., Evans ,EM. ,Fiander , AN. ,Borysiewicz ,LK. , Cerundolo ,V. , Man , S. 2000, Use of fluoresceinated HLA-A*0201/HPV 16 E7 peptide complexes to isolate rare human CTL recognising endogenous HPV antigens. Cancer Research 60:365-371.

27.Banchereau, J., and Steinman , RM., 1998 , Dendritic cells and the control of immunity Nature 392 (6673) :245-52.

28.Mayodormo , I.,Zorina, T.,Storkus ,WJ. , Zitvogel ,L , Celluzzi ,C., Falo , LD., Melief ,C., Ildstad ,ST., Kast ,WM. , Deleo , AB. , 1995. Bone marrow –derived dendritic cells pulsed with sythetic tumour peptides elicit protective and therapeutic anti-tumour immunity. Nature Medicine 1 (12) :1297-1302.

29 .Nestle ,FO. , Alijagic , S., Gillet ,M. , Yuansheng ,S. , Grabbe , S. , Dummer , R. ,Burg , G. , and Scadendorf ,D., 1998. Vaccination of melanoma patients with peptide or tumour lysate pulsed dendritic cells. Nature Medicine 4(3): 328-332.

30. Navabi ,H. , Jasani , B., Adams , M., Mason , M. 2000. In vitro evaluation of cervical tumour lysate as a source of antigen for Dendritic Cell (DC) based immunotherapy of cervical cancer. Proceedings of AACR Abstract No 5569 p876.

31 Grabbe S .,Kampgen E., Schuler G. Dendritic cells : multilineal and multi- functional. Immunology Today 21(9) :431-3.

32. Dhodapkar , MV., Steiman ,RM. , Sapp , M. , Desai H. , Fossella C., Krasovsky J,Donahoe , SM., Dunbar , PR.., Cerundolo ,V., Nixon , DF., 1999 Rapid generation of broad T cell immunity in humans after a single injection of mature dendric cells J Clin Invest 104:173-180.

34. Steinbrink , K., Jonuleit. , H, Moller. ,Schuler. ,G. ,Knop J. , and Enk , AH. 1999 Interleukin 10 treated human dendritic cells induce a melanoma –antigen –specific anergy in CD 8+ T cells resulting in a failure to lyse tumour cells. Blood 93 (5): 1634-1642.

Flow cytometric cytotoxicity assay with GFP gene modified target cells

DARIUSZ IŻYCKI*, KATARZYNA GRYSKA*, PIOTR GRABARCZYK*, PIOTR J. WYSOCKI*, ANNA JAROSIŃSKA*, SERGIUSZ NAWROCKI# DARIUSZ W. KOWALCZYK* AND ANDRZEJ MACKIEWICZ*.
*Department of Cancer Immunology GreatPoland Cancer Centre Poznań, Poland. #Dept. of Radiation Therapy, GreatPoland Cancer Centre, Poznań, Poland

1. INTRODUCTION

The cytotoxicity assays have been one of the essential tools in studies of effector functions of the immune system. In order to avoid use of radioactive materials many groups have developed alternative ways to quantitate cell mediated lysis. These methods include release of target cell cytoplasmic enzymes (1), dye inclusion or vital dye uptake reduction (2-4). In most of the assays target cells have to be labeled prior analysis which albeit easy to perform is unnecessarily time consuming. Here we describe the measurement by flow cytometry killing activities of human NK cells against K562 cells stably transduced to express enhanced green fluorescent protein (EGFP). After short incubation with effector cells killed EGFP positive K562 cells can be later easily identified by propidium iodide (PI) staining. Since EGFP is expressed in every target cell it requires no further cell labelling, cell purification, or extra washing steps thus, it is more time efficient than current assay methods.

Progress in Basic and Clinical Immunology, Edited by Mackiewicz *et al.*
Kluwer Academic/Plenum Publishers, New York, 2001

2. MATERIALS AND METHODS

2.1 Target cells

The human NK target K-562 erythroleucemic cell line (ATCC), was maintained in continuous suspension culture in standard conditions.

2.2 Construction of bicistronic retroviral vector pMINV-EGFP and transduction of the K-562 target cells

Construction of the bicistronic retroviral vector were performed using pMINV-EGFP retroviral vector. The EGFP encoding sequence was excised with SmaI-XbaI from pEGFP-1 vector (Clontech), blunt ended and cloned into HpaI site of pMINV. The constructed pMINV-EGFP vector was introduced into PA317 packaging cells by electroporation, followed by 14 days of selection in G418 (500μg/ml). The infectious medium from above confluent PA317 pMINV-EGFP cells was harvested and stored in –70°C. K562 target cells were transduced by 24h incubation in MINV-EGFP containing medium suplemented with polybrene (4μg/ml). The transduced cells were selected with G418 for 14 days, what resulted in 97% of EGFP-positive cells as confirmed by flow cytometry (Fig.1c).

2.3 Effector cells

Mononuclear cells isolated from peripheral blood of healthy adults were incubated in plastic cell culture plates for 60 min. at 37°C. After gentle rinsing, nonadherent cells were harvested and re-suspended in a complete medium at a density of $1x10^6$ viable cells/ml and used immediately for cytotoxicity assays.

2.4 Target cells labeling

K-562 cells were labeled with lipophilic carbocyanine membrane dye 3,3' – dioctadecyloxacarbocyanine perchlorate (DiO) as described previously (5). Briefly, $5x10^4$ viable target cells were incubated with 3mM DiO for 20 min. in a complete medium at 37 °C, and then washed twice with PBS and re-suspended in a complete medium at a density of $1x10^6$ cells/ml.

2.5 NK functional test

The cytotoxic activity was tested in a rapid flow cytometric assay as decribed previously (5). Effector, DiO labeled cells or K-562/EGFP target cells were placed in triplicates in 12x75 assay tubes to yield E:T ratios of 40:1, 20:1, 10:1, 5:1. Then propidium iodide (PI) solution (0,1mg/ml) was added into each tube and after 4 hours incubation cells were analysed by flow cytometry. DiO labeled and EGFP gene modified K-562 target cells without effector cells were placed into separate tubes to set background spontaneous cell death.

2.6 Flow cytometric data analysis and acquisition

EPICS XL flow cytometer was used to assess two parameter flow histograms. EGFP and DiO labeled target cells emit a green fluorescence (FL1) while PI stained compromised cells emit far red fluorescence (FL-3). For the mixture of DiO labeled target cells and effector cells the percentage of a specific lysis was assessed using a quadrangle analytical gate and calculated according to the formula published earlier (5).For the mixture of K-562/EGFP gene modified an alternative method of data analysis was examined. Two analytical gates were established to gating EGPF modified target K-562 cells. First, FS vs FL1 analytical gate shown single positive EGFP modified target K-562 cells and unstained effector cells. The original amorphic gate were replaced into elliptical cell-seeker (autogating) regions that was drawn around the population of K-562/EGFP positive cells with the border set at 0.1% of the peak height of the processed population. K-562/GFP target cells were analysed then in two-parameter quadriangle analytical gate that was performed on the FL1 (EGFP) vs FL3 (PI) "dot-plot" type. The display area showed i) double positive IP+EGFP modified K-562 target died cells and ii) K-562/EGFP intact cells.

3. RESULTS

The typical results of experiments are shown on Fig.1. K-562/EGFP positive cells with high expression of GFP protein were gated and analysed by flow cytometry (Fig. 1a, Fig. 1 b).

The quadrant analysis of two fluorescences of target K-562/GFP cells displayed in Fig.1c identifies two populations of target cells: i) EGFP positive intact target cells and ii) EGFP/PI double stained K-562 dead cells.

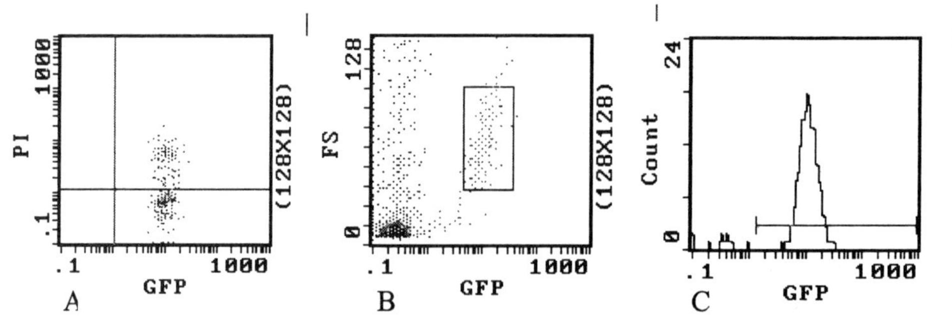

Figure 1. K-562/EGFP target cells were analysed in two-parameter quadriangle analytical gate that was performed on the FL1 (EGFP) vs FL3 (PI) "dot-plot" type. The display area shows double positive IP+EGFP modified K-562 target died cells and K-562/EGFP intact cells (Fig1a). More that 98% of K-562 EGFP gene modified target cells used in NK cytotoxic activity assay express EGFP (Fig.1b-c).

The NK cytotoxic activity measured by both the DiO method and K-562/EGFP assay gave similar results, as shown in Fig. 2. Kinetics of the NK flow cytometric assay have shown that the mean value of lysis for healthy donors was the highest after 4 hrs incubation for each of the assays (Fig.2) and was 71.4 % (E:T= 40:1) as measured by K-562/EGFP assay and 69.8 % (E:T= 40:1) using K-562/DiO labeled target cells. Statistical data analysis showed no important differences in values of cytotoxic NK cells activity between the assays ($p<0.05$). Moreover, reproducible measurements after 4 hrs incubation showed the best correlation ($r=0.73$ for 2 hrs vs. 0.92 for 4hrs) with the DiO assay .

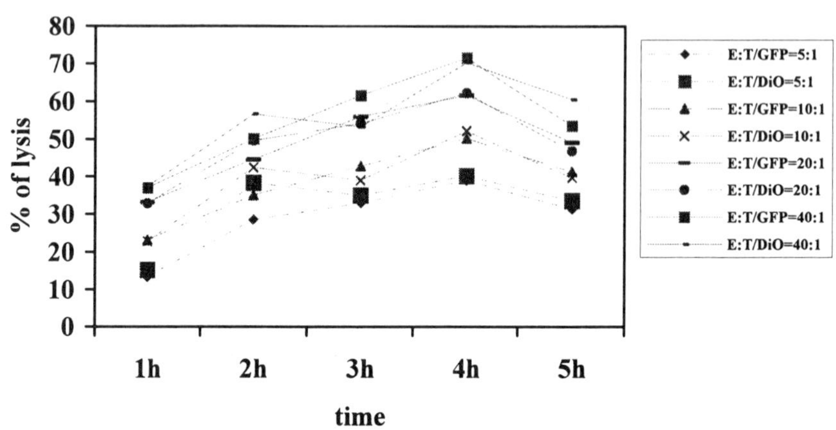

Figure 2. Comparison of lysis in different E:T ratios. Percent cytotoxicity obtained after 1, 2, 3 and 4 hrs EGFP flow cytometric assay are compared to values obtained from DiO flow cytometric method.

4. DISCUSSION

Assays measuring cell mediated toxicity are one of the most often performed tests in immunological studies. Considering that routine tests especially those designed for clinical settings should be reliable, reproducible and easy to perform, we tried to entirely simplify the procedure. The principle of our method is to quantitate by flow cytometry the percentage of killed target K562-EGFP cells after short incubation with effector NK cells. K562 cells expressing EGFP upon contact with NK cells undergo cell mediated lysis, their cell membranes become permeable allowing entry of added propidium iodide which binds to DNA and stains affected cells in red.

These two dyes effectively discriminate between effector cells which are double negative or stained with red only (dead cells) and target cell populations. Thus, killed targets can be easily distinguished from unaffected K562-EGFP cells according to their double (green/red) fluorescence. Our method showed comparable high specificity, sensitivity and reproducibility to another well established non-radioactive assay based on target cells stained with DiO and propidium iodide. Moreover, the presented assay is extremely easy to perform. Since K562-EGFP cells can be utilised for the assay immediately from a culture dish thus it offers a great advance over methods requiring prior cell labelling either with radioactive isotopes such as 51 Chromium or alternatively with fluorescent dyes. Real work time may be reduced at this step by at least one up to two hours. Although not tested in our system, elimination of additional washing steps might be beneficial for overall target cells viability which may influence their susceptibility for cell mediated lysis. Moreover, stable EGFP expression in every cell eliminates problems due to inefficient cell labelling which later greatly affect signal to noise discrimination and its uniform labelling pattern literally eliminates presence of unlabeled cells which might falsely decrease observed cytotoxic values in cold target inhibition manner. Similarly to other flow cytometry based NK assays, assessment of specific lysis is very straightforward estimated from a histogram set on gated EGFP positive cells. This direct evaluation eliminates additional calculations thus even further reduce analysis time. The described method has been used routinely in our laboratory and proved to be consistent over many separate experiments.

ACKNOWLEDGEMENTS

This work was supported by grant from Polish State Committee For Scientific Research (PBZ-K002/PO4/99).

REFERENCES

1. Korzeniewski C, Callewaert DM. An enzyme released assay for natural cytotoxicity. J Immunol Methods. 1983. 64: 313-320
2. Mossmann T. Rapid colorimetric assay for cellular growth and survival: Application to proliferation and cytotoxicity assays. J Immunol Methods. 1983, 65 : 55-62
3. Green LM, Reade JL, Ware CF. Rapid colorimetric assay for cell viability: Application to the quantitation of cytotoxic and growth inhibitory lymphokines. J Immunol Methods 1984, 70:257-268
4. Wierda GW, Mehr DS., Kim YB. Comparison of fluorochrome labeled and 51Cr-labeled targets natural killer cytotoxicity assay. J Immunol Methods. 1989, 122: 15-24.
5. Chang L et al. Rapid flow cytometric assay for the assessement of natural killer cell activity. J Immunol Methods. 1993, 166:45-54

Flow and video-imaging cytometry – usefulness of DNA ploidy measurements in diagnosis of malignant melanoma

JANUSZ SKOWRONEK[1,2], ZBIGNIEW KARAŚ[2], ROMAN M.KRENZ[3], JERZY B. WARCHOŁ[2]
[1]Department of Radiotherapy, GreatPoland Cancer Center, Poznań, [2]Department of Radiobiology and Cell Biology, University of Medical Scienses, Poznań, [3]Department of Neoplasms Pathology, University of Medical Scienses, Poznań, Poland

1. INTRODUCTION

DNA content detected by video-imaging and flow cytometry in malignant and premalignant cells becomes more and more often routine adjunct to clinical and histological diagnosis. It seems that the presence of abnormal DNA in many neoplasms is correlated with the poor clinical course (1,4,5). However, diploid cell population was found also in such malignant cell transformations as leukemia, lymphoma, and aneuploidy in such benign transformations as thyroid adenoma, mastopathy and premalignant cutaneous lesions. It is clear that DNA ploidy is not always an adequate parameter to differentiate benign from malignant lesions.

Recent results of DNA ploidy measurements in malignant melanoma cells are contradictory. There are relatively few conflicting studies, which describe DNA content of malignant melanoma and pigmented nevi.

The aim of this study is to present the results of DNA ploidy analysis in malignant melanoma cells in comparison with choosen prognostic clinical and histopathological factors and to present results of DNA ploidy analysis in randomly chosen nevi removed surgically. We compared both cytometric methods.

Progress in Basic and Clinical Immunology, Edited by Mackiewicz *et al.*
Kluwer Academic/Plenum Publishers, New York, 2001

2. MATERIAL AND METHODS

The study material contained 103 malignant melanomas and 61 nevi. In the group of pigmented nevi 21 Spitz nevi, 2 congenital nevi, 27 compound nevi including 3 with significant proliferation, 6 dysplastic, 4 intracutaneous and one junction nevi were identified.

Measurements of DNA ploidy in cell nuclei were done using two cytometric methods: flow cytometry and video-imaging cytometry. Suspension of cells from paraffin blocks, and for image cytometry, additionally fresh cells smears were stained for DNA. About 1000 cells of study population (image cytometry) or 10000 cells (flow cytometry) and 100 cells of human lymphocytes (internal control) were analysed. Results were achieved in form of histograms reflected percentage of cells in respective phases of cell cycle. The histograms were scaled using diploid references where diploid is equal 2n and is defined by the presence of cells differing from diploid by less then 10%. The tumor was considered as aneuploid when the histograms showed a distinctive peak differing from standard by at least 10%.

3. RESULTS

In whole population of malignant melanoma diploid DNA content was detected in 33 tumors (32,0%) and aneuploid DNA content in 70 tumors (68,0%) [$p<0,01$]. Correlation between aneuploidy rate, sex, age and localization did not show significant differences. Aneuploidy rate was higher in II and III clinical stage, significant correlation was shown between aneuploidy and tumor thickness greater then 1,50 mm and in Clark Level III,IV and V. There was no correlation between aneuploidy and clinical type, lymph node involvement, inflammatory infiltration, ulceration, cell type and regression.

In the whole population of nevi aneuploid or tetraploid DNA content was identified in 14 nevi (23,0%) and diploid in 47 nevi (77,0%) [$p<0,001$]. Aneuploidy was found in one of 2 congenital nevi, in 3 of 24 compound nevi, in one of 3 compound nevi with proliferation, in 3 of 6 dysplastic nevi, in 5 of 21 Spitz nevi. In one Spitz nevi the tetraploid profile of DNA was found).

4. DISCUSSION

In whole group of malignant melanoma aneuploid DNA content was significantly greater then diploid DNA content. In examined group correlation between DNA ploidy and sex, age and localization of primary lesion was not observed. Female sex and localization of primary lesion in lower limbs prognoses better but in multivariate analysis (this features are occurring often connected), considering a fact that in women ulceration (worse prognostic factor) occurs rarely, prognostic meaning of both features is not so unequivocal. Higher clinical stage is connected with poor prognosis (higher tumor thickness according to Breslow, higher Clark level and positive lymph node status). Own results show higher aneuploidy rate in tumors with thickness greater then 1,50 mm, with Clark level III, IV and V. Difference in aneuploidy rate between clinical stages II-III and I was not statistically significant. Comparison of another histological factors with DNA ploidy did not show correlation. Small group of published results did not allowed to draw conclusions.

So far DNA ploidy results in melanocytic nevi have been contradictory (2,3). Some authors observed certain percentage of aneuploidy and tetraploidy in benign melanocytic lesions. It can indicate a higher risk of proliferation and melanoma development.

Both our own results and the results reported by many other authors concerning the DNA ploidy in the cells of different nevi, which are benign, nonneoplastic lesions, indicate the occurrence of a certain amount of aneuploidy and tetraploidy. It may indicate an increased tendency towards proliferation and associated increased risk of malignant transformation. It suggests the need for measuring DNA ploidy in nevi considered as premalignant and should qualify such patients for more frequent prophylactic examinations. The nevi cannot be used as diploid control in DNA ploidy determination.

The present study confirmed the usefulness of video-imaging and flow cytometry method for the routine DNA content analysis (*table 1*). The results obtained from both methods were identical. Flow cytometry is a fast cytometric method, great number of cells and many of cell parameters can be measured at the same time. Defect of this method is lose of morphological identification of cells and complicated preparing of cell solution. Advantage of video-imaging cytometry is the possibility of morphological identification of cells using microscope and possibility to selection of artefacts and regular normal cells. Defect of this method is small group of measured cells and time-consuming measurement. By small population of obtained tumor cells video-imaging cytometry is a method of choice.

Table 1. Comparison of both cytometric methods

Flow – cytometry	Video - imaging cytometry
Advantages	Advantages
1. possibility of measurements with a speed of thousands of cells per second 2. possibility of detecting one atypical cell in thousands of normal cells 3. possibility of measurements even tens of parameters simultaneously	1. possibility of morphological identification measured cells 2. possibility of assessment cell fractions described using flow cytometry 3. makes possible selection of default cells and artifacts 4. makes possible use of additional measured parameters, like surface area, shape factor, cells circumference, etc.
Defects	Defects
1. lack of direct observation of measured cells 2. necessity of long-term preparation of cell suspension 3. necessity of achieving total dispersion of cell without disturbing of structure 4. possibility of false results arise from place more cells one on another or partial dispersion	1. small number of measured cells 2. time - consuming measurement 3. necessity of internal standard and standarization of measuring equipment

5. CONCLUSIONS

1. Both, the video-imaging cytometry and flow cytometry, can be employed for DNA ploidy measurements in cells.
2. The determination of cellular DNA content in cell does not differentiate between benign and malignant lesions.

REFERENCES

1. Barlogie B, Raber MC, Schumann J, Johnson TS, Drewinko B et al. Flow Cytometry in Clinical Cancer Research. Cancer Res 1983; 43: 3982-3997
2. Barnhill RL, Aguiar M, Cohen C, Kang S, Kennedy J, Schmidt B, Sober AJ, Solomon AR. Congenital Melanocytic Nevi and DNA Content. An Analysis by Flow and Image Cytometry. Cancer 1994; 74: 2935-2943
3. Bartkowiak D, Schumann J, Otto FJ et al. DNA Flow Cytometry in the Prognosis of Primary Malignant Melanoma. Oncology 1991; 48: 39-43
4. Buchner T, Hiddemann W, Wormann B et al. Differential pattern of DNA-aneuploidy in human malignancy. Pathol Res Pract 1985; 179: 310-317
5. Skowronek J, Adamska K, Filipiak K, Karaś Z, Krenz RM, Rutkowski R, Warchoł JB - DNA ploidy in malignant melanoma, skin cancer and pigmented nevi, Neoplasma 1997; 44: 282-288

Author Index

Subject Index